D1558642

Practical Clinical
Hypnosis

Scientific Foundations of Clinical Counseling and Psychology

Eugene Walker, series editor

Practical Clinical Hypnosis

Techniques and Applications

Robert G. Meyer
University of Louisville

Lexington Books
An Imprint of Macmillan, Inc.
NEW YORK
Maxwell Macmillan Canada
TORONTO
Maxwell Macmillan International
NEW YORK   OXFORD   SINGAPORE   SYDNEY

Library of Congress Cataloging-in-Publication Data

Meyer, Robert G.
    Practical clinical hypnosis : technique and applications / Robert
G. Meyer.
        p.   cm. — (Scientific foundations of clinical and counseling
psychology)
    Includes index.
    ISBN 0-669-27729-0
    1. Hypnotism.   2. Hypnotism—Therapeutic use.   I. Title.
II. Series.
    [DNLM: 1. Hypnosis.   WM 415 M613p]
    RC495.M45   1992
    615.8'512—dc20
    DNLM/DLC
    for Library of Congress   92-20250
                                                                    CIP

Lexington Books
An Imprint of Macmillan, Inc.
866 Third Avenue, New York, N.Y. 10022

Maxwell Macmillan Canada, Inc.
1200 Eglinton Avenue East
Suite 200
Don Mills, Ontario M3C 3N1

Macmillan, Inc. is part of the Maxwell Communication
Group of Companies.

Printed in the United States of America

printing number
1   2   3   4   5   6   7   8   9   10

To Peggy
who enchants me

Contents

Preface

Clinical hypnosis is an area that is useful and interesting yet replete with potential and controversy. This book discusses the potentials and controversies, though the major focus is on practical clinical applications. Hypnotherapists (novice and expert) will find it useful in everyday practice. My goal was to be both practical and thorough yet to cite and use the empirical and clinical literature wherever appropriate. Although lodged in the context of available research, it offers an ample discussion of a wide range of clinical techniques and applications, many of them exemplified by suggested scripts, detailed suggestions, and case examples.

The book starts with a short introductory chapter, with facts and discussion placed within the context of a history of hypnosis. Following are the seven chapters that comprise part I of the book. These chapters provide techniques for assessing susceptibility and the applicability of hypnosis to a particular client; induction and deepening techniques; direct, posthypnotic, and indirect (including Ericksonian) techniques; age regression; and self-hypnosis. Part II has ten chapters that detail applications of clinical hypnosis with habit disorders, psychological disorders, pain management, dentistry, medical problems, performance enhancement, and forensic cases. It also has a substantial chapter on applications with children. The last chapter discusses issues hypnotherapists will face in related legal matters, including detailed advice on how to cope with associated legal challenges.

Numerous individuals made a significant contribution to this book. They are each listed after the chapter to which they made their contribution: 2, James Walker; 3, James Walker and James Bloch; 4, James Walker and David Connell; 5, David Payne; 6, David Connell; 7, Vicki Ragsdell; 8, Debbie Scheer; 9, Quinn Chipley; 10, David Kelley; 11, Sheldon Levinson; 12, Linda Douglas; 13, Michael Phillips; 14, Patricia Wolff; 15, Kathy Walker; 16, Lori Gibson; 17, Curtis Ohashi and Steven R. Smith.

Thanks are owed to reviewers who read the manuscript and made helpful comments that led to improvements in quality and usefulness.

Special thanks are due to my editor at Lexington Books, Margaret Zusky. A major acknowledgment and thank you goes to Sandy Hartz, who helped with much of the typing and coordinated that phase of production. I also thank Jennifer Yurt, Tonia Dean, Suzanne Paris, Lou Black, and Kathi Eberle for their helpful contributions.

1

Introduction

> "Who are *you?*" said the Caterpillar. . . . Alice replied, rather shyly,
> "I hardly know, sir, just at present—at least I know who I *was*
> when I got up this morning, but I think I must have been changed
> several times since then."
> —Lewis Carroll, *Alice's Adventures in Wonderland*

Hypnosis has been a fascinating and controversial topic for centuries, with many attempts to define it and numerous theories to explain it. Most could agree with the common assertion that "hypnosis is an altered state of consciousness," but beyond that, agreement is hard to find.

It is quite clear that hypnosis has proved effective as a primary or adjunct technique for a wide range of medical and psychological disorders and conditions (Morgan, Darby, and Heath, 1992; Levitan, 1991; Sarbin, 1991; Yapko, 1990; Wester, 1987). The current popularity of clinical hypnosis results from a variety of factors, including professional and cultural interest in altered states of consciousness, beginning in the 1960s; a resurgence of interest in and acceptance of cognitive phenomena, beginning in the 1960s; the specific work of Milton Erickson, Ernest and Josephine Hilgard, T. X. Barber, Martin Orne, Harold Crasilneck, Gail Gardner, and many others; the integrative work of D. Corydon Hammond, Erika Fromm, Jeffrey Zeig, and numerous others; the ascendance of electicism in psychotherapy; the increasing interest in effective and economical ways to treat psychological and physiological disturbances; and increasing support for its effectiveness in specific areas and for the effectiveness of psychotherapy in general.

From an overall perspective, clinical hypnosis can potentially help in any one case in a number of ways: by mobilizing resources and strengthening motivation, developing and amplifying a relaxation response, providing access to material not usually accessible, confronting and dissolving suppressed mental contents that are blocking progress, putting the client in touch with newer, more effective ego states, enhancing imagery for hypnotic or other techniques, and providing for vicarious rehearsal of more effective behaviors and cognitions.

Discussing and detailing the varied techniques of applying hypnosis within the context of the diverse applications for which it has proved useful is the subject of this book. Before moving on, however, a brief survey of the historical developments within which these clinical techniques and applications have evolved will be useful.

Since ancient recorded history—and even in the glimmerings of prehistory—various methods of influence that are clearly hypnotic in nature have been easily detected; references to "temple sleep" and to being enchanted by the "evil eye" can be traced back to 3000 B.C. In the Talmud, hypnotic-like maneuvers as a method of controlling certain animals, including poisonous snakes, are described and specifically allowed on the Sabbath.

A stone stele from Egypt in the reign of Ramses XII of the Twentieth Dynasty is said to be the earliest record of a hypnotic session, and Lewis Wolberg (1972) suggests that the earliest description of hypnosis is in Genesis 2:21–22: "And the Lord God caused a deep sleep to fall upon Adam, and he slept, and he took one of his ribs, and closed up the flesh instead thereof. And the rib, which the Lord God had taken from man, made he a woman, and brought her unto the man."

Following are major landmarks in the history of hypnosis:

Ca. 1525: Paracelsus (1493–1541), a Swiss physician, asserts that the stars exert a magnetic force and that magnets can influence the human body.

Ca. 1625: Robert Fudd (1574) and Johann Baptist Van Helmont (1577–1644) assert that people possess a magnetic force, that two proximate people create a magnetic field, and that magnets can be manipulated to generate cures.

1636: Daniel Schwenker, a professor of mathematics and oriental studies at the University of Altdorf, publishes *Deliciae physico-mathematicae,* in which he asserts that wood shavings on the beak immobilize a bird as it fixates on them.

1646: Father Kircher, a Jesuit priest, observes in his book, *Die Vorstellungswelt des Huhnes* (The fowl's world of ideas), that gently pressing a bird to the ground and drawing a line forward from its beak will cause it to remain immobilized, usually until it is directly startled. Father Kircher believed this was a result of the bird's "phantasy" in concert with "wonderful magnetic" effects and termed it "animal bewitchment."

Ca. 1650: Valentine Greatrakes, who healed patients by stroking them, became known as the great Irish Stroker. Many kings and princes were said to heal through a "royal touch."

Ca. 1750: Father Maximilian Hell (1720–1792), a Viennese Jesuit priest, gains fame from his magnetic cures, accomplished by using steel plates applied to the naked body. Johann Gassner (1727–1779), also a

Catholic priest, promotes the viability and visibility of the healing power of exorcism.

1704: Richard Mead, in *De imperio solis ac lunae in corpara humana et morbis inde oriundis,* argues a physicochemical hypothesis wherein tides in the atmosphere change the "gravity, elasticity, and pressure" of the air, which in turn produces bodily changes, including disease.

1766: The dawn of a scientific approach to clinical hypnosis is found in Franz Anton Mesmer's (1734–1815) medical dissertation at the University of Vienna, "De Planetarium influxu" (On the influence of the planets). Plagiarizing the concepts and words of Mead but eliminating the concept of the air as a mediator, Mesmer writes of his attempts to study physical effects in humans by the planets, especially the sun and moon (which were then referred to as planets, though Mesmer specifically repudiated the concepts of astrology). His unique contribution was the idea that "cosmic" and "planetary magnetism" could be contained in the bodies of specific people and animals ("animal magnetism") and then be transmitted by magnetic passes and/or a "magnetic bath." In the magnetic bath, people sat in a circle and held hands, with cures being signaled by individuals' suffering a "magnetic crisis," crying out loud, and convulsing (similar to certain group therapy and/or religious experiences and to primal scream therapy). When Mesmer discovered that objects other than magnets could generate the same rate of cures (60 to 70 percent), he argued that this type of magnetism could be transferred. He also argued that people differ in their ability to store up and transfer magnetism. Not surprisingly, he thought he was close to tops in this ability. However, few scientists agreed with him. Indeed, he received the continuing support of only one establishment scientist, Charles d'Eslon, physician to the brother of the king of France. Eventually a commission of nine eminent scientists, including Benjamin Franklin, Dr. Guillotine, a strong advocate of punishment theory, the chemist Lavoisier, and the astronomer Bailly, said there was nothing to support his theories. Mesmer objected that they had tested only d'Eslon's individual abilities, not Mesmer's theory, as Mesmer refused to participate himself. In 1774, Mesmer successfully treats F. Oesterlin's conversion hysteria with metallic magnets.

1784: A. M. J. Chastenet, the marquis de Puysegur (1751–1825), a member of Mesmer's secret society Harmonia (but a much better observer and recorder of data than Mesmer), discovers "artificial somnambulism" with the characteristics of responsiveness to the mesmerist's commands, lucid speech, and amnesia for trance events. Puysegur, who adopts as his motto *Croyez et voulez* ("believe and will"), recognizes psychological characteristics of the operator as important, though he ignores the relevance of such factors in the subject. Nevertheless, he did recognize that the subjects could not be "magnetized" against their will.

Ca. 1800: José Custodio de Faria (known as abbé Faria) (1755–1819), a Portuguese priest and sometime student of Puysegur, is the first to point to and then highlight the importance of characteristics in the subject. In addition to "liquidity" of the blood and a propensity to perspire, he also notes psychological characteristics like "psychic impressionability" (apparently suggestibility) and the ability to relax and go to sleep easily. He is the first to assert that subjects can be rendered insensitive to the pain of surgery—and is the first recorded case of a hypnotist's being duped into believing he had successfully hypnotized someone. In 1816, a Parisian actor pretended to go into a somnambulistic state but later said he was fully awake, ridiculing the abbé. This same actor later appeared as Soporito, a caricature of the abbé, in a popular stage play, *Magnetisomanie.* The abbé eventually lost his credibility and died a pauper.

Early 1800s: Marquis de Lafayette delivers the first paper in the United States on mesmerism.

1813: First reported relief of dissociated traumatic grief memories using hypnosis, by the Dutch physicians Wolthers, Hendriksz, De Waal, and Bakker. They attributed this to magnetic influences.

1821: Under the direction of Dr. Recamier, moxas are burned on the bodies of two patients who show no apparent pain while in a "mesmeric coma."

1829: After a woman is put into a trance by her physician, the surgeon, Cloquet, removes an ulcerated tumor of the breast.

1831: Foissac is the first to use hypnosis in obstetrical medicine.

1836: Oudet performs the first recorded tooth extraction under trance-induced anesthesia.

1842: James Braid (1795–1860), a Scottish collery doctor and surgeon, who practiced in Manchester, proposes the term *neurohypnotism,* which is soon shortened to *hypnotism,* from the Greek word *hypnos* for "sleep." He also puts an emphasis on the term *suggestion* and the importance of psychological factors but actually introduces no theories or discoveries of great import.

1843: John Elliotson, a professor at the University of London, produces the first volume of *Zoist,* a journal devoted to cerebral physiology and mesmerism. Thirteen volumes are eventually published.

Ca. 1845: The Phreno-Magnetic Society flourishes in Cincinnati, and the Société du magnetism is active in New Orleans until the Civil War.

Ca. 1850: James Esdaille (1808–1859), a Scottish surgeon practicing in India, extensively integrates the use of hypnosis into his practice, performing at least 1,000 minor and 300 major operations using hypnosis. In 161 cases of scrotal tumor, in which the mortality rate had been 50 percent, the use of hypnosis reduces the rate to 5 percent. Esdaille was persistently berated by his medical colleagues with the accusation that the "natives" who were his patients were actually in pain but were not telling him out of deference or politeness. (Apparently these colleagues were also assuming they were dying at a markedly lower rate in order to please him.)

1851: Andries Hoek, a Dutch physician, is the first to use a psychological uncovering technique in his treatment of Rita van B., who experienced what would probably now be termed posttraumatic stress disorder. She had suffered several traumatic experiences, including repeated abuse, rape, and the witnessing of the accidental death of one of her uncle's servants.

Ca. 1880: Jean Martin Charcot (1825–1893), the most distinguished neurologist of the nineteenth century, makes a number of contributions to theories of hypnosis—virtually all of them erroneous (the most notable being that deep hypnosis is a pathological phenomenon). Charcot saw hypnosis as a kind of artificial neurosis comparable in some ways to conversion hysteria. His errors are explained in part by the fact that he never hypnotized anyone. The hypnosis was done by residents, whereupon Charcot would come in and give suggestions or try other manipulations. This is an excellent example of where an eminent researcher in one area dabbles in another, but the strength of his reputation lends weight to the inaccurate findings that result from dabbling as opposed to focused, consistent study.

1890: Pierre Janet (1859–1947) is appointed by Charcot as director of the Psychological Laboratory at Saltpetrière. He explains and corrects many of Charcot's errors and, with Charcot, is a force in bringing the scientific method into the study of hypnosis. At approximately the same time Hippolyte Bernheim (1837–1919) calls attention to Ambroise-Auguste Liebault's (1823–1904) book *Sleep and Related States*, originally published in 1866. This book and Bernheim's renown focus attention on the role of suggestion in hypnosis and provide some counterweight to Charcot's view of deep hypnosis as pathological. The followers of Liebault and then Bernheim are referred to as the Nancy school.

1893: Josef Breuer (1842–1925) and Sigmund Freud (1856–1939) publish the original chapters of *Studien uber hysterie,* which discusses using hypnosis to encourage spontaneous verbalizations that lead to catharsis. This work marked a shift from the traditional direct suggestion approach to an approach reflecting the later psychoanalytic concepts of repression and catharsis. Freud later abandoned hypnosis, influencing many mental health practitioners in the years hence. Paradoxically, his rejection of hypnosis led to his discovery of psychoanalytic technique and theory. Certainly the authoritarian brand of hypnosis that was in vogue in Freud's era was a factor here, as was Freud's shock when one of his female clients spontaneously awoke from a trance and threw her arms around him in a romantic manner.

1897: *People v. Ebanks,* the first clearly documented forensic case in the United States. The defense attempted to show through hypnotically enhanced testimony that Ebanks's alleged amnesia for the events of the crime was simply a result of his not being at the crime scene. The court denied the admissibility of the evidence, and Ebanks was convicted.

Ca. 1900: Morton Prince (1854–1929) emphasizes personality as a factor in hypnosis and pioneers the use of hypnosis in reintegrating multiple personality clients.

1919: In "Turnings in the Ways of Analysis," Freud states that in "the application of our therapy to numbers . . . hypnotic influence might find a place in it again, as it has in war neurosis."

1923: Milton H. Erickson (1901–1980) (at the request of Clark Hull, the noted behavioral therapist, and while Erickson was still an undergraduate premedical student at the University of Wisconsin) leads a graduate seminar on his informal but interesting research on hypnotism. This event marked the beginning of Erickson's career in hypnosis and apparently helped stimulate Hull's interest in hypnosis.

1933: Clark Hull (1884–1952) publishes *Hypnosis and Suggestibility.* Although the particular behavioral-based theory Hull promoted received little acceptance, he fueled an emphasis on the use of systematic and controlled experimentation, in part spurred by the development by mathematicians of the null hypothesis statistical model. In approximately 1900, he had been the first to use this method in hypnosis research. Like Charcot, Hull was influential in promoting controlled hypnosis research. His theoretical concepts lingered longer than would have been the case based on their truth value because of his reputation.

1949: The Society for Clinical and Experimental Hypnosis is founded and expands to an international society ten years later.

1955: The British Medical Association endorses hypnosis as an acceptable modality of treatment.

1957: The American Society of Clinical Hypnosis is founded.

1958: The American Medical Association recognizes hypnosis as a legitimate treatment technique in medicine and dentistry.

1961: The American Psychiatric Assocation endorses hypnosis as an acceptable treatment modality.

1965: Ernest R. Hilgard's original text, *Hypnotic Susceptibility,* gains broad recognition when it is republished as *The Experience of Hypnosis.* As with Clark Hull, hypnosis gains increased credibility when a renowned researcher in traditional learning theories turns his attention to hypnosis.

1969: The American Psychological Association creates an interest-affiliation section for psychologists interested in hypnosis.

1981: In *State v. Hurd,* the New Jersey Supreme Court adopts six procedural rules or safeguards for hypnotically enhanced testimony. Known as the Hurd rules (see chapter 18), they are the precedent for most procedural safeguards.

1987: In *Rock v. Arkansas,* the U.S. Supreme Court holds that it is a violation of constitutional rights to arbitrarily preclude testimony in a criminal trial about memories recalled during hypnosis. The Court asserts that the recognized difficulties with such testimony can be handled through cross-examination or by adopting appropriate rules of evidence.

This brief history underscores the controversial aspects of hypnosis and hints at the emerging importance of hypnosis as a clinical tool. The rest of this book highlights the importance, and the breadth of technique and application, of hypnosis as a clinical tool.

Part I
Techniques

Part I discusses the wide range of techniques available to hypnotherapists: preliminary approaches and considerations, induction and deepening techniques, direct and indirect (especially Ericksonian) techniques, posthypnotic and age regression techniques, and self-hypnosis. The discussion will touch on applying these techniques to various disorders, but in the main in this part, technique subsumes application.

2
Hypnotic Susceptibility and Preliminary Considerations in Hypnosis Cases

An acquired taste
But hell, aren't they all
—Anton Myrer, *The Last Convertible*

Hypnotic Susceptibility

Need to Measure Susceptibility

Hypnotherapists are aware that individuals differ in their ability to experience hypnotic phenomena. Some people go much more deeply into a trance than others, and some may not go into a trance at all. Some will be highly responsive to suggestions made by the clinician; some will not. Hypnotic susceptibility is this capacity of the individual to enter a hypnotic state and experience hypnotic phenomena (Weitzenhoffer, 1980; Nadon et al., 1991; Balthazar and Woody, 1992).

It is important to assess how deeply the client is in a trance, and usually this is done as part of the induction process. The client's overt response to suggestions can be observed, and after the session is complete, the client can be asked to describe his or her experience during the suggestions. Often clinicians use one of the standardized scales designed to measure hypnotic susceptibility, permitting a quantitative and reasonably thorough and precise description of hypnotic ability.

It can be quite helpful to take some measure of susceptibility with each client. There is little sense in attempting such hypnotic techniques as age regression or amnesia if the client is unable to experience even relatively simple hypnotic tasks. In such cases, hypnosis could be abandoned, with another, likely more useful, treatment strategy adopted instead. In some cases, such as the use of hypnosis for anesthesia in surgery or dentistry or for hypnotic refreshment of memories for forensic purposes, thorough testing is even more helpful. Testing for hypnotic susceptibility also can be used to confirm to the client his or her abilities. Such confirmation is useful because positive expectancies serve to heighten responsiveness (Saavedra and Miller, 1983), especially if these expectancies result from personal experience (Wickless and Kirsch, 1989).

The usefulness of standardized scales in clinical settings is at times debatable, and the clinician will wish to make trial uses of them to ascertain whether they will be helpful with a given population or treatment plan. The major drawback to their use is their length, although more economical scales have been developed. Another concern is that they may not tap the classic suggestion effect, that is, the experience of involuntariness that is thought by many to be the hallmark of a true hypnotic response (Weitzenhoffer, 1980). The fear is that the client may be observed performing the tasks of a given scale and receive a high score yet may be doing so voluntarily, with no real experience of involuntariness. This concern can be addressed by thorough questioning of the client following the completion of the scale. Furthermore, scores on the standardized scales are typically highly associated with the classical suggestion effect.

Another concern with using standardized scales is that because of their format, they may screen out an individual who is truly responsive and result in excluding that person from potential benefits to be gained through hypnosis. Certainly in many cases, a personalized induction succeeds where the standardized scale does not (Edmonston, 1986). Consequently, in cases in which hypnosis may present a unique benefit to a client, the clinician should use multiple methods and repeated attempts before abandoning hypnosis.

A benefit of using standardized scales, particularly taped versions, is that they may engage subjects who are initially resistant to hypnosis. The impersonal characteristics of a standardized induction or a taped version can often circumvent personal resistance issues, especially among highly educated populations, compulsive individuals, or those who fancy themselves to be above gimmicks and tricks. The use of a "scientific" scale, labeled as such, that allows the clients to rate their own abilities often provides an acceptable way for the wary intellectualizer to engage in hypnosis.

Common Tests of Susceptibility

Each of the more common tests of hypnotic susceptibility and responsiveness can be used to evaluate an individual's susceptibility and may be incorporated into an induction procedure.

Hand Drop and Levitation. The subject is told to extend one or both arms, and then the suggestion is presented that one hand will become either lighter or heavier, resulting in vertical movement of that limb. The drop suggestion is easier to achieve, since gravity will contribute to the effect. The levitation technique is less likely to succeed but is more of a true test.

Sway Test. The therapist stands behind the standing subject, with hands on or near the subject's shoulders or back or to the side, and suggests that the subject will sway toward the clinician. It may be advisable initially to have the client sway normally, so that the clinician can circumvent any fears of the client of falling. Wright and Wright (1987) point out that this technique may also serve as a metaphor to acclimate the patient to surrendering to the therapist's suggestions.

Finger Lock. The subject is given the suggestion that it will not be possible to separate his or her clasped fingers once they are intertwined, success being indicated by the inability to do so.

Eye Catalepsy. Subjects are told that their eyelids will be "heavy" or "glued shut." Success is measured by their inability to open their eyes when challenged to do so.

Hallucination. This more difficult test (Lubar et al., 1991) may be given within any sensory modality. For instance, the client may be presented with a strong unpleasant odor, with the suggestion that it smells like flowers. A common auditory sensation to use is that a fly is buzzing near the client's head, and the client is encouraged to shoo it away.

Posthypnotic Suggestion. Subjects are given the suggestion that they will perform some action in response to a signal after they have been awakened—perhaps touching a part of their bodies or changing chairs in response to a noise produced by the hypnotist.

Amnesia. In one of the more difficult tasks, subjects are directed not to recall the events that have occurred since their induction or not to recall a particular event that occurred during the session until a prearranged signal is given.

Standardized Susceptibility Tests

Scales for measuring hypnotic susceptibility and hypnotic depth have been in existence since the nineteenth century. In the late 1950s and early 1960s, the hypnotic research program at Stanford University created the first of the modern scales, which are still used. The scales were created primarily for research purposes, although their use in clinical practice is not precluded. More recently, standardized scales that are more amenable to clinical use have been formulated.

Stanford Hypnotic Susceptibility Scale, Forms A, B, C (SHSS). These individually administered scales (Weitzenhoffer and Hilgard, 1959, 1962) form the backbone of most of the research literature on hypnotic susceptibility. Forms A and B are similar sets of tests intended to yield equivalent results for research purposes. The following test items are contained on these scales:

1. Postural sway.
2. Eye closure.
3. Hand drop.
4. Arm immobilization.
5. Finger lock
6. Arm stiffness.
7. Moving hands together or apart.
8. Inability to speak.
9. Insect hallucination.
10. Eye catalepsy.
11. Posthypnotic suggestion.
12. Posthypnotic amnesia.

Form C of the SHSS was designed to be used with or without a formal induction procedure. In general, it contains more tasks of a cognitive nature than Forms A & B (such as suggested dreams), more hallucinations, age regression, and fewer ideomotor items.

The SHSS forms have a wealth of research available on them and are well documented and easy to use. Depending on the clinician's style, some problems may occur with the stronger, authoritative, and hypnotist-centered language of each of these scales compared to more recent ones. Also, each of these scales is very time-consuming. The clinician or researcher who wishes to test for responsiveness in the absence of an induction will not be able to choose Forms A or B because they are integrally tied to a standardized induction procedure. Form C is more flexible in this regard. The tasks on Form C also seem to be more likely to be experienced as involuntary, thus perhaps better tapping the classic suggestion effect.

Harvard Group Scale of Hypnotic Susceptibility (HGSHS). This scale (Shor and Orne, 1962) is an adaptation of the SHSS Form A so that it can be group administered. The postural sway item is replaced by a head-falling task, and the inhibition of speech is replaced by a suggested inability to shake the head. This scale has excellent reliability and a wealth of research. More recent versions of it provide for subjects to rate their subjective experiences during the administration. It is worded in an authoritative manner.

Children's Hypnotic Susceptibility Scale (CHSS). Another adaptation of the Stanford scales, this one (London, 1962) is directed toward assessing the hypnotic abilities of children. The wording has been adapted for ease of comprehension, with alternate sets of wording for young children and teenagers. Like the other Stanford-type scales, this one is very time-consuming.

Stanford Profile Scales (SPS). These scales (Weitzenhoffer and Hilgard, 1963) were designed to permit a more qualitative assessment of an individual's hypnotic abilities. In contrast to the SHSS, which simply yields a classificatory number indicating susceptibility, the SPS yields a qualitative profile that attempts to assess the subject's abilities regarding analgesia, anosmia, deafness, regression, and personality change. By providing the clinician with a broader picture of the subject's abilities, it has some advantage over the other scales.

Stanford Hypnotic Clinical Scales (SHCS). These scales (Morgan and Hilgard, 1978/79), with both adult and child versions, are an attempt to provide standardized but time-conscious means of measuring susceptibility in a clinical setting. They are very worthy of consideration in this regard. Although they, like the other Stanford-based scales, are worded rather authoritatively, this thrust is less evident than in the others. Their time economy will appeal especially to clinicians. They also include age regression and dream suggestions, which are more likely to be useful to clinicians. A revised version of the scale for children has shown some improvement in application and reliability (Plotnick, Payne, and O'Grady, 1991).

Hypnotic Induction Profile (HIP). Another scale developed especially for clinicians, the HIP (Spiegel, 1974) is very brief, usually requiring less than ten minutes. It includes such items as eye roll, dissociation of limb, and limb levitation. One potential negative of this measure, depending on the clinician's level of comfort with physical contact with the client (especially a new client), is that this procedure requires the clinician to touch and stroke the client's hand. Its use of the eye roll test may also be of concern to some clinicians, since its value as a susceptibility test has been questioned.

Creative Imagination Scale (CIS). This is a very permissively worded scale (Wilson and Barber, 1978). No standardized induction is included. It is subjectively scored by the hypnotic subject. Its procedures much more closely approximate the style of clinical hypnosis commonly practiced today than the HIP. Drawbacks are that it requires more time to administer than the HIP and does not include a specified induction.

Intrapersonal Factors Related to Susceptibility

Hypnotic susceptibility is very stable within individuals over time, and this fact has naturally led to a search for intrapersonal factors with which it is associated. Clinical lore is replete with ideas that certain personality types are especially susceptible or resistant; however, except in a few studies, research has not yet borne out these observations.

General Personality Correlates. It has long been known that hypnotic susceptibility has not been reliably associated with any major personality factor, including anxiety, hysteria, neuroticism, and extroversion (Barber, 1964). Nor has it been associated with any personality inventory scales to date, although many of the more recent scales on the Minnesota Multiphasic Personality Inventory-2 (MMPI-2) and other newer personality inventories have not yet been substantially addressed. Null results have also been found with such constructs as locus of control (Saavedra and Miller, 1983), cognitive style (Bergerone, Cei, and Ruggieri, 1981), and even sophisticated electroencephalogram measures (Lubar et al, 1991). Some research suggests a possible relationship between persuasibility and hypnotic susceptibility (Malott, Bourg, and Crawford, 1989; Edmonston, 1986), but this concept seems more like an alternative definition of hypnosis than a true personality factor. In summary, clinical lore to the contrary, clinicians should not assume on the basis of personality variables that an individual will not be amenable to hypnosis.

Absorption, Attention, and Dissociation. One promising set of intrapersonal characteristics is the individual's attentional and fantasy abilities. Observations with highly susceptible individuals suggest that many of these persons reported vivid and frequent fantasy experiences. Tellegen and Atkinson (1974) developed the Absorption Scale to measure this construct and found that it was reliably associated with hypnotic susceptibility. Since that time, numerous studies that have been performed suggest that absorption is associated in varying ways with hypnotic susceptibility (Nadon et al., 1991; Crawford, 1982). For example, Balthazard and Woody find that a high level of absorption is more strongly correlated with the ability to perform difficult rather than easy tasks.

Some recent studies have cast a shadow on some of this research, however. Researchers have failed to replicate these findings consistently if subjects are unaware that they are involved in an experiment involving hypnosis. This suggests that much of the supposed relationship between absorption and hypnotic susceptibility may have been due to the fact that highly hypnotizable subjects are simply more acquiescent or adept at conforming to demand characteristics (Radke and Stam, 1991).

Resistance

Resistance (either conscious or unconscious) is designed to protect the client from anticipated or perceived threat. It is different from lack of hypnotic capacity. Resistance should not be attacked and will often respond to interpretation and working through, utilization in induction, or support, reassurance, and education. Common sources of resistance include the following:

- The client's preference for controlled experience or avoidance of receptive or novel experience.
- Fear of "having to change"; avoidance of change.
- Sensitivity to interpersonal influence and authority.
- Fear of one's own emotional experience.
- Fear of a rapid consciousness shift.
- Defense against dynamic uncovering.
- Distrust of the therapist.
- Perception of the therapist's lack of confidence.

Trance Depth

Depth of hypnotic response lies on a continuum from light to deep/somnambulistic. Experts in hypnosis would consensually agree that about 80 percent of the population can achieve at least a light trance, which is sufficient for most therapeutic work, and 5 to 15 percent are capable of deep trance, which is necessary for age regression, anesthesia, and uncovering of primary process. Clients often experience fluctuations of trance depth during hypnotic work.

Manipulable Factors and Modifying Susceptibility

Assuming that at least 5 to 15 percent of the population are strongly resistant to hypnosis, it will not be unusual in a clinical situation to encounter someone who apparently cannot be inducted. Although hypnotic responsiveness is thought to be a fairly stable aspect of personality (Barber, 1964; Weitzenhoffer, 1980), this does not mean that attempts to induct should cease after a single unsuccessful attempt. A number of techniques increase the likelihood that unresponsive subjects will respond more positively.

Repeated Attempts. Frequently hypnotic susceptibility increases with repeated attempts (Edmonston, 1986). Many clinicians report that they make five to six attempts before ceasing efforts. Bramwell (1903) reports that one patient was hypnotized on his sixty-eighth attempt.

Attitude toward Hypnosis. The subject's attitude toward hypnosis has been shown to be related to hypnotic susceptibility. In general, the more positive information the subject has available about hypnosis, the greater is the hypnotic susceptibility that can be expected. Failure to produce responsiveness in a subject should signal the clinician that some concerns about hypnosis may remain for the subject, and further assessment should be pursued.

Expectancies. The subject's expectancy that hypnosis will be effective seems to be a potent factor in hypnotic susceptibility (Saavedra and Miller, 1983; Wickless and Kirsch, 1989). This is probably why many of the most popular induction methods serve to increase subjects' expectancies. Especially with the person of questionable hypnotic susceptibility, everything that the clinician can do to increase the expectancy that induction will be successful should be performed.

Rapport and Status. The nature and quality of the relationship with the clinician may exert strong effects on the patient's hypnotic susceptibility. Rapport and trust are quite important. Gfeller, Lynn, and Pribble (1987) found that 50 percent of poorly responsive subjects made significant gains in their hypnotizability following a training program focused on trust and rapport factors. The expert status of the hypnotist also may be important, although research findings are mixed. One particular study of interest (Pereira and Austrin, 1980) indicated that subjects with an external locus of control experienced greater responsiveness with a high-prestige hypnotist than internals, although for both groups, prestige at least mildly improved their responsiveness.

Motivation. The patient's motivation to submit to induction is a factor in hypnotic susceptibility, as indicated by research studies (Barber, 1964) and clinical reports. Crasilneck and Hall (1985) say that for hypnotherapy to be most effective, the patient must feel that the suggestions being given by the hypnotist "echo in a profound way the patient's own deeper inner voice." Motivation is not a factor that is easily manipulated by the clinician; it depends far more on the patient, the nature of the presenting problem, and the patient's history.

Training Programs. One formal training program developed to increase hypnotic susceptibility is the Carleton Skills Training Program (CSTP) (Gorassini and Spanos, 1986). This program consists of four elements: a videotape in which a subject models hypnotic responding, a description of methods of absorption in hypnotic imagery, instruction about responding to suggestion, and practice by viewers of what they have learned. Administration of the program seems to increase the hypnotic susceptibility of the subjects, although there are some indications that it is not as powerful as once thought (Bates and Brigham, 1990; Gfeller, Lynn and Pribble, 1987).

The CSTP's experimental nature and time-consuming format probably preclude its use by most hypnotherapists. Nevertheless, consideration of its elements is useful in planning inductions of resistant subjects. Preparation of written materials addressing common misconceptions about hypnosis and orienting the individual to the hypnotic situation are recommended in any case.

The Decision to Employ Hypnosis

For clinicians dealing with behavioral problems, hypnotherapy is only one of many methods to consider. It could be argued that therapeutic responsiveness, whether in a hypnotic context or not, is often the first goal of an office visit with the client and is a product of the client's own needs and the rapport with the therapist. The decision of the clinician to attempt to add hypnotic responsiveness to the "normal" responsiveness that should already exist requires a careful weighing of risks and benefits to the treatment. In most cases the following steps are guidelines for the production of an effective hypnotherapeutic experience:

1. Assessment/selection.
2. Formulation of rationale.
3. Client preparation.
4. Trial hypnotic induction and debriefing.
5. Hypnotic induction.
6. Deepening of trance and trance ratification.
7. Trace utilization and presentation of suggestion.
8. Dehypnotization, reorientation, and debriefing.
9. Integration of trance work into the broader therapeutic focus.

It is true that a hypnotic induction is likely to provide the client with an experience of involition and a heightened sense of suggestibility. It is also possible that the hypnotic experience can lead to a disruption of treatment, and clients should be informed of that possibility, even if it is considered a remote possibility in that particular case.

Hypnosis can be a powerful tool, and like any other tool, it can be misused. Ethical use of hypnosis requires knowing the limits of one's skill and knowledge; clinicians should seek consistent consultation and supervision until they have experience with this technique, and they should keep informed of developments in the field. Participating in the education process and in research is useful, and taking continuing education courses is vital. It is important to be affiliated with a professional group with a primary interest in hypnotherapy—for example, a division of a professional organization, such as the American Psychological Association or the American Psychiatric Association—or with one of the two major respected groups in this area:

American Society of Clinical Hypnosis
2200 East Devon, Suite 291
Des Plaines, Illinois 60018
(708) 297-3317

Society for Clinical and Experimental Hypnosis
128-A Kings Park Drive
Liverpool, New York 13090
(315) 652-7299

One critical ethical issue in hypnotherapy, as in any other treatment profession, is being aware of the limits of one's practice. *If there is any question as to whether any significant, active component of the disorder being treated is outside the clinician's areas of competence, a prior clearance or a consult with and/or referral to an expert in that area is essential.* I emphasize this caveat because it potentially applies to all disorders discussed in this book.

MacHovec (1988) reviews empirical and clinical reports of complications and side effects of hypnosis, dividing them into three major factors:

1. Subject variables: Characteristics of clients that make them vulnerable to negative effects—such as repressed or unconscious issues tapped by the hypnosis, personality dynamics such as resistance or secondary gain, and misunderstanding of suggestions, attitudes, and expectations of the hypnotist.
2. Hypnotist variables—both personal factors, which are the same as those listed for subjects, with the addition of unmet sexual or social needs, chemical dependence, and personal bias, and professional factors, which include weaknesses or deficiencies in training, experience, or skill and theoretical biases that lead to an insufficiently broad view of dynamics or other factors operating with a particular client.
3. Environmental variables, which may include aspects of the physical environment that have some effect on the client in a negative or affect-laden way, either by association with some memory or by conscious or unconscious misinterpretation.

The use of hypnosis must have a therapeutic rationale and goal, and the therapeutic relationship must be the context. Hypnosis is a transactional process and generally will occur only in a relationship of trust and positive motivation in the client. Not all clients are good hypnotic responders, and the timing of hypnosis in the therapy process is crucial, so selection and pacing are important.

Client Selection

Positive indicators of client responsiveness include the following:

- Client intelligence—an approximate r of .60 of hypnotizability and intelligence.
- Client's childhood and adulthood skill in imagery production.
- Client's history of strict punishment in childhood.
- Client's report of imaginary playmates in childhood.
- Client's openness to new experience and to risk taking.
- Client's motivation to change and to solve problems (nonconscious motivation).
- Client's capacity and willingness to participate in a therapeutic alliance.
- Client's trust in his or her own psychological processes.
- Client's suffering from intrapsychic conflict, anxiety/phobia, psycho-physiological symptoms, stress, or similar problems.
- Experience with dissociative states (for example, meditation, religious induced).

Negative indicators include the following:

- Subnormal intellectual functioning.
- Psychological concreteness and absence of symbolic thought.
- Alexithymia (no labels for feelings) or strong psychosomatic or schizoid/schizotypal presentation—that is, clients who are psychosocio-avoidant.
- Active substance abuse or dependence.
- Paranoia, extreme compulsivity, and fear of loss of control.
- Agitation, mania, delirium, dementia, or severe attention deficit (organic states).
- Masochistic, self-defeating pattern (although these clients will submit to trance).
- Severe characterologic depression.
- Rejection of hypnosis for religious or other reasons (although the therapist may educate the client to accept hypnosis).
- Lack of motivation in treatment.

Particular caution should be used when the client:

- Shows fragile ego strength and/or reality testing.

- Exhibits intensive primitive impulses or affects, unless these are recentered on sensory boundaries rather than in free fantasy.
- Has strong ambivalence about therapy in general or hypnosis specifically.
- Exhibits significant indicators of acute suicidality.

Let us consider some related issues and concerns in more detail.

Treatment Factors

Efficacy in Achieving Treatment Goals. The patient's own goals for treatment should be an initial guiding principle for using hypnosis. However, regardless of whether the patient presents for a physical or psychological problem, he or she is trusting the clinician to formulate a treatment plan to restore health or ease distress. Therefore, the clinician's first task is to consider whether hypnosis can provide a benefit. Although there are not numerous well-controlled outcome studies of hypnotic treatments for specific disorders, there are numerous disorders for which hypnosis is clinically reported to be used with good effect.

The scarcity of outcome research often leaves the decision of whether to use hypnosis to the clinician. Like most other psychotherapeutic techniques, hypnosis is beneficial to some clients, with some problems, with a given therapist, some of the time. In the absence of clear outcome research, clinicians need to self-evaluate the efficacy of their treatments, through single-subject designs or otherwise, and use hypnosis only for clients for whom it is likely to be beneficial and practical.

Rationale. The induction of hypnosis should be placed in the context of the entire treatment plan for a patient. The clinician keeps the perspective of what hypnosis is supposed to accomplish and how it can be integrated with the rest of the intervention. The nature of the planned suggestions should be considered in advance, and it is well to be prepared to be able to communicate this rationale to the client, as the following case shows.

> Ted was a client at a small-town mental health clinic. He had initially presented with a major depression, which had followed a lengthy period of marital conflict and a divorce. Both of his parents and his former wife were verbally abusive, and Ted was a sensitive individual who accepted their derision at face value. Soon after the depression had resolved, Ted received a new manager at work who was sarcastic and insulting, and his depression began to return. The therapist, unsuccessful at helping Ted to develop a more critical, distant attitude toward his boss's statements, suggested to the client that they try to approach his memories of his parents' abusiveness hypnotically. After this suggestion, Ted missed two sessions. A telephone

call revealed that he had interpreted the therapist's changing of strategies as an indication that he had failed, and his depression had also significantly increased. He needed significant encouragement to return to treatment, and attempts at hypnosis were abandoned.

Meaning of the Induction. The decision to use hypnotherapy often represents far more than is apparent on the surface. Referral to a hypnotherapist may mean that other treatments have failed. The clinician's decision to use hypnosis may indicate to any patient that therapy up to that point has been a failure. To some patients, particularly in mental health settings, hypnosis may represent an opportunity to focus counterproductively on methods rather than on a more central issue. And for patients with strong dependence transference, hypnosis could reinforce that reaction.

Clinician Discipline. There are frequently issues surrounding the patient's expectations about the clinician's discipline or "school of therapy." For a somatically oriented patient who is seeing a physician for supposed treatment of gastric upset and "nerves," a recommendation of hypnosis may be met with outrage that the doctor would suggest that "it's all in my head." The psychotherapist is less likely to encounter such surprises. Such problems are also less likely as clinicians keep in mind the expectations for their discipline in any subculture and, especially, the expectations of their patients in this regard.

Therapist Factors

> Even if we ascribe to him superhuman virtue, since he is exposed to emotions which awaken such desires, the imperious law of nature will affect his patient, and he is responsible, not merely for his own wrongdoing, but for that he may have excited in another.
> —Bailly and others, in their secret report on mesmerism presented to the king of France, 1784

Training and Study. All clinicians must be adequately trained. Although almost anyone can learn the basics of hypnotic induction, training and experience are required for the ability to adapt the procedure to the problem at hand, to place the hypnosis in the context of the total treatment approach, and to appreciate the importance of the context of the problem. In general, this means formal, supervised, long-term mental health training, as well as supervised training and experience in hypnotic techniques. The current trend toward associate- or bachelor-level persons, such as physical therapists, using hypnotic techniques is inappropriate. Indeed, many master's-level programs do not provide the depth or sophistication needed to allow the use of hypnosis in clinical treatment. The unsupervised practice of hypnotherapy by such persons should be a rationale for granting compensation in the event of negative effects on the client.

In addition to formal training, hypnotherapists should keep up on current literature on the application of hypnosis. Although hypnosis has been used therapeutically for many years, a critical mass of well-controlled empirical research is just starting to emerge. Yet in many ways the phenomenon itself is not understood, let alone how it works clinically and how it can be made to work better. Awareness of these issues and of progress in the field can assist clinicians in providing the best possible care for patients.

Awareness of Limitations. Good hypnotherapists have an awareness of their limitations. A nonmedical hypnotherapist seeing a patient for a physically related condition should regularly consult with a physician. Additionally, through experience, individual hypnotherapists will find they do not work well with certain types of clients and should refer these clients.

Awareness of Clinician's Own Issues. Hypnotic techniques can be especially appealing to clinicians who still struggle with authoritarian or control issues; such clinicians need constant self-examination to prevent abuse. Clinicians who drift toward a seducing manner with attractive patients may find the transference issues raised by hypnosis difficult to deal with. Hypnosis can also be misused by using it to satisfy the therapist's curiosity rather than restricting oneself to addressing only therapeutic issues.

Empathic Perspective. Hypnotherapists' skills are enhanced by the ability to empathize with and understand the subject's experience. Appreciating the subject's point of view prevents many problems from emerging and allows enactments to become a source of therapeutic help rather than counterproductive power struggles.

Tolerance of Failure. Good hypnotherapists lack defensiveness and have a healthy tolerance for failure. It may be easy for a therapist to imagine and plan a successful intervention for a patient, but the success of any approach, hypnotic or otherwise, is dependent on many factors out of the clinician's control. The ability to accept failure, swallow disappointment, and try something else is critical.

Patient Factors

Many clinicians report that they do not hypnotize individuals with certain disorders because of the dangers thought to be involved—for example, persons with a psychotic diagnosis, persons thought to be in a highly weakened ego state, and suicidal individuals. To my knowledge, no systematic, definitive research has been performed that addresses the question of potential danger; however, from a clinical and practical point of view, there are general issues that contraindicate the use of hypnosis for these persons.

The individual's susceptibility to hypnosis should be taken into account; it can be aided by administering some of the tests described or even by a standardized scale. Low hypnotic susceptibility does not necessarily preclude a positive treatment response, but clinicians will carefully weigh the possibility that engaging in repeated hypnotic attempts with little success may reduce the economy of treatment in general.

Overall Concepts

The following concepts reflect both therapist and patient factors:

Educate before the session and debrief afterward.

Even successful hypnotherapy does not generate instant change. Persistent repetition of suggestions over time, consolidation of gains, and working through are necessary.

Identify and respect the defensive "accomplishment" of symptoms and dysfunction.

Avoid dynamic uncovering or emotional evocation with clients with low ego strength or who show risk of decompensation or disorientation.

Avoid using hypnosis for symptom removal until careful interview and assessment has identified the "accomplishment" or "secondary gain" of the symptom. The goal of treatment is not to strip the client of available coping strategies. When symptomatic behavior is the most effective strategy in the client's behavioral repertoire, it is important to develop more effective response alternatives before removing symptoms through hypnotic or other treatment.

Be gradual in uncovering work to avoid overwhelming the client's defenses and to allow the client to develop greater affect tolerance.

Take care always to bridge the hypnotic section of a therapy session into the overall session itself.

Introducing hypnosis into therapy can often interrupt resistance-based stagnation in treatment. The client's sudden failure to generate meaningful material is a sign of resistance that can be circumvented by hypnotic dreaming or internal inquiry about the function of the resistance.

The hypnotic state allows the client's development of a vivid subjective reality. The therapist can suggest imagery to foster this constructive process, avoiding overly detailed images that will interfere with the client's own imagery generation.

When giving direct suggestions, repeat several times to optimize reception.

In addition to the specific utilizations of hypnosis in meeting therapy goals, the very experience of the altered state of consciousness serves a catalytic effect, contributing to flexibility in the client's experience. The client who initially is a poor responder to hypnotic induction often shows considerable improvement with practice, which will mirror improvement in the therapeutic alliance and participation in therapy.

As the last point indicates, the process of hypnotic induction is the point of entry into a process that can have powerful effects on a client. The next chapter examines induction in detail.

3
Induction Techniques

Clinical hypnosis can fit within a broad definition of psychotherapy—that is, the use of psychological methods to help people make desired changes in behavior, somatic symptoms, thought processes, perception, and affect. This includes a focus on psychodynamics (nonconscious influences, conflict states), learned behavior (habits, conditioned responses), cognition (expectancies, meanings, distortions, appraisal processes, attributions), interpersonal behavior (patterns of interaction), and psychophysiological patterns.

For clinical purposes, hypnosis is defined as an altered state of consciousness, characterized by receptivity and focused concentration, with a heightened access to nonconscious experience, response strategies, and behavioral potentials. In this altered state of consciousness, the cognitive-associative structures that characterize the normal state are not operative, so a flexibility is introduced into the client's experience, as is heightened suggestibility (Schumaker, 1991). This flexibility of experience, suggestibility in behavior, and the receptivity in perception that is part of the hypnotic state are characteristics utilized in treatment. One's normal state of consciousness is maintained by an appraisal of events or experience (reality testing), as well as an array of monitoring and executive functions. In the hypnotic state, these functions are at least partially suspended due to induction procedures (Edmonston, 1986; von Kirchenbaum and Persinger, 1991).

Preparing the Client for Induction

General Principles of Induction

Timing and pacing are critical to successful hypnotic induction (Edmonston, 1986). A relaxed, confident, fluid manner of presentation serves to place the hypnosand at ease, allowing the reduction of cognitive and perceptual vigilance that is essential for development of the passive, receptive mental set upon which the trance state is based. Dramatic and rapid induction techniques have been developed and are often useful, yet when the hypnotic state is to be used for therapeutic purpose, it is usually best to minimize the risk of failure by being slow and careful, allowing for the gradual shift from normal consciousness to trance (Gravitz, 1991).

A permissive style of induction requires the therapist to attend closely to signs of hypnotic response in the client (Strauss, 1991) and then use those cues to proceed further (for example, by suggesting imminent eye closure only upon observing signs of relaxation and eyelid heaviness). In a sense, the hypnosand controls induction through the pace and nature of response to suggestion. Once eye closure is obtained, the therapist can lead and pace the process more fully, since the receptive state is then present to some degree. Allowance for the gradual development of hypnotic phenomena remains important, though, throughout the entire induction process.

The use of repetition is a central element of induction style at all points in the induction, both to create a soothing, monotonous atmosphere (reducing vigilance) and to maximize receptiveness to suggestion. The use of simple messages and suggestions allows the client to suspend monitoring and appraisal and thus develop the receptive, passive state characteristic of hypnosis.

When an eye fixation–eye closure induction is used, some clients fail to show eye closure even though other signs of hypnotic response may be present (fixed stare, immobility, muscular relaxation, and shallow breathing, for example). With these persons, the therapist should directly request eye closure, proceeding with the induction and testing for trance depth.

The induction of the hypnotic state is certainly an acquired skill, and increasing practice leads to greater facility and trance depth. The client who shows minimal response in a first or second induction may well develop greater response subsequently. There should be no implicit or explicit pressure to "succeed," since this will elicit performance anxiety, which will lead to arousal, inhibiting hypnotic response. The therapist should typically communicate acceptance and support of any response (including no response) shown by the client, as if it is exactly what is expected.

Apart from clear ineptitude on the part of the therapist, whether a hypnotic response occurs is primarily under the control (nonconscious as well as conscious) of the client. Communicating this clearly to the client may circumvent resistance to being controlled or influenced.

Successful and ethical use of hypnosis in treatment is based on the full and informed consent of the client (Gravitz, 1991). If, after open discussion of hypnosis and its expected benefits in treatment, the client is unwilling to participate, this should be respected. Yet numerous clients who initially refuse hypnosis agree to it later if they do not feel pressured by the therapist.

Introduction of Induction

Once the decision to attempt a hypnotic induction has been made, the patient must be readied for the process. Mention has been made of the potential effect of the patient's reaction to hypnosis. The idea at this point is to introduce the idea of an induction in a way that will not be threatening or frightening. I prefer to introduce the idea at a point in treatment when the treatment and treatment goals are an issue. Often this is appropriate at the first session if the patient is open at that time to a variety of approaches to dealing with the problem. Nevertheless, it may be difficult to assess all the necessary factors at the first session, so the idea is best addressed following the assessment phase or at a time in treatment when a summary of treatment progress is being made. Consider the following example:

> *Therapist:* Patty, it sounds as though you have improved a lot but that you still feel frightened when you are around other people. You need to decide if you wish to continue therapy and work on this. If you'd like to work on this some more, there are a few things we could try. One that is likely to help is hypnosis, and I have some other ideas as well. Why don't you give this whole idea some thought, and we'll talk about it more next session.

When hypnosis is brought up, it should always be introduced as an option, which is one of "a number of ways" to address the patient's concerns. This reduces pressure on the patient to assent, it prevents overinvestment in hypnosis as the only answer to the patient's problems, and it minimizes the adverse effects on the patient's attitude (and hence the treatment) if induction fails.

A patient's attitude toward hypnosis is a strong predictor of his or her eventual response to suggestion (Saavedra and Miller, 1983; Gravitz, 1991). Once the topic of hypnosis has been broached, the clinician will want to assess the patient's attitude toward it thoroughly. From a practical point of view, such an assessment is indispensable, and the clinician should not take initial denials of a negative attitude at face value. The patient may initially deny any concerns for a variety of reasons—perhaps lack of assertiveness, embarrassment, or a reluctance to question an authority.

Often a clinician who has mentioned hypnosis to the subject subsequently will find that the subject has been formulating many questions. *Hypnosis* is a strong word in our culture, and subjects frequently remember the initial mention of the topic and reflect a great deal upon it. Following is a typical exchange:

> *Therapist:* Patty, I mentioned the other day that hypnotism is one method that is often helpful to people with concerns like yours. How do you feel about the idea of being hypnotized in order to deal with your problem?
>
> *Subject:* I've thought a lot about it, but I don't really understand. How could that help my problem?

Occasionally a clinician will encounter an immediate, strong, negative reaction from the subject. This should always be met with validation of the patient's feelings, assurance that the clinician will not pressure the subject to engage in hypnosis, and provision of an opportunity for the subject to air concerns. Usually this approach results in the patient's relaxing and asking questions of the clinician, providing an opportunity for any myths or concerns to be dealt with more effectively than if the clinician attempts to confront the issue immediately.

More frequently, however, the potential subject does not have a negative reaction but does have some questions or misconceptions. Recognition and validation of these concerns is recommended, followed by addressing them in as straightforward a manner as possible. If the patient begins to ask broad or rambling questions, the clinician should ask, "What are your real concerns about being hypnotized?" in order to ascertain the specific fears of the patient rather than getting involved in lengthy dissertations.

Specific Concerns

Involuntariness. One of the most frequent questions is, "Can I be forced to do something against my will?" Taken at face value, this is a difficult question to answer; it is a matter of debate whether a hypnotized person can be so forced (Perry, 1979; Edmonston, 1986). In terms of the client's experience, many theorists believe that the nonvolitional sense during hypnosis is the hallmark of hypnotic response (Weitzenhoffer, 1980).

An immediate negative response to this question is not recommended for a number of reasons. Rapport with the patient may be harmed or the client may be confused if the clinician assures him or her of complete volition and then the subject has a nonvolitional experience. Furthermore, and more likely, denial of involition by the clinician may impugn the effectiveness of hypnosis in the patient's mind.

Most important, the question about coerciveness is almost always an expression of deeper and more specific concerns, and an immediate negative response may discourage the client from expressing these. Often it is asked by a shy or self-conscious subject who has seen a stage hypnotist suggest silly actions to a subject and who is afraid of being embarrassed. Or he or she may have seen a movie or read a novel in which hypnotized subjects were manipulated in some criminal manner, as in the 1991 movie *Dead Again*. A deeply moral or religious person may fear that some of the planned suggestions or interventions will involve shunned behavior or ideas. In each of these cases, the clinician can offer assurances to the patient that whatever concerns the subject has will be respected. If this is insufficient, then clearly greater trust between the patient and clinician needs to be established before induction is attempted.

Doubt. Many subjects immediately express doubt that they can be hypnotized. This possibility can be acknowledged but minimized by assuring the patient that the achievement of even a light trance or relaxed state is often helpful. This response has the advantage of circumventing a sense of failure should the client truly not be hypnotizable.

Fear of Being Stranded in Hypnosis. Potential subjects often ask if there is a danger that they will remain in hypnosis—for instance, if the therapist becomes incapacitated or dies. They can be reassured that this is not a possibility; the decision to become hypnotized and to remain in hypnosis will always be their own. The clinician may wish to reveal that many subjects find hypnosis so pleasant that they are reluctant to leave it and that this may be true of the subject. Often this type of statement helps to allay fear with a positive expectancy.

Religious Issues. Some potential patients have negative attitudes about hypnosis as a result of their religious beliefs; they may be afraid of antireligious or antimoral suggestions. For these clients, this is more of a trust issue than one specifically dealing with hypnosis. However, patients who come from conservative Christian traditions may object to hypnosis not because they are afraid of antimoral suggestions but because they have been taught that hypnosis is evil or dangerous in and of itself. Indeed, such fears are on the increase because of the use of hypnosis or hypnoticlike techniques in the new age movement and Eastern religions, each of which many conservative Christians view as direct threats to a Christian worldview.

Clinicians who encounter such problems probably should abandon any attempts at hypnosis, at least at that time. But if hypnosis appears indispensable to the patient's welfare, some further attempts can be made. The development of a trusting relationship may help matters, as may the invitation of a religious leader who is respected by the patient. It may even be possible to find a pastoral counselor as a cotherapist who has some proficiency in hypnosis and can cast it in religious terms acceptable to the patient.

Assessing Subjects' Preferences for Imagery

Some time should be spent assessing the images the subject prefers to day-dream about or that are especially pleasant to enable the clinician to tailor an induction that will be pleasant and likely to be well received. One should not assume that any specific image is pleasant, since these preferences may be highly idiosyncratic. For example, suggesting that the subject imagines lying on the beach may seem quite pleasant to a clinician who is an ardent sunbather but upsetting to a subject who is extremely self-conscious about body image or who is hypochondriacal (or even just realistic) about skin cancer.

An interesting case of failure of induction further underscores several of the points mentioned on induction.

> Betty is a rather shy forty-nine-year-old white female, a homemaker, and an active deaconess at her Baptist parish. She was referred to a physical therapist by her orthopedic surgeon following an injury to her back in a fall. The surgeon was unable to relieve the patient's discomfort and suggested to the therapist that he felt that anxiety was contributing to Betty's pain and that a hypnotic induction with suggestions of progressive relaxation would be helpful, in addition to the planned physical therapy. The doctor had previously discussed the possible contribution of anxiety to Betty's problem with her and met with stiff resistance to this notion.
>
> Without informing the patient that an induction attempt was imminent, during one of the therapy sessions the physical therapist began a hypnotic induction with the progressive relaxation method. The therapist told Betty to imagine that a man was massaging her toes, then her calves, thighs, and so on up her body. Unknown to the examiner, the sexual implications were extremely distressing to Betty. As the physical therapist reached Betty's scalp and continued with suggestions of relaxation, Betty calmly opened her eyes, looked at the therapist, and stated, "You think I'm crazy too." Neither Betty's pain nor her anxiety was helped by her treatment, and she terminated with both the surgeon and the therapist following the incident.

A number of mistakes were made in Betty's case:

- The physical therapist was not qualified to practice hypnotherapy, to assess Betty's psychological condition, or to formulate a treatment plan.
- Informed consent was not obtained. Betty did not understand or consent to the rationale for using hypnosis.
- Betty's attitude toward hypnosis was not assessed, and the therapist clearly failed to anticipate her expectations.

- Betty's preference for imagery was not assessed, which resulted in great embarrassment for her.
- No one recognized that this patient viewed hypnosis as meaning that she was "crazy."

A Preinduction Preparation Exercise

Billie Strauss (1991) has developed an approach, called the Apple Technique, that helps clients become more responsive to a hypnotic induction. In addition to anecdotal support, she collected data indicating improved responsiveness on the Stanford Hypnotic Clinical Scale for Adults (SHCS:A) from the use of the Apple Technique as an introductory device.

The technique is an exercise that takes one to three minutes and involves imagination (of an apple) and ideomotor ideation (hand levitation). Strauss reports choosing the apple for her technique because it is familiar and benign, although she does note general cultural associations to apples (as in "Snow White and the Seven Dwarfs" and sayings like "an apple a day keeps the doctor away"), as well as the unique associations to apples that individuals carry. Other fruits, or even other objects, could be substituted for apples if these show any indication of causing difficulties for a client. As adapted from Strauss (1991), the basic procedure is as follows:

1. After discussing the client's abilities and understandings in the areas of concentration and imagination, suggest a "test" or "check" for the client's ability to use the imagination. Explain that although this is not the hypnosis phase of treatment, the client may allow himself to go into hypnosis.
2. Ask the client to close his eyes and hold out his hand. Say, "I'm putting an apple in your hand; now describe it to me." Although some clients immediately respond with a description of the apple, others may need more urging or cues—for example, touching the hand in a manner that might suggest an apple has been placed there. Clients typically describe the apple in various ways (for example, it is yellow-gold, mushy, big, has a hole in it). Some of these comments can be followed up by logically sequential questions—for example, "Is it mushy all over, or just in spots?" But, move fairly soon into asking about sensory modalities that the client has neglected to mention, e.g.; "What color is the apple?", "Is it a soft or hard apple?" "What does it smell like?"
3. Ask, "Would you care to take a bite out of the apple?" If the client communicates having taken a bite, ask something to strengthen the image, perhaps, "How does it smell now?" or "What does it taste like?"

The basic concept is that the modalities the client responds to in this exercise—sight, sound, taste, texture, weight, even movement—are the modalities he or she will be most responsive (or nonresponsive) to in hypnosis. Also noteworthy is how much structure, cues, and open-ended questioning the client needs. Particular attention must be paid to cues to which the client responds strongly because this same pattern is likely to be found in hypnosis, and if it is a consistent pattern, the therapist may need to explore why the client cannot go into these areas without help.

If the client is responsive to the apple image and in some fashion indicates a willingness to proceed directly into hypnosis, the weight of the apple can be focused on. If the client is able to imagine the weight, the therapist suggests that in a moment he or she will take the apple out of his hand and that he will then notice that his hand feels lighter. If he responds at all, the therapist suggests increasing lightness and arm levitation. Then using a modified Chiasson (1973, p. 14) technique, the therapist suggests that as the client's hand reaches his face, he will find himself in a comfortable and relaxed but focused state of hypnosis.

If at any point the client shifts to nonresponsiveness or noninvolvement, technique direction can be shifted. For example, if the client denies the weight of the apple or a lightness response in the hand, it can be suggested that he continue to focus on the therapist's voice, breathe calmly but deeply, continue feeling contented and comfortable in this state, and return to the images and cues he showed strength with in the earlier phases to see if that works. Finally, the client is aroused with suggestions of alertness, comfort, and control and congratulated on whatever success he attained.

After using this technique, the therapist questions the client about the degree to which he was absorbed in the experience, how vivid the imagery was, how comfortable he was, and whether he had any unusual experiences or associations. The therapist can use the responses to these inquiries in his or her adaptation to the upcoming prototypical induction technique.

Strauss (1991) cautions that virtual or complete failure to imagine an apple is rare but suggests concreteness, limited capacity for imagery, and, by inference from her empirical data on the SHCS:A, limited capacity for a therapeutic response to hypnosis. Nevertheless, the great majority of clients respond positively, and in such cases, it leads either directly to hypnosis or facilitates a later induction.

The Induction of Hypnosis

There are almost as many different methods of inducing hypnosis as there are hypnotists. Strict memorization of an induction technique is not recommended, since induction strategies must be molded to each patient's characteristics and preferences for imagery.

Treatment can often be facilitated by using the induction as well as the process of hypnosis itself to suggest that the client will be eagerly receptive to new ideas and understandings, eager to experiment with new behaviors, more acutely aware of his or her own thoughts, feelings, and actions, find new solutions to problems, and so forth. Even without these explicit suggestions, the fact of inducing hypnosis itself may soften up the client's resistance to treatment somewhat by providing the experience of a pleasant, nondangerous yielding to the therapist's influence and providing a perspective-shifting experience of an altered state of consciousness.

Issues in the Induction Technique

Patient Relaxation and Comfort. Even experienced patients frequently arrive at the clinician's office with anxiety. It is best to provide a few minutes for this to pass and to allow the patient to reacclimate to the setting and relax a bit. Reclining chairs or couches are often used to provide a relaxed and comfortable setting for the subject.

Seating. Differing seating arrangements may be used to increase the client's comfort and decrease distraction. The clinician will want to sit behind or beside the client who is self-conscious and likely to be distracted by the clinician's gaze and in front of clients with mistrust issues unless a very strong rapport exists with the client.

Freedom from Distraction. The hypnotic setting should be as quiet and distraction free as possible. This is not a necessary condition for a successful induction; I have observed successful inductions even in the presence of numerous distractions, such as great traffic noise or building construction. Nevertheless, it is recommended since distractions may prevent a marginally responsive subject from entering a deep state and might be unwittingly incorporated into the trance by the subject. One of my first hypnotic subjects was a depressed and highly anxious woman who was hypnotized to provoke a relaxation response. In the midst of her first induction, she was asked where she would like to go that was pleasant and safe for her. She chose to go home and immediately upon entering the front door of her home, via trance, a patient in an adjacent office began screaming in anguish at the top of her lungs. My patient began sobbing uncontrollably, and she related in trance repeated sexual abuse at her home by her parents and grandparents. This revelation eventually was useful for the patient, but it resulted in a difficult and unpleasant first induction and reluctance to engage in hypnosis again.

Using Language Appropriately. Modern inductions rely on verbal induction techniques, client cooperativeness, and formation of mental events. Consequently, the language of the induction is becoming increasingly important in creating a hypnotic response.

Wright and Wright (1987) provide some useful suggestions about the language the clinician uses during the induction. They suggest that suggestions be framed positively, rather than proscribing actions or using *no* or *not*. For example, instead of giving the following suggestion to a dental patient, "You will *not* be able to put the tip of your tongue into the empty socket left by the tooth that was removed," they recommend a positive suggestion that the tongue will be drawn to the front of the mouth away from the socket. This avoids using language that implies a struggle of wills. Similarly, they suggest that the word *try* not be used for positive suggestions, since it implies uncertainty. Finally, they recommend using language that is familiar and understandable to the patient.

Timing of Statements. Some hypnotherapists (Jencks, 1984) recommend that the induction patter be timed in accordance with the breathing pattern of the patient. At the least, the induction should proceed soothingly and rhythmically.

Duration of Induction. Little is known about the optimal length of the induction process. Some hypnotic induction techniques are meant to be virtually instantaneous, and some require a much greater length of time. A general rule is that the induction should be long enough to yield the greatest degree of hypnotic susceptibility and depth possible without extending it beyond which there are no appreciable gains in hypnosis. If anything, it may be best to err on the side of length, since as London (1963) points out, an induction that is too short runs the risk of reducing responsiveness, while a long induction presents no problem other than the possibility of putting the patient to sleep. Unnecessarily lengthy inductions also present a cost in time and money.

Tests of Nonhypnotic Suggestibility

As a matter of course, many hypnotherapists use hypnotic tests of suggestibility before attempting an induction to screen patients for expected depth of hypnosis. These are usually low-difficulty tasks from one of the hypnotic susceptibility scales, such as hand drop or head falling. These may be useful to acclimate the patient to the hypnotic situation prior to presentation of an actual induction and may, if used carefully, increase the subjects' belief in their own hypnotizability, an important factor in hypnotic susceptibility. Since induction tends to increase hypnotic response, clients should not be ruled out on the basis of their reaction to one of these tests.

Specific Induction Techniques

> No one was ever hypnotized by looking at a lark-mirror, until Luys
> borrowed that lure from the bird-catchers and invested it with
> hypnotic powers. On the other hand, any physical method will
> succeed with a susceptible subject who knows what is
> expected of him.
> —J. Bramwell, 1903

Progressive Relaxation. Some form of relaxation technique is one of the most frequently used methods of induction; it can be used by itself or in conjunction with other techniques. There appears to be much greater time distortion (usually reporting a much longer duration than actually occurred) in hypnosis than in the progressive relaxation phase (von Kirchenbaum and Persinger, 1991). In the form of relaxation termed progressive relaxation, the subject is instructed to obtain a comfortable position and then to relax muscle groups, usually sequentially beginning at the head or the feet and slowly moving across the rest of the body. One author recommends a spiral pattern (Venn, 1984). The subject may be directed to count during this procedure. Some hypnotherapists direct the subject to tense the muscles prior to relaxing them, although some subjects report this to be distracting.

Eye Fixation. The subject is asked to focus on a specific point with the eyes while the clinician goes through the induction talk. Usually a point is chosen that will induce speedy eye strain, such as a point above eye level, a light, or a spot on the ceiling. The natural symptoms of strain are suggested to the subject as part of the induction, reinforcing the idea in the subject that responsiveness is occurring. Finally the eyelids are suggested to close, and the deepening procedure continues.

Chiasson's Method. This process can be quite effective with some more resistant subjects or even standard subjects (Page and Handley, 1991). Chiasson (1973) had patients place one hand in front of the face with the palm facing away and the fingers pressed together. This position creates considerable tension on the arm and hand muscles, inclining the arm to move and the fingers to spread. The patient is given the suggestion that these natural responses will signal the fall into a hypnotic state.

Pendulum Technique. The patient is instructed to hold a pendulum, such as a necklace pendant or a coin attached to a chain, in front of the eyes. As the patient focuses on it, the therapist suggests that the pendulum will move, which it indeed does as a result of involuntary muscle movements. The subject is told that the increasing swing of the pendulum indicates a deepening trance, until the pendulum is dropped altogether as the subject goes into trance.

Hand Drop Method. This test of suggestibility is also often used to induce hypnosis. The subject is instructed to extend the arm, with the therapist suggesting that the fall of the arm indicates a movement into trance. Sometimes this method is combined with eye fixation, such as by holding a coin in the hand in front of the eyes or by focusing on a spot on the hands or a fingernail. Suggestions of hand levitation may be used.

Other Techniques. Numerous other techniques abound. They are not used typically in standard inductions but may be employed as last resorts.

The eye gaze method is frequently encountered in historical accounts of hypnosis (Bramwell, 1903). The subject is directed to look into the hypnotist's eyes while the hypnotist repeatedly directs the subject to go into a trance. This method is very authoritarian and can evoke strong transference reactions, so extreme caution should be used.

Erickson (1964) and Kroger (1977) describe the confusion method, in which the subject is presented with a barrage of conflicting images and contradictory suggestions, while the suggestion of entering a trance is repeated over and over. Presumably the conscious mind is overwhelmed by attempting to deal with all the conflicts and acquiesces into a trance state. This method may be especially useful for very compulsive subjects who are resistant to trance.

Kroger (1977) recommends the nerve center method for resistant subjects. The subject is told that there are certain "nerve centers" that facilitate trance. A less sophisticated client might even be told that pressure on these points "induces trance," whereas more sophisticated clients would probably need to hear that they "facilitate trance." The clinician grasps the back of the neck and the upper portion of the nose and exerts pressure while engaging in hypnotic patter informing the patient that the beginning of trance will be indicated by the head's falling forward. As the induction continues, the clinician increases pressure on the back of the head and neck and releases the pressure on the nose, causing the head to fall forward. This induction uses direct subterfuge but may be useful in last-resort types of cases if the clinician is comfortable with this kind of interaction.

Components of an induction technique that are useful for a specific disorder are discussed in the chapter that addresses that disorder. Additionally, many of the techniques discussed in chapters 5, 6, and 8 can be useful in the induction process.

Prototypical Induction

The prototypical induction described here should not be memorized and then used in a rote fashion. Mastery of it allows a therapist to use the prototype as a core method, with modifications made to suit the individual client. The induction is based on eye fixation, progressive relaxation, and hand drop techniques. It seeks to allay client fears as much as possible in case there are concerns that the client has been unable or unwilling to relate.

Therapist: Now I would like for you to make yourself comfortable in your chair. You may experience the need from time to time during the session to adjust yourself and make yourself more comfortable. That will be fine. Now I would like for you to choose a spot up there where the ceiling meets the wall. Just find one spot that you can keep your eyes on. I'm going to ask you to keep your eyes focused on that spot, wherever you might choose for it to be. Find a spot; focus your eyes on that spot. You may find your eyes will wander from that spot from time to time. That is natural. But each time, bring your eyes back to that spot.

Let me remind you, as you focus, that you will not be asked to do anything embarrassing. You are in control. Just as you are choosing right now to focus on that spot, you will always be able to choose what to do. Right now, let those kinds of worries go, and focus more and more on that spot. Your eyes may wander or stray, but you always bring them back. Just keep looking at the spot and listening to my voice.

As you focus your eyes, it may be easier for you to relax more and more and not think about anything but keeping your eyes focused. That's right. Just let yourself become more relaxed and comfortable, always focusing your eyes and comfortably listening to my voice.

It may be that your eyes are feeling somewhat tired. That is all right. It is quite natural for them to be tired when hypnosis is beginning. They will get more and more tired, more and more relaxed, and you will become more and more comfortable and at peace. Soon your eyes may just close of themselves. If you feel them starting to close, just comfortably allow them to, and become more and more comfortable and relaxed.

Let yourself enjoy this experience. This is your time. In a moment, as your eyes become heavier and heavier, they will want to close of themselves. When they do close, that will signal that you can become even more comfortable and relaxed.

As the therapist observes signs of response—increasing eye blink; eyelid drooping; upward eye roll; slack facial muscles; slow, shallow respiration; a blank facial appearance—he or she feeds these back within the hypnotic patter and suggests increasing "alert drowsiness," which will reduce the likelihood of the client's slipping into sleep. The next suggestion is to let go and enjoy the drowsiness. When there are eye signs of responsiveness, the therapist suggests eye closure: "As you become more relaxed, be aware of the growing heaviness in your eyelids, which want to close to let you slip more fully into this alert and focused, but drowsy and relaxed state." When there is increased eye response, closure is suggested more directly: "Within a few moments, your eyes will naturally and easily drift shut, as if they have a will of their own, and you will slip easily and smoothly into this deeply relaxed, alert drowsy state of focused concentration; as your eyes close, you will feel a wave of relaxation flowing over your body, taking you deeper and deeper." The next suggestion is an increasing narrowing of awareness: "With your eyes closed, you can let your attention shift more and more within your body, letting the world outside, other than my voice, fade away as you become more and more aware of the sensations within your own body."

This patter continues until the client's eyes are closed or until it becomes clear, perhaps after five to ten minutes, that they will not. If the latter occurs, I direct the client to close her eyes. If that becomes necessary, it will be important to cast this as a success for the client, emphasizing how well she is doing. Once the client's eyes are closed, the induction continues with progressive relaxation:

> *Therapist:* Now, if you'd like, think about your muscles and how they could become more relaxed. They could become so much more relaxed and comfortable. Think about the muscles in your feet. Just allow all the tension to be released from them. That's right, this is your time. Just allow those muscles to relax. When you feel that your feet are just as relaxed as you want them to be, focus on your ankles. Let all the tension go from them. That's right . . .

This patter continues, addressing each major muscle group. An option is to suggest a focus of attention upon breathing for awhile:

> *Therapist:* Focus your awareness upon your breathing, feeling the air as it flows in and out of your body. Imagine your body as an air sac, filling completely as you inhale, all the way to the tips of your fingers and your toes and emptying completely as you exhale, each exhalation taking you one step deeper into this pleasant, relaxed, alert but drowsy state.

Suggest letting the tension from within the body flow out, using metaphor.

Therapist: Imagine the tension in your body to be a fluid, like water. Let this tension flow out of your body, as if the chair that you're in is a sponge, absorbing and soaking up the tension from your body. [or, "Imagine turning on a faucet, letting the tension drain out of your body."]

Internal sensations of relaxation can be suggested: "Feel your body becoming loose, limp, and relaxed, as if your body were made out of rubber," or, "Feel the heaviness developing throughout your body as you sink deeper into the chair, feeling the contact between your body and the chair become stronger," or, "You may feel numb, or tingling sensations within your body as you become relaxed.

In the first induction, the client's preference for imagery may be assessed:

Therapist: Now that you're feeling very relaxed, very comfortable, I'd like for you to imagine some places outside of this room where you feel very comfortable. Maybe you'd like to think about walking through the woods, rocking gently in a boat, or lying quietly in a room by yourself. Imagine being wherever you'd like, and as you're thinking about these, I want you to choose one place and imagine yourself there.

As the patter continues, the client is "rewarded" by allowing her to enjoy imagining being in this chosen place.

Then suggestions are given of deepening:

Therapist: As you continue to drift deeper and deeper, imagine yourself slowly walking down a wide, spiral staircase, deeper and deeper down. Every breath you exhale takes you one more step down, deeper and deeper. [or, "I'm now going to count from one to ten, and with every number I count, you will slip deeper and deeper down into this drowsy, alert, relaxed state of focused awareness . . . one . . . two . . . three . . . ten. Now deeply, deeply relaxed, drowsy but alert."]

Other imagery that can be used for deepening includes descending in an elevator or escalator, with counting, and imagining a leaf high in a tree that is gently floating down to the ground. The therapist's own imagination and/or the natural imagery revealed by the client can be drawn upon.

At this point, the therapist can further the induction by fractionation: bringing the client out of trance rapidly with prior suggestion as to reentering trance to a deeper level upon opening her eyes or hearing a cue:

Therapist: I am going to count backward from three to one, and when I reach the number one, you will feel wide awake, opening your eyes. As soon as you open your eyes, you will find the words *calm and tranquil* being repeated in your mind and, closing your eyes, will quickly and easily slip into an even deeper state of drowsy, alert relaxation than you are experiencing right now. Three . . . two . . . one . . . Calm and tranquil . . . calm and tranquil.

The therapist may proceed now with therapeutic utilization of the hypnotic state or offer tests of trance depth. Testing is advisable if there is reason to suspect failure to develop trance or if it seems important that the client accepts the fact of having been hypnotized. Since the client's failure to experience the test phenomena reduces the level of suggestibility, it is best to be cautious and conservative in induction and trance testing, avoiding prematurity in testing. Testing can range from limb catalepsy (immobility) to positive and negative hallucination formation. Yet since most desirable treatment effects occur with relatively light trance depth, a few simple tests usually suffice to demonstrate a therapeutically adequate level of trance development.

Therapist: Focus your awareness on the feelings within your right arm, noticing that with every passing moment your right arm is becoming heavier and heavier . . . feeling your right arm pressing more and more heavily against the arm of the chair, as if your arm is made of wood . . . heavier and heavier with every moment . . . as it rests more heavily on the arm of the chair, your arm feeling so very heavy that if you were to try and lift it, you would be unable to do so. I'm going to count from one to three, and when I reach the number three, I want you to try and lift your right arm, which will be so heavy that you won't be able to lift it. One . . . two . . . three . . . All right; relax and let your arm go loose, slipping into an even deeper state of alert, drowsy relaxation and focused attention.

Arm rigidity is another test:

Therapist: I want you to slowly raise your right [left] arm in front of you, so that it is straight. Make a tight fist, tighter, your arm becoming stiff and rigid. [Heighten response by lighting stroking the client's extended arm, from the shoulder toward the hand.] Your arm is becoming so stiff and rigid that if you

were to try to bend it, you would be unable to do so . . . I am
going to count from one to three . . .

It is essential with testing, as with the rest of hypnotic experience, to
allow sufficient time for the suggested phenomenon to be developed. Psychomotor retardation is a central characteristic of the hypnotic state, so the
client will generally appear sluggish in response to any suggestion. To avoid
the risk of test failure, the therapist can suggest the test phenomenon without completing the challenge. This may lead to the client's subjectively
experiencing the phenomenon (thus increasing subsequent response) while
not actually risking noncompliance.

Since therapeutic trance utilization does not require great trance depth
and since test failure reduces subsequent response, the therapist may choose
to proceed with utilization following trance deepening, without testing. This
is the point of utilization, typically the goal of using hypnosis in treatment.

Following utilization, the next step is dehypnotization: helping the client return to normal waking consciousness in a gradual manner that avoids
disorientation:

Therapist: I'm now going to count backward from five to one, and as
I count, you can lift up slowly from this deeply relaxed state
which you are experiencing, so that by the time I reach the
number one you are feeling wide awake, rested, relaxed, and
refreshed, ready to open your eyes. Five . . . let the energy
slowly flow back into your body . . . four . . . feeling the
energy . . . three . . . slowly feeling more awake, being more
aware of sounds outside of yourself . . . two . . . one . . .
Feeling wide awake, refreshed, rested, and relaxed, and
opening your eyes.

The return to full waking consciousness is generally gradual, lasting
several minutes past formal trance completion, which then gradually disappears within several minutes. Sufficient time should be allowed for this
decompression before the session is ended. The therapist may wish to employ some imagery to facilitate dehypnotization: ascending an escalator or
elevator, swimming up "from a deep lake within yourself, toward the sunlit
surfaces above," or something else.

After the trance has lifted, the clinician can assess what kinds of images
were pleasant for the client and use them in subsequent sessions when a
pleasant, relaxed state needs to be invoked. Debriefing upon dehypnotization should inquire about the client's experience of the induction; problems
encountered; particularly vivid, beneficial, affect-arousing aspects of the
induction; idiosyncratic imagery or metaphor (to be used in subsequent

work); awareness from utilization, and interesting or suprising cognitive or perceptual associations.

The following case illustrates the induction of a difficult client.

Sherry is a twenty-three-year-old female civil engineering student who has been experiencing severe test anxiety, and this problem is threatening her progress in her training program. She has a rather compulsive personality style, and the therapist has observed that her primary defenses are rationalization and intellectualization.

Prior to and during Sherry's tests, she had recurring images of her instructor's shaking his head while reading her papers and images of herself being unable to answer any questions. Her therapist suggested attempting to replace these images with self-efficacious ones via hypnotherapy, but Sherry described an experience of attending one hypnotic session for smoking cessation in which the induction failed. She considered hypnosis a "gimmick," and, at any rate, it was an experience that she could not have.

The therapist did not argue with her but gave her some literature that described hypnosis and addressed several misconceptions. When she was also asked to describe her previous experience, it became clear that the clinician had made no attempt to form a rapport with her. Her current therapist suggested that a more "scientific" approach toward hypnosis was very likely to be successful.

Without attempting an induction and with her eyes open, the therapist began the hand drop technique, telling her to extend her arm, then relax her arm muscles, and demonstrating that relaxation resulted in her hand's dropping. The therapist stated that, "scientifically," it was not possible for her arm to remain extended when her muscles were relaxed.

The therapist explained that people differ on hypnotic susceptibility, and Sherry was administered the Harvard Group Scale of Hypnotic Susceptibility via tape recorder, with the therapist explaining its creation and use. Sherry scored in the medium-high range in susceptibility and reported a strong sense of involuntariness on her responses. In this same session, a hypnotic induction was attempted, and Sherry achieved a deep level of trance.

Treatment proceeded with no further difficulties, and her test anxiety was greatly relieved.

4
Deepening Techniques

The Concept of Deepening

There is a lot of confusion surrounding the concept of hypnotic depth. Invariably hypnotherapists include in their induction procedures phrases such as, "You are going deeper, deeper and deeper," and so forth. Some books on hypnosis include separate chapters on deepening techniques. Yet it is often left unclear how "deepening" differs from induction. Further, little research exists on deepening techniques, and the research literature typically uses the terms *hypnotic depth* and *hypnotic susceptibility* as synonyms. Hypnotic susceptibility scales are often referred to as "depth" scales, and some susceptibility scales actually contain the word *depth* in their titles.

Although different authors quibble regarding the actual definition of hypnotic depth, the fact is that as popularly used, it is not a distinct and separately measurable construct. In its popular usage, the term subsumes many different constructs, each reflecting certain dimensions of the hypnotic experience.

Hypnotic Susceptibility

One of the constructs subsumed under "depth" is hypnotic susceptibility. Historically, the terms have been closely associated (Edmonston, 1986; Berrigan et al., 1991). The term *hypnotic susceptibility* seems to imply an either-or condition that a subject either is or is not hypnotizable. In fact, it is used to refer to the relative capacity of an individual to experience hypnotic phenomena. Thus, it is almost identical to the idea of depth. The distinction in usage is that hypnotic susceptibility is usually employed in the context of assessment and classification of individuals in research or in screening them for future hypnotic attempts; *hypnotic depth* is typically used to refer to the experience of a hypnotic subject who is undergoing clinical hypnosis.

In discussing hypnotic depth, then, the focus is on the hypnotic experience of an individual for the purposes of enhancing that experience and for facilitating treatment. Deepening procedures are ways of enhancing the subject's capacity to experience hypnotic phenomena. In the context of treatment, the assumption is (and research is generally supportive) that the individual's increased capacity to experience difficult hypnotic tasks such as amnesia or hallucinations will also indicate an increased capacity to respond therapeutically to hypnosis. One of the goals of deepening, then, is to facilitate the individual's ability to experience hypnotic phenomena.

One method of measuring the success of the deepening procedures being used is to employ the hypnotic susceptibility tests such as hand drop, catalepsy, and amnesia to determine the level of depth. The hypnotherapist can refer to any standardized hypnotic susceptibility scales to determine which items are of greater or less difficulty. Hypnotic susceptibility tests are usually organized as Gutman scales: the passage of a test implies that all the tests below that level also may be passed by the subject. In any hypnotic session, as the subject is able to do more and more difficult tasks, the hypnotherapist is made aware that the deepening procedure is working.

Responsiveness to Suggestions

Deepening refers more to specific instances of hypnosis rather than to a person's overall abilities. Although an individual may be quite susceptible to hypnosis in terms of natural capabilities, in any particular session, he or she may be quite resistant to entering as deep a state as he or she is capable of. Consequently, clinical deepening procedures focus on enhancing the client's hypnotic abilities at one specific time with one given therapist. *Hypnotic depth* is thus a more situational and clinically relevant term than *hypnotic susceptibility*. It refers to what is happening with the client regardless of the client's abilities.

Hypnotic Sleep or Trance

Hypnotic depth also refers to the degree that the subject is able to disregard external stimuli other than the hypnotherapist and focus on the inner experience of the process. This perceptual narrowing is often referred to as "hypnotic sleep" or "trance." It is this aspect of hypnosis from which hypnotic "depth" most likely received its name (Edmonston, 1986). For those familiar with hypnosis, it seems natural to talk about the experience as one of sleep or diminished awareness (although it has characteristics quite opposite from true sleep). The eyes are closed, and the subject is often told that they are so heavy that they cannot be opened. There is often a feeling of profound heaviness and torpor, with relaxation and regular breathing. Vertical imagery of going down into trance is usually used. Some talented subjects achieve somnambulism, in which they are consciously unaware of their activities during hypnosis and usually cannot recall them. The feeling after emerging from the trance is generally one of having been asleep.

The deepening procedure is intended to enhance this subjective experience of perceptual narrowing and relaxation. As this experience becomes stronger, the subject becomes ever more able to ignore distractions and not be troubled by anxieties. This results in the hypnotherapist's communicating more effectively and also making it more likely that the hypnotherapist will be able to circumvent any defenses that are present.

Specific programs have been developed to increase hypnotic depth or responsiveness. One of the most notable is the Carleton method. However, like many other endeavors of this sort, the early promise of significant gains in hypnotic response has met with mixed success at best when scrutinized by researchers who have little investment in the success of the method (Bates, 1990; Bates and Brigham, 1990). Spanos, DeBrevil, and Gabora (1991) do provide some empirical support for their skill enhancement approach to increasing hypnotic depth.

Absorption

The converse side of this relaxation and narrowing phenomenon is an increased awareness of the inner experiences of the client. As trance becomes deeper, the client is able to become increasingly absorbed in images, fantasies, and the interventions of the hypnotherapist. At deeper levels, images and suggestions come to be experienced as reality, as evidenced by the ability to have directed hallucinations or perceive illogical or impossible situations. Dissociations such as hallucinations of leaving the body or assuming different personas may be experienced.

Specific Deepening Procedures

Hypnotic depth is a multidimensional construct, and enhancing it involves manipulating a number of factors (Spanos, DeBrevil, and Gabora, 1991). Each of the factors mentioned regarding facilitation of induction, such as rapport building, enhancing expectancies, and minimizing distraction, applies equally to the deepening process. Every factor that affects the individual's hypnotic experience has a potential impact on the depth achieved.

Provision of Information

In order to achieve a deep level of hypnosis, subjects need to know what is expected of them. Often hypnosis is treated as an entity that exists apart from the person and that, when achieved, will invariably result in the same phenomena. This is not the case. Client knowledge and understanding facilitates depth. The hypnotherapist needs to explain hypnotic depth to the subject. Consider the following example:

Therapist: Joe, I'd like to let you know what to expect as you and I continue to use hypnosis in our sessions. As time goes on and you get more and more accustomed to being in hypnosis, you are going to find yourself able to go even deeper into hypnosis than you have been, if you wish to go deeper. This means that you will be able to let yourself be even less aware of what is going on around you. You will be less aware of your body and less aware of any thoughts that aren't helpful to your treatment. And it will be easy for you to have some experiences that I suggest, like imagining things in your mind or remembering things very clearly. If you allow yourself, you will even be able to not feel discomfort or even not remember things that happened while in hypnosis. These things may or may not happen right away; I will allow you to set the pace.

Merely telling clients that they are going deeper into hypnosis may well be useless unless they understand what this means. Remember that all of the hypnotic responses are contingent on the individual. Hypnosis is not automatic.

Facilitating Involvement

This requirement for the subject to aid in creating the phenomenon needs to be communicated to the subject to facilitate deepening. The previous example stressed to the client that hypnosis was contingent on the client's wishes and willingness to experience them. It is helpful to explain to clients, especially those who are more sophisticated, that hypnotic phenomena are made possible by their own actions. For example, they cannot hold their eyes open if their facial muscles are completely relaxed. This explanation lets them know that they are in control of their experience. Paradoxically, this empowerment of the client also helps to circumvent resistance—for example:

Therapist: Joe, as you wish to go deeper into hypnosis, you can allow this to happen by letting yourself relax more and more. I cannot do this for you; it's up to you. As I use the phrase *deeper and deeper,* let this remind you to let yourself relax as much as you would like.

Client Reinforcement

Another method of deepening is to generate practice of and then reinforce the behaviors of the client that are consistent with the deepening experience (Spanos, DeBrevil, and Gabora, 1991). This allows the client to understand better which behaviors are appropriate and helpful in achieving deeper states, and it provides added incentive for doing so.

The reinforcements used for any given client can be determined by the therapist on the basis of what is most likely to be reinforcing for that person. The most common reinforcement is praise and recognition, for example, "Lisa, your hand began dropping very quickly. You are doing very well." For some clients, touch may be reinforcing. While performing a glove an-esthesia test with a client, the therapist can pat the client's involved hand and praise him or her for success. For children, reinforcers are even more important to hold their attention and let them know what is expected. Praising, touching, and giving rewards are very effective—and, of course, M&Ms always seem to work.

Observation. Successful reinforcement requires that the hypnotherapist be sufficiently aware of depth-consistent behaviors to reinforce. Careful obser-vation of the client is required. For hypnotherapists who like to seat them-selves behind their clients, this may present a problem; a better vantage point is recommended until the client learns the hypnotic deepening re-sponse. Behaviors to monitor include increased regularity of breathing, re-duced muscle tone, myoclonic jerks, decreased fidgeting, and any positive responses to suggestions.

Signaling. Even careful observation cannot always inform the hypnothera-pist of the client's experiences, especially with subjective experiences that are not outwardly observable. For example, the therapist has no way of knowing if a client has achieved an image without asking. This is also often true of relaxation; although the therapist may observe external behaviors that indicate relaxation, this too is actually an inner experience. Conse-quently, ideomotor signaling is usually necessary for deepening techniques. Ideomotor signaling is the client's use of a movement, usually a finger lift, to communicate with the hypnotherapist during hypnosis. Simple speech may be used, and speech is necessary for more complex communications, but many individuals find speech to be distracting while under hypnosis, and others have difficulty speaking at all because of muscle relaxation. Clients can be trained in ideomotor signaling by telling them prior to the induction that, for example, a lift of the right forefinger during hypnosis will indicate "yes" and a lift of the opposite finger will mean "no." This is then played out and reaffirmed while the client is in hypnosis. Any system can be used as long as it is simple and does not create distraction. Consider the following illustrative case:

> Bud was a rather shy, self-conscious accountant who presented for hypnotherapy for pain control. He had been involved in a skiing accident that injured a nerve in his neck, and he experienced constant, acute pain in his left arm. It was necessary for him to type at a keyboard at his job, but medications of sufficient strength to make his pain bearable caused him to become so drowsy that he could not maintain attention at work. Consequently he sought hypnotherapy.
>
> Bud was very cooperative with the hypnotherapist but found it difficult to reach a sufficient depth of hypnosis to achieve analgesia. Upon careful questioning, it became apparent that recurrent, anxious, self-focused thoughts were interrupting his participation in deepening attempts. These thoughts involved fears of failure and images of his losing his job.
>
> After becoming aware of this, Bud's hypnotherapist did not attempt induction for four sessions. Instead, he oriented Bud to techniques to monitor his anxious thoughts and worked with him supportively to normalize his fears. Prior to attempting hypnosis on the fifth session, the hypnotherapist asked Bud to raise his right finger if he began experiencing the anxious thoughts during hypnosis. When Bud indicated that he was doing so, the therapist allowed him to express these thoughts openly and encouraged him to approach his troubling images in the trance. Soon this led to a normalization of his fears, and Bud achieved an effective level of trance. After he was thoroughly trained in hypnotic analgesia techniques and was able to control his pain sufficiently to continue working, he went on to seek psychotherapy to deal with his general anxiety.

Ratification

Deepening is also facilitated by ratifying the client's experiences. Many clients have a fear of failure in hypnosis, and confirming to them that they are truly exhibiting a hypnotic response is important. Using hypnotic tests such as eye closure or hand drop, which are very likely to result in a positive response, even with a minimal level of trance, is one way of ratifying the experience to the client. Another effective method is to ask the client following the trance to describe any sense of involution during the trance, which signals a substantial, effective level of hypnosis at those times. Reports of deep relaxation and absorption should also be encouraged. Some clients who do not achieve a deep level of trance will not report these types of experiences. For these clients it is especially important not to disparage their experience but to choose aspects of their experience that were more consistent with depth and reinforce them:

Therapist: Wanda, I know that your hand did not raise much when I suggested it would, but I am glad that you say that it did feel very tired. The fact that it was feeling different at all shows that you were open to suggestions. As you get more practiced at hypnosis and more comfortable with your control of this experience, you will find it easier to experience your arm lifting.

Expectation

Along these same lines, the therapist should do everything possible to create a positive expectation that hypnotic depth will occur. Expectancy is a powerful part of hypnotic phenomena (Silva and Kirsch, 1987). During efforts to allay client fears about hypnosis, one should be careful not to disparage hypnosis or minimize its power. Use of "when" language while orienting the client and during the induction and deepening is useful: "When you feel even more relaxed than you do now, signal me." "When you feel that your arm is getting lighter all by itself, let it rise." It is also important for the hypnotherapist to maintain an unruffled, positive attitude. Client failures should be reframed as successes as much as is possible.

Using Client's Motivation

A procedure that can be effective is to remind clients during the deepening procedure of their motivation for treatment. Clients who are ambivalent about treatment because of short-term discomfort can be reminded about their long-term goals. For example, a smoking cessation client presenting because smoking is an obstacle to her succeeding at tennis can be reminded that her ultimate goal is good physical health. Forensic clients can be reminded about their need to cooperate with the attorney.

An important consideration here is not to be coercive or goading with such statements, particularly with resistant clients, or they can serve to increase resistance. Statements must be carefully phrased to avoid patronizing language.

Paradoxical Intention

For clients who are consciously or unconsciously resistant, their resistance needs to be dealt with as much as possible by improving the therapeutic relationship, recognizing their concerns, allowing them to express their concerns, and normalizing them. Clients who are more passively resistant and unlikely to respond well to a direct approach of their resistance can often be remediated through paradoxical intention. The following example is of a thirty-eight-year-old salesman who presented for smoking cessation therapy.

> While loudly asserting that treatment was something that he wanted, Bob admitted that he had originally come for treatment at his wife's insistence. He was intrigued by hypnosis and could be induced but consistently achieved only light levels of trance. Attempts to question him about his resistance were met with strong denials. After two unproductive sessions, his therapist announced that the next two sessions would involve only practice in hypnotic techniques and that "relaxation is all that is necessary." Bob was told that these sessions would involve imagery and fantasy that he would choose and that hypnotic depth would not be particularly useful during these sessions.
>
> During the two sessions, the hypnotherapist avoided focusing on Bob's smoking behavior and after induction guided him through neutral images. At the end of the second session, when it was apparent that Bob was much deeper in trance than he had been previously, antismoking therapy continued.

Vertical Imagery

A method many hypnotherapists use is vertical imagery. A common technique is to ask clients to imagine an elevator or escalator (or staircase, as in the 1991 movie *Dead Again*) and to imagine themselves descending and noting that as they do they will go deeper into trance. Descending imagery is probably more useful than ascending because it is more constant with the other metaphors used in hypnosis—depth, going deeper, feeling heavy, and so on. For example:

> *Therapist:* Imagine that you are waiting for an elevator. It is waiting to take you where you want to go—deeper into trance, deeper and closer to the good health you want. It will not arrive until you wish for it. It is getting closer, but it is up to you when it arrives. Lift your finger when the elevator door opens. Good. Step into the elevator when you are ready, and make your selection as to how far down you wish to go. Signal me when you are ready. That's good. As you begin down, you will find yourself becoming more and more re-

laxed and feeling more and more comfortable. That's right— farther and farther down.

Fractionation

Some hypnotherapists use fractionation: taking clients in and out of hypnosis very quickly, with the hope of achieving successively deeper levels of trance. Repeated experiences do improve hypnotic skill, but some clients find fractionation confusing and distracting, so its usefulness has been questioned. Research reports support these observations. Hammond and associates (1987) found that, on the average, fractionation did not improve depth, although some patients showed significant gains with it. Fractionation may be helpful in the idiosyncratic case but should not be used for every client.

Touch

Touching is another deepening technique that can be helpful but is questionable for general use. In the early days of hypnosis, stroking and "laying on of hands" were invariably used to induce and deepen patients. Repeated "passes" of the hands over the body were thought to deepen the trance. When it was discovered that it was not a necessary procedure, touch was abandoned and even censured.

The use of touch can result in negative effects for some clients—either by causing distraction or by eliciting transference issues. If the hypnotherapist does use physical contact, it is recommended that it be used out of a specific therapeutic rationale on a case-by-case basis, that the client be questioned carefully with regard to its beneficiality, and that any opportunities for client misunderstanding be circumvented by careful explanation. Sessions using touch should at least be audio recorded. If feasible, acceptable to the client, and not distracting, video recording is recommended.

Sensory-Enhanced Imagery

Hypnotherapists are acutely aware of how important imagery can be in effecting change. For example, when working to increase performance by visualization (whether administered hypnotically or not), quality and intensity of imagery is a critical predictor of how useful the visualization exercises are.

Some individuals easily generate imagery; for others, it is more difficult. Bringing detail into the hypnotically suggested images can be helpful, and this is the tack most hypnotherapists use. However, for a number of patients, standard approaches are not enough to help them develop effective imagery. One reason that this may be so is that the stimuli typically used to enhance the imagery come through only one sensory modality, the auditory mode. And even when extra and detailed suggestions are provided, this is also through the auditory modality. A technique for enhancing imagery (especially when in hypnosis) that I gradually developed and have found to be useful can be logically termed sensory-enhanced imagery (SENHI).

Visual and auditory stimuli predominate in our society. Hypnotherapists often implement auditory stimuli to enhance imagery and sometimes add visual stimuli (slides and videotapes, for example). But I have not found these stimuli to be especially useful. Visual stimuli tend to define and even constrict images rather than enhance or stimulate them. Moreover, we have rather constant training—from television, for example—to be passive in the face of visual imagery. Finally, using visual imagery requires clients to have their eyes open yet be hypnotized, a counterproductive strategy with many clients. And except in rare cases, I have not found the payoff from auditory stimuli—for example, musical passages played through earphones (Walker, 1990)—to be worth the effort. Kinaesthetic stimuli are theoretically useful but offer overwhelming logistical and liability issues.

On the other hand, tactile and olfactory stimuli are very useful in developing SENHI. Indeed, William Dember (1991), an experimental psychologist at the University of Cincinnati, has shown that scents can produce signifiant behavior change over a substantial duration of time. He proved empirically that a peppermint scent improves mood and work performance.

The range of potentially useful stimuli, including those that are not especially pleasant, is enormous. The more "stuff" of this sort that is available, the more enhancing stimuli can be presented to clients. I have found that presenting scents easily elicits images in most image-resistant patients. This is not surprising since olfaction is considered the most primitive of the senses.

Presenting tactile stimuli is also effective in eliciting images in people who usually have difficulty here. Fabrics of various textures have been useful, as are pieces of wood, coral, and a small soft doll or teddy bear figure. I have found that stones of various shapes and surfaces have been the most helpful. A collection of stones I picked from a beach has proved to be especially pleasing and useful for most clients. They look like a set of miniature Henry Moore sculptures.

I ask the patient, while hypnotized, to take each stone and thoroughly feel it and try to "experience" it. With some stones, there is little reaction, so I ask the patient to handle another one. On occasion, I see a patient show a facial or body response to a stone, even while the patient says he or she is getting no images. I ask patients to "keep at it for awhile" and often find they eventually break through to important images that have heretofore been resisted. Such images are often the key to getting through a therapeutic impasse.

A variation of this approach is to give the patient a glob of a gelatinous substance, like clay or plasticene, and ask him or her to "feel it and work it into some shape that feels right" or "into a shape that feels like it's in there." Patients can be asked to associate with images while doing this or instructed, analogous to automatic writing, to just hold the substance and let their unconscious mind guide their hands: "Your unconscious will form the clay in a way that will then release thoughts and images that it will, at some point, want your conscious to know about. Just relax as your unconscious may want to do this slowly or quickly. Either way is fine."

Like many other therapeutic techniques, developing SENHIs is a skill that grows with experience. It is a useful ancillary deepening technique, especially with clients who have difficulty developing images from auditory cues.

Extrasession Techniques

A number of techniques that can be used outside the hypnotic session can also be implemented to deepen in-session hypnotic response. Practice with progressive relaxation or some form of meditation or with a technique that combines physical work with meditation, such as yoga or tai-chi, can be effective. One especially useful technique for this purpose is autogenic training (Schultz and Luthe, 1959; Luthe, 1969; Van Dyck et al., 1991). Some people have noted that autogenic training is analogous to hypnotherapy (Korn, 1984). While autogenic therapy can be applied to specific disorders with effectiveness, it primarily and efficiently improves various psychological self-regulatory functions. This not only enhances one's overall capacity for psychophysiological adaption and increases resistance to the negative effects of various kinds of specific stress but makes the individual more responsive to other interventions. As such, it is also an ideal technique to help the individual reach deeper levels of hypnotic response.

My own approach to autogenic training has evolved over years of practice with it. When I moved to Louisville, I was using variations of the traditional "overall formula" "I am at peace," rather than the overall formula that I discuss later in this chapter, "I am calmness throughout." The reason for changing was a negative reaction by my first client, which served to remind me that the primary private psychiatric hospital in Louisville at that time was Our Lady of Peace; being "at Peace" was not a desired image. Of course, other overall formulas can be used, for example, "I am centered in calmness."

From this point up to the final commentary on this technique, I use a wording that can be directly presented to a client—for instance, in a handout that is then supplemented by office practice and/or tapes.

Autogenic Training

Autogenic training is a technique based on a significant body of research supporting the idea that psychological factors strongly influence physiological factors and also that autogenic training can change processes such as the general stress syndrome as well as more specific psychophysiological processes in the body. The basic ideas on autogenic training were developed in the early 1900s in Germany and were subsequently thoroughly researched, particularly in Europe; they have spread throughout the world.

Positions

Prone Position. The great majority of people find that the most efficient way to learn and experience results from autogenic training is to do the exercises while lying on a couch or a bed. (The following suggestions help most people maximize their results, but these comments are not to be read as hard and fast rules and can be modified to individual needs.) While lying down, the legs are usually slightly apart and relaxed so that the feet are inclined outward at a V-shaped angle. Some support (a folded blanket) under the knees helps many people to relax the muscles of both legs. The trunk, shoulders, and head are most easily relaxed when kept in a symmetric position. The arms should lie relaxed and slightly bent beside the trunk of the body. The fingers remain slightly spread and flexed and generally do not touch the rest of the body.

Particular attention should be given to determining the most relaxing position for the head, neck, and shoulders. It is advised to try different pillows to see which is most comfortable for these exercises. Most people have found that foam rubber pillows are not the most effective. It appears that preference should be given to semiresilient or nonelastic materials for the pillows and even, if possible, the upholstery of the training couch or bed. If there is a continuing of stiffness in the neck or shoulder muscles during the exercises, consider whether the head has been kept symmetrical and whether the pillow is in a reasonably comfortable position.

While doing the exercises in the prone position, it is always advisable that the shoes be removed. When a blanket is used for cover, it should not be tightly wrapped around any part of the body since restriction or pressure may have a somewhat distracting effect during the exercises. Another point, and one frequently overlooked, is that certain people relax more completely and perform the exercises more effectively when given some support under the knees.

Reclining Chair Position. The autogenic exercises can also be performed in a reclining chair that has a high enough back so that the trunk and head can rest passively and comfortably. Most of the suggestions made for the prone position are also relevant here.

Often reclining chairs provide postures that are not as comfortable as may first appear. Pillows and other means can be used to adjust the contours of the chair so that it becomes a comfortable position. There should also be support throughout the length of the arms and the legs.

Straight Chair Position. Attaining some comfort and mastery of the straight chair position is helpful because it allows clients to practice the exercises in a great many places, including at work or even in public places such as airports.

In this posture, the edge of the seat should not exert pressure on the legs, and the feet should rest solidly on the ground. In order to attain a position of maximal relaxation in this position, the client first straightens up completely while in a sitting position. Then, with both arms hanging down at the sides, he or she suddenly relaxes completely, which results in a kind of collapse of the trunk, shoulders, and neck, with the body supported primarily by the skeleton and ligament structure. It is best to keep the back relatively straight; in other words, the trunk collapses downward without bending forward. To the degree possible, the body should feel as if it is hanging loose. Most people find it ideal to have the underside of the forearms rest on the upper thighs. The head has dropped forward, and the arms, although touching the legs, generally feel as if in a loose position. One way to test the state of relaxation in this position is to lift one's hand and then let it drop of its own accord, or else have a trainer do this.

Training Elements

Passive Concentration. Autogenic training proceeds most efficiently for people when they approach it with an attitude generally conceived of as passive concentration, which may best be explained by contrasting it to active concentration. The decisive difference between active and passive concentration is the attitude toward the functional results to be achieved. Passive concentration implies a casual attitude and a passivity toward the intended outcome of the autogenic exercises on that particular day. (This does not mean that there is no hope for positive results as an outcome of the exercises, but during the exercise, there is no need to see results occurring.) Active concentration, on the other hand, is characterized by a concern and attention and even active efforts to try to make the result come about during that particular exercise. This attitude of active concentration often generates mild anxiety about performing well or achieving results, which is counterproductive to the overall training and should be avoided.

Autogenic training produces results over a gradual period of time. It is good practice to take the attitude, "During this particular session I really don't care whether my particular goal [such as warmth] happens. I know it will happen sometime, so I'm calm about it now." The client might be instructed to meditate on achieving passive concentration before actually going into the exercises and then, after finishing, look back to see if he or she achieved it. If not, the exercise can be viewed as a learning experience for the next time. Those who suceed can congratulate themselves and commit to trying to achieve the same attitude of passive concentration the next time.

Steady Flow of Images. A second important element in autogenic training is maintaining a steady flow of mental images, allowing no lapses of time to occur between repetitions. This steady flow may be provided by an "inner voice" or by visualizing the particular formulas as if they are in print or as if they are a neon sign in the mind that can be switched on and off at will. It is not particularly critical which modality or which method is used to maintain this steady flow of images other than speaking the words aloud. The form (inner voice, visual image, and so forth) that is most comfortable should be used throughout the later phases of therapy to enhance the conditioning effect.

Mental Contact. Mental contact refers to putting the attention of one's mind in touch with the particular body part that is the focus of the particular formula that the client is imagining verbalizing at that time. For example, a client using the formula "my right arm is heavy" should try to imagine being mentally in touch with that arm. Some people even imagine themselves as being their arm. Whichever way works best is fine; what is important is to try to gain that mental contact over time while proceeding through the exercises.

From both experimental and clinical observations, it is clear that the functional value of these various formulas is markedly enhanced to the degree that the person not only maintains a steady flow of images but at the same time can gain mental contact with the part of the body that is the area of focus. This flow of images should be kept in pace with the formula being repeated.

Reduction of Stimuli. Autogenic training is always most succesful when external stimuli are reduced to the lowest possible level during the procedures. To the degree available, the exercises should be practiced in a quiet room with very low lighting, if any, with all restrictive clothing (glasses, belt, girdle, or necktie, for example) loosened to a point of comfort or removed.

A further reduction of external stimuli is gained by closing the eyes. It is desirable to do this as soon as the posture is taken. A number of studies point to a functional relationship between the phenomenon of eye closure and the facilitation of more passive states of mental activity.

Preparing for the possibility of other types of external distractions is also helpful in facilitating exercises—for example, by taking the telephone off the hook so as to avoid having a call occur during the exercises. Nor should the exercise be performed when there is time pressure.

Time in Practice. A practice period is generally made up of four or five subunits of practice. During the initial phases of autogenic therapy, each subunit of the exercises should take approximately one minute. That is, all of the formulas being worked on up to this point are practiced for approximately sixty seconds. After each subunit of the exercises, the trainee brings himself or herself back to a normal feeling by opening the eyes, flexing the arms and legs somewhat vigorously, and breathing deeply. Then he or she returns to the position chosen and carries out another subunit of the exercises, again for approximately sixty seconds. This is repeated until he or she has carried out four or five subunits to make up the practice for that day.

It is very important to practice at least once a day, if at all possible; in most situations, two times a day may be comfortable. It is best not to practice more than two times a day as this generally indicates a need to try to achieve results very quickly, and practicing much more than a couple of times a day does not seem to increase the efficiency of the exercises. After practicing the autogenic exercises for a month or so, some people feel comfortable in increasing the length of the subunits of exercises up to two to five minutes, while cutting down on the overall number of subunits of exercise. This is an individual decision.

The Exercises

The Overall Formula. Most of the formulas gradually introduced into training are specific to a part of the body, but one overall formula, "I am calmness throughout," is interspersed throughout the repetition of the other formulas. With this formula, the mental contact is made with the body as a whole, possibly by the trainee's feeling as if he or she is in a "central core" of the body or up above the body looking down and watching it relax.

Standard Exercise 1: Heaviness. The induction of a feeling of heaviness in the limbs is particularly conducive to overall relaxation. This exercise is carried out by the use of the following formula repeated in a steady flow while maintaining mental contact with each part: "My right arm is heavy," "My left arm is heavy," "Both arms are heavy," "My right leg is heavy,"

"My left leg is heavy," "Both legs are heavy," and, finally, "My arms and legs are heavy." These need not always be repeated in the same sequence. Occasionally (possibly after three or four other repetitions), "I am calmness throughout" is used, while returning the mental contact to the overall body and person. After some months of practice, many trainees find that they gain a result relatively quickly by simply using the formula, "My arms and legs are heavy." But certainly in the initial stages it is important to use all of the formulas.

Standard Exercise 2: Warmth. Just as with heaviness, the induction of warmth in most body parts induces the relaxation and restorative effect that is sought in autogenic training. The formulas used in standard exercise 1 of heaviness are repeated but with *warm* substituted for *heavy*. During the initial training, these are interspersed with the formulas on heaviness—for example, "My right arm is heavy," "My right arm is warm," "My left arm is heavy," "My left arm is warm," and so forth. After some weeks of training, when the trainee notices consistent results upon repetition of the formulas, he or she can experiment with collapsing some of them and using phrases such as, "My right arm is heavy and warm," or even, "Both arms are heavy and warm."

Standard Exercise 3: Respiration. Allowing oneself to breathe naturally is a critical step toward achieving the autogenic effect. The goal is not necessarily trying to achieve a slow and deep breathing pattern during the exercises but to let the breathing eventually take over at its own rate. The phrase used here, "My breathing just naturally happens," emphasizes that breathing happens regardless of the conscious control of the individual and this gives many trainees a sense of being in touch with the most basic forces in their body and in the world. Passive concentration is particularly important here, although most trainees find it initially difficult to avoid trying to breathe slowly and deeply. The goal, nevertheless, is to let it just happen. The mental contact in this exercise is usually with the general chest area, although some people find it helpful to allow mental contact with the overall body.

Standard Exercise 4: Abdominal Warmth. The phraseology used in this exercise is, "My solar plexus is warm." The mental contact for this exercise is with that area approximately two to three inches below the navel. Attainment of warmth in this area effectively counteracts some of the internal disruption from anxiety and strongly furthers the autogenic aims. Many trainees find it difficult at first to visualize this area, but they gradually feel more comfortable with it and note the positive benefits when they achieve it.

Standard Exercise 5: The Cooling of the Forehead. Whereas warmth is conducive to relaxation throughout most parts of the body, the induction of a sense of coolness is most helpful when focusing on the forehead. The term used in this exercise is, "My forehead is cool and smooth." The mental contact is usually made with the overall area an inch or so above the eyes up into the scalp.

In all of these exercises, trainees may occasionally note fleeting images related to the effect desired—for example, regarding the cooling of the forehead, they may fleetingly envision a cool breeze passing over the forehead. Such images can be helpful if they are not allowed to continue very long and disrupt the mental contact or the steady flow of the formulas.

A Comment on Autogenic Training

Autogenic training is useful as a deepening technique. When time is not of the essence, the client can be trained in it in an initial session and then practice it at home for several weeks before schedulingr the first hypnosis session. A log of responses and associations to autogenic training provides a wealth of information that can be productively used in hypnosis.

Autogenic training provides the side benefit of being a technique clients can easily integrate into their life-style, similar to yoga, tai-chi, or certain religious-meditational practices. In fact, it was originally designed to be applied in this fashion (Schultz and Luthe, 1959). It is an effective long-term strategy to enhance immune responses, lessen chronic anxiety, and facilitate cognitive reprogramming.

Autogenic Neutralization

Wolfgang Luthe, an original contributor to autogenic training (Schultz and Luthe, 1959), also developed autogenic neutralization (Luthe, 1969). Unlike autogenic training, autogenic neutralization has gone virtually unnoticed since its original presentation. Autogenic neutralization can be thought of as a supervised but largely self-administered psychodynamic-meditative therapy. It is effective with clients inclined to self-analysis and who can discipline themselves to practice the technique (which requires much more home practice time than autogenic training does).

It assumes prior training in autogenic training and asks the client to engage in free-association-meditative sessions (often of duration of an hour or more) at home, which are best utilized if audio recorded and listened to by the client and occasionally by the therapist. Autogenic neutralization practice serves to deepen any concomitant hypnosis sessions and directly facilitates cognitive insights, imagery-dream experiences, and emotional abreaction and age regression techniques, in or out of the hypnosis. Luthe (1969) provides a number of issues and cautions that should be considered here.

Music-Enhanced Hypnosis and Self-Hypnosis

Music can stimulate therapeutically useful images. It has been used effectively in hypnosis (Walker, 1991), as well as in other therapies. In the LSD mind expansion therapies pioneered in the 1950s and 1960s by Walter Pahuke, Stavislav Grof, and others, their subjects, who had ingested LSD, were blindfolded and put in a comfortable, monitored environment. Music was presented to them through earphones in sequences designed to stimulate certain types of religious and emotional experiences. One assumption in their work was that pieces of music had become "classical" because they appealed to and elicited the most important, and basic, emotional-cognitive responses.

Musical pieces can be used at specific junctures in hypnotherapy. This can be enhanced by a structured program of musically facilitated self-hypnosis, presented here as adapted from Walker (1991). The basic instructions, given while the person is still in hypnosis, would be something like this:

Therapist: You've done a good job with hypnosis. Now I want to talk to you about also using hypnosis at home to [state the goals, depending upon both the needs and the abilities of the client. For some the goal may be no more than tension reduction. Others may be capable of associative dreaming and/or abreaction]. Every day, when [choose a time—for example, "you are getting ready to go to sleep"], you will take fifteen minutes to a half-hour. You'll select music that you feel is right for you that day, music that may take you where you want to go. You'll make all the preparations you need in order to cut down the chance of being disturbed. You start the music, put yourself in a position you find comfortable, close your eyes, relax, and say to yourself, "I'm relaxing and going into hypnosis." Let your whole body relax and focus on the music just like you will do in our sessions here when you use music as a pathway into hypnosis and toward [state some goals]. Quietly, almost automatically, in rhythm with [the life force, God's universe, or whatever else is appropriate], you will let your body relax and your mind go quiet, feeling this experience deepen as you breathe. Focus your attention as you listen to the music, and let the music become a pleasant pathway leading you deeper into hypnosis.

The further down the pathway the music takes you, the more focused on it you become. At the same time, other things going on that you usually would notice fade into the background of your awareness. As you lose awareness of those other things around you, your body becomes even more deeply relaxed, and the music may stimulate various images or fantasies in your mind. These experiences will generally be positive because the music will structure the experience in such a way that will rule out any consistent negative thinking. If you have some negative thoughts, the music will pull you back into a positive vein. [This may need to be modified somewhat if the goal is abreaction.] Also, as the music keeps going, you will go further into the hypnosis.

Then, whenever the music comes to an end, you will take direct notice that the music has ended. At that time, you will calmly and peacefully, yet with increasing alertness, bring yourself out of hypnosis, by counting backward from five to one: five . . . four . . . three . . . two . . . , one. You will feel alert and refreshed.

Even though you took some precautions, it's still possible that something or someone could interrupt you during the session. If that happens and it does absolutely require your immediate attention, you'll just think, "I have to wake up," and you'll be fully alert and feel refreshed. In fact, you can awaken yourself from this self-hypnosis by just deciding to wake up. The following formula just helps you do it quicker and more efficiently. As I already mentioned, the words you can use to quickly awaken yourself from hypnosis are to count backward from five to one: five . . . four . . . three . . . two . . . one, and you will then awaken—this is the same procedure we use when I hypnotize you here in the office. Now remember that if you are disturbed by an interruption and it's not necessary to wake up, you will not be distracted by the interruption, and soon it will just fade into the background.

Your ability to relax and to [include goals] is a skill, and like all other skills, you will be better at it, and go deeper in hypnosis, the more you practice this technique. So each time you practice this, the positive effects will accumulate. Much of this beneficial buildup will be in your subconscious, so you don't have to, and should not try to, create the effects or be disappointed if they don't seem evident right away.

It's important that you understand this is a special way of listening to music and that you will never accidentally go into hypnosis while listening to music, even if it's a piece of music you listened to while in hypnosis. It will never happen while driving a car, and you should never try to use it in any situation where you need to be alert. You will only go into hypnosis when you make a conscious decision to go into hypnosis and say the words, "I'm relaxing and going into hypnosis." Remember this is an experience that has the special purpose of [speak of goals]. You will not be able to use it for nontherapeutic purposes.

Now I'm going to count backward from five to one, and you will awaken and feel refreshed.

After awakening the client, the therapist reinforces the suggestions that he or she should use this only for therapeutic purposes, only when he or she can exert some adequate control over interruptions, when in a safe place, and never while driving a car or doing other tasks that require some alertness to the outside. It works best if the therapist then sets up some music and has the client practice the self-hypnosis in the office. Occasionally checks in future sessions can be made to see if there is anything that should be corrected.

Prolonged Hypnosis

Prolonged hypnosis (PH) is related to deepening in a symbiotic fashion; standard deepening techniques are used in prolonging hypnosis, and in turn PH can be used as a deepening technique.

PH is seldom addressed in the literature. Kuriyama's (1968) article is probably the most important early work in this area, and Kleinhauz (1991) has more recently discussed it. Nevertheless, those who do use it consistently report its usefulness. It has been used most often in chronic medical conditions, especially if they include substantial and chronic pain, and it offers some potential in certain chronic psychological conditions as well, such as posttraumatic stress disorder and agoraphobia.

The basic structure of a PH treatment plan includes (Kleinhauz, 1991) the following:

1. Individualized induction.
2. Training in self-hypnosis, with chosen signals for induction and dehypnotization. They should be developed such that the same signals can be used by the therapist or by the client, with the client practicing each signal in the session until a reasonable degree of mastery and confidence is obtained. These signals help the client develop a sense of self-control and confidence in the procedure. Depending on the individual client's situation, family members or friends or other treatment staff may be instructed in specific induction and dehypnotization procedures for this client.

3. Suggestions concerning the client's capacity to fulfill basic physiological needs while under prolonged hypnosis.
4. Suggestions to increase motivation and to change the perceptions and meanings toward the symptom and toward symptom reduction, cessation, or substitution.
5. Other hypnotic techniques (age regression, time distortion, use of metaphors, abreaction, and so forth).
6. Audiotapes that repeat or amplify the session work.
7. A plan as to how long the client is expected to stay in hypnosis each day and how this is to proceed and a formulation that relates techniques to goals.

As most practitioners are aware (sometimes painfully aware), liability issues can arise with even the most benign techniques. PH is a benign technique, but some psychological functions can be compromised while in the hypnotic state. It is recommended this procedure be used only where there will be consistent, immediate supervision, ideally by inpatient staff but at least by family members or friends. Implementing PH requires a substantial outlay of effort at the onset. However, if the patient is able to respond, the results are worth it, especially since the disorders it is usually applied to are severe.

Summary

While hypnotic depth is not easily separable from hypnotic susceptibility, it is a useful clinical concept. It refers to the increased responsiveness and increased absorption that occurs as the person surrenders more and more to the hypnotic trance. Facilitating this process is the goal of deepening, and any method that serves to increase the client's trust in the therapist, increases expectation that hypnosis will occur, minimizes distration, and serves to circumvent resistance is beneficial. The clinician is encouraged to experiment with clients who present in different fashions to determine what methods are most likely to facilitate their experience.

5
Indirect and Ericksonian Techniques

Types of Suggestions

The two major techniques of giving suggestions in hypnosis are direct and
indirect. Direct techniques are those that directly attack a problem or symptom by suppressing them with orders (suggestions), bringing about a condition designed to lead the subject to evaluate more productively the
effectiveness of the symptom or life-style and resulting in a demonstrable
behavioral change. Erickson, Hershman, and Sector (1961) believe that
directive hypnotherapy will be successful in only a small minority of cases
because direct techniques do not address the natural defenses of the client.
They suggest that resistance increases in proportion to neurotic needs; the
more neurotic the client is, the more problems there are in psychological and
neurophysiological functioning; individuals with less neurosis will comply
better to direct techniques.

Indirect techniques are more widely used in hypnotherapy, because they
are believed to treat the underlying causes of the problems (Erickson, Rossi,
and Rossi, 1976). In comparison to direct suggestions, where stimulus leads
directly to response, the stimulus of indirect suggestions bears no obvious
relation to the response (Masters, 1992). The suggestions are covert in
indirect approaches, overt in direct approaches, as indirect suggestions are
moderated by internal processes that the subject is unaware of. Erickson,
Rossi, and Rossi (1976) assert that a problem with direct approaches is that
it is difficult to ascertain if the subject is complying; however, direct approaches ensure that any response to the suggestion may be due to the
demands of the situation or to the prestige of the hypnotist rather than in
response to the suggestion. It follows that since an indirect suggestion cannot be mediated by conscious awareness, because of its covert nature, any
response to an indirect suggestion will be due to the intervention and not to
situational or prestige factors.

Erickson, Hershman, and Sector (1961) contrast direct and indirect suggestions for induction of hypnotic deafness. A therapist using the direct approach might say, "When I count to ten, you will experience yourself getting more and more deaf, until finally, at the count of ten, you won't be able to hear anything at all." For the indirect approach, he or she might say, "I wonder how it feels to a person who is about to lose his hearing? I wonder if he notices that sounds seem to grow very, very slightly less distinct at first, if he finds that they seem to be more vague or fading off into the distance? I wonder if the person then gets more attentive and leans toward the sound. Does he cup one ear or both ears, or maybe test his hearing by putting a finger in one ear to see if there is a blockage there? Does he notice that despite the fact he can see the speaker's lips moving, that he is unable to hear anything except an occasional noise coming through?" The indirect approach will produce hypnotic deafness that will stand up to all of the physiological tests of deafness because it allows the subject to utilize unconsciously all of his or her own feelings, sensations, and knowledge in order to limit the ability to hear. The indirect approach did not arouse the subject's defenses by ordering him or her not to be able to hear. Yet it is also true that direct suggestions have a long tradition of value in the hypnotic armamentarium, either as a primary or adjunct approach (Brown and Fromm, 1987).

Indirect suggestions do not overtly attack the symptom; in some cases, they cannot even be readily identified as pertaining to the presenting symptoms. They are used primarily because most therapists agree that much of the work done by the client is accomplished subconsciously. Usually indirect suggestions bear a resemblance to direct suggestions but avoid the tone of instruction so as to avoid the pitfalls of resistance. For example, if the therapist believes the client would be more comfortable in trance with closed eyes, an indirect suggestion might follow this example:

Therapist: Some people feel more comfortable during hypnosis when they have their eyes closed. You may decide you would feel more comfortable with your eyes closed. You may decide you would feel more comfortable with your eyes closed. On the other hand, you may choose not to close your eyes. I am confident that you will do what is best for you to be the most comfortable during our session. So, as I count from ten to one, your eyelids may become heavier and heavier, and you may completely close your eyes if you choose. Ten, nine, . . .

On the other hand, a direct approach might resemble this example:

Therapist: You will feel much more comfortable during hypnosis if you have your eyes closed. I want you to fix your gaze on a spot on the ceiling. Now, as I count back from ten to one, your eyes will become heavier and heavier, and when I reach one, your eyes will be completely closed. Ready? Ten, nine, . . .

As the examples suggest, the major difference between direct and indirect techniques is in the form of the suggestion rather than the content. In actuality, a difference between indirect and direct methods may simply be the subject's understanding of the suggestion. Direct and indirect suggestions may be viewed as existing on opposite ends of a continuum, although most actual suggestions contain varying degrees of directiveness. In contrast to the direct approach, which is overt and takes advantage of the client's motivation and interest in learning ways to solve problems, the indirect approach is covert and seeks to address the unconscious mind and avoid natural resistances. Indirect suggestions place distance between the suggestion and the symptom, reducing the need for resistance (Masters, 1992). Theoretically, when the symptom is purely neurotic and not consciously mediated, the use of indirect suggestions may allow the therapy to operate on the same level as the neurosis; indirect suggestions speak directly *to* the neurosis rather than to the symptom, which is only an outward manifestation of the neurosis (Erickson and Rossi, 1981; Otani, 1990).

Therapy works on many levels, and the use of indirect suggestions may allow the healing process to occur on many levels. Indirect suggestions may work to free the psyche from battling aspects of itself through resistance and encourage integration. When the meaning of a suggestion is ambiguous, the client can project his or her own meaning on it and use it in the most positive way. This may be why metaphors have such clinical usefulness: they allow each person to ascribe individual meaning to them and find the best way to apply them.

But there are some problems with indirect suggestions, as there are with direct suggestions. Some clients may find the treatment mysterious and unrelated to their concerns, and this may lead to greater anxiety about therapy and even increase resistance. With some clients, establishing a therapeutic alliance may be tenuous. If the client feels initially that the therapist is not addressing his or her concerns or misinterpreting what he or she is presenting, the therapeutic alliance may be damaged; the therapist may lose credibility, and the potential for influencing the client toward positive change may be lost.

In contrast to traditional direct methods of hypnotherapy, the methods developed by Milton Erickson favor the use of paradoxical and indirect techniques. These provide a useful alternative to more direct methods, and most of the concepts described in this chapter have influenced the development and use of indirect techniques.

Milton Erickson has stimulated advances in psychological treatment on a number of fronts. Notably, his pioneering efforts have contributed to family therapy, brief therapeutic approaches, theories of communication, and hypnotherapy (Otani, 1990; Lankton and Zeig, 1988; Zeig, 1982; Erickson and Zeig, 1948/1980; Haley, 1973). Trained as a psychiatrist, Erickson, despite waning professional interest in the legitimacy of hypnotherapy, began in the early part of this century a lifelong exploration into the benefits of altered states of consciousness. Ironically, his early efforts in part came to fruition because of help and encouragement from Clark Hull, the classic behaviorist.

It is likely that Erickson's original interest in altered states as well as in communication developed as a result of his early struggle with polio and the subsequent period of confinement. During recuperation from this illness, which left him partially paralyzed, he became acutely aware of the communication patterns of those about him. His subsequent professional growth capitalized on this early learning, which certainly influenced his views of hypnosis. Later career development strengthened his early interest in altered states of consciousness, and he was instrumental in bringing the use of hypnotherapy into the consideration of clinicians and academics. He was a cofounder of the *American Journal of Clinical Hypnosis*.

Through this developmental process, he postulated attitudinal differences between classic hypnotherapeutic approaches and the process that would become uniquely associated with him and his followers. Ironically, Erickson's disdain for writing (and, to many observers, his lack of talent as a writer) may have helped fuel both the legend and the legacy of his work. Others moved to organize, amplify and develop his many original contributions.

It is useful to keep in mind the zeitgeist of psychiatric thought at the time that Erickson began his forays into hypnotherapeutic interventions. In 1896, Freud denounced the use of hypnosis on the grounds that not every patient was susceptible to hypnosis; total symptom relief did not seem possible; there was often an increase in repression brought about by post-hypnotic suggestions; and the transference relationship was adversely affected by the use of hypnosis (Brill in Freud, 1938, pp. 8–9). Many of Erickson's underlying assumptions about the process of trance induction and utility are direct refutations of these criticisms.

Unlike many of his contemporaries, Erickson was never firmly wedded to theory-driven interventions. Instead, espousing a concept of the individual's implicit and idiosyncratic psychology, he stated, "Each person is a unique individual. Hence, psychotherapy should be formulated to meet the uniqueness of the individual's needs, rather than tailoring the person to fit the Procrustean bed of a hypothetical theory of human behavior" (Erickson, in Zeig and Lankton, 1988, p. vii). As a result, Ericksonian therapy is more typified by the use of therapeutic interventions that are adapted to meet the needs of clients than to fit within an underlying theoretical framework.

Among the three most notable intervention strategies used by Ericksonian therapists are indirection, conscious/unconscious dissociation, and utilization of the client's natural behavior (Lankton and Lankton, 1983).

Erickson's use of indirection is in direct contrast to the direct suggestion used by earlier proponents of hypnosis, such as Charcot and Freud. As Erickson stated, "People come for help but also . . . to have face saved. I pay attention to this and I'm likely to speak in a fashion that makes them think I'm on their side" (Haley, 1973, p. 206). Erickson felt that direct suggestions would mobilize clients' defensiveness and thwart the therapeutic process. Instead, he was more likely to use indirect suggestions, double binds, metaphors, and naturalistic inductions.

The concept of the unconscious and conscious mind is a foundation of both hypnotherapy and psychodynamic theories. Whereas the goal in psychodynamic therapies is to achieve understanding and thus mastery over the elements in the unconscious, Erickson was not often focused on the achievement of insight in controlling nonconscious processes. Erickson would assist clients in understanding how their unconscious is another avenue of communication to which they can choose to attend. Instead of seeing communication as simply a linear, verbal mode, he chose to adopt the view of multiple channels of information, which would include mental and physical processes and to which it may be possible to only attend a small portion. Another way of looking at this is in terms of dominant and nondominant hemispheres (Erickson and Rossi, 1979, p. 247).

Utilization is an especially unique contribution of Ericksonian thought to the therapeutic understanding and more specifically to hypnosis. Erickson tailored his therapy to the client and individual idiosyncrasies and as a result attempted to utilize every response clients bring into the therapeutic milieu. Viewed from this context, concepts such as resistance (an important concept in hypnotherapy) dissolve into meaninglessness or simply point to the rigidity of the therapist in refusing to adapt the therapeutic approach. Erickson believed that individuals know more than they think that they know and that change is simply a matter of evoking that knowledge to bring about new and creative responses to their environment. Erickson said, "Whatever the patient brings to you in the office, you really ought to use" (Erickson and Rossi, 1981, p. 16).

Attitudinal Differences in Ericksonian Approaches

Erickson radically departed from the recognized approaches to therapy in general and hypnotherapy in particular. Although he never operated from a theoretical understanding of individuals that was codified in any rigid fashion, there are nonetheless certain attitudes that underlie his view of the nature of change and guide the structuring of the hypnotherapeutic process. These have been channeled into eleven treatment principles that are typical of Erickson's approaches (Lankton and Lankton, 1983) and appear embedded in most indirect approaches to hypnotherapy.

1. Individuals operate out of an internal schema as opposed to depending on sensory experience. Each person understands the world from an idiosyncratic perspective, and therefore the first goal of therapy is to understand this individual's worldview. Although he attempted to see the clients' world as they did, he also recognized the difficulty in this and frequently encouraged clients to alter or transform his words so that they would be most effective—for example, as applied in hypnotherapy, "You make your own sense out of my words. My voice can turn into the sound of a friend or a stranger, someone from your past, your own voice."

2. At any point, individuals are making choices based on what seems optimal for them. People often make choices that are not objectively the best possible for them, but the operative element in this principle is that people are choosing what seems to be the subjectively best choice at that time. Looking at clients' behaviors from this perspective leads to the dismissal of concepts such as resistance and encourages the therapist to see the client as an active participant in attempting to improve the quality of his or her life.

3. An explanation of a person's behavior is not necessarily an explanation of that person. Erickson eschewed formal theoretical formulations of personality functioning. This tenet suggests that whereas a theory may be of some help in understanding a client's behaviors, it does not represent the totality of that person.

4. All messages that the client gives are important. All too often, therapists focus on the verbal modality as primary. Ericksonian approaches see the verbal as only one of many channels of communication and as such find merit in attending to nonverbal modes of communication, including facial and body movements.

5. Offer choice rather than limiting it. Erickson stated, "You realize that the first thing in psychotherapy is not to try to compel him [the client] to change his ideation; rather, you go along with it and change it in a gradual fashion and create situations wherein he himself willingly changes his thinking" (Erickson and Zeig, 1948/1980, p. 335). Instead of focusing on change as the therapist conceives of it, the therapist must accept the client and provide interventions that will allow for modification in his or her worldview.

6. Each individual possesses the resources he or she needs. Erickson empowered his clients with the view that they contained all the elements in their personal histories that would bring about the wanted changes, including memories, learnings, or skills.

7. Understand the client through their model. A unique view of Ericksonian approaches is to accept and utilize the client's idiosyncratic worldview. This allows for the rapid development of rapport, for it signals to the

clients an implicit understanding of their universe. This may be accomplished by modeling their speech or by listening to the underlying messages and reflecting these back to the client.

8. The individual with the most flexibility will be the change or control agent in any system. Erickson felt that rather than rigidly adhering to a model of therapeutic interaction, meeting clients at their level was more beneficial. For example, after meeting a psychotic client who talked in word salad, Erickson mastered the individual's idiosyncratic speech patterns and "talked" back to him. Eventually the client coherently asked Erickson to stop talking "crazy."

9. It is not possible not to communicate. This principle reiterates the notion that the verbal mode, although often overemphasized, is not the only mode of communication. It challenges the therapist to look for the subtle, nonverbal ways in which clients communicate and to be guided by these messages.

10. Break down change into small parts. Realizing that change is a difficult and complex task, Erickson recognized that clients may have to go at a relatively slow pace and accept small realizations before others are accepted. This pace and subsequent success help clients achieve a sense of self-worth and self-efficacy.

11. The psychological communication is most important. Among the levels of communication are the social (the things that people say) and the psychological (what they think that may or may not be expressed in words). Erickson believed that when there are conflicting messages, the psychological message will be the most salient and driving. Therefore, it is important for the therapist to attend to the congruence between these two levels of communication and to realize that the psychological message has primacy.

These operating assumptions are in many ways different from those of other therapeutic modalities. The acceptance of a mind-set suggested by them, however, is crucial to the development of the Ericksonian approach to hypnotherapy.

Therapeutic Hypnotic Induction

In the traditional model of hypnosis, the induction is merely the overture that leads to the real therapeutic work. In contrast, Ericksonian induction is not discrete from the process of therapy and is itself considered therapeutic. Rather than simply providing a framework for hypnotherapy, the induction is an integral part of the process. In the traditional model, there are specific standard induction methods that are memorized and used for any client. Ericksonian inductions are situation and person specific and therefore may differ dramatically from traditional inductions. The traditional induction is ritualized so that it lasts as long as the practitioner's preconceived script, whereas Ericksonian hypnotic induction may be relatively brief and merely looks for consistent minimal responding on the part of the client, signaling that the induction is complete. Finally, in traditional hypnotherapy, the end of the induction is quite clearly defined and controlled by the therapist. In the Ericksonian model, the induction blurs into the therapeutic work, and thus deepening and therapy are often by-products of the induction procedure.

From their experience with Milton Erickson, Lankton and Lankton (1983) condensed a seven-stage process that can be utilized in effecting a conscious/unconscious dissociation induction. Although these are represented as seven discrete steps, there is often considerable overlap between the stages. During this explication, I provide specific examples as to how the process might be applied. These do not represent definitive or exclusive means of obtaining the desired effect of trance; rather, they serve to offer general suggestions about what might be effective. It is in the spirit of Ericksonian hypnotherapy for the individual practitioner to develop induction techniques that fit not only him or her but also are most consistent with the personal psychology of the client.

1. Prepare the client for trance. Assess the client's previous experience with hypnosis and provide appropriate information to supplant faulty assumptions. Also, the therapist at this time provides a brief overview of what the client is likely to experience during the induction and trance in order to allay any fears. Following this discussion, the therapist could give the following directive:

Therapist: Would you turn your chair slightly and lean back in your chair with your hand on your thighs and look in this general direction. Don't move. Don't talk. But let yourself listen to me, and we'll go where you feel ready.

2. Focus attention and establish rapport. According to Erickson (Erickson and Rossi, 1981), the establishment of rapport is essential. He advocated three techniques for this: (1) matching the client's language use and structure, (2) using metaphors for further matching, and (3) matching the client's facial expression, body language, and breathing patterns and timing verbal statements to coincide with these. In order to focus the client's attention, Erickson would begin with an interesting or puzzling metaphor, thus capturing the client's focus—for example:

Therapist: And I'm gonna talk about something that occurred in your childhood and first went to school. And had to learn to write the letters of the alphabet. It seemed like a terribly difficult task. All those letters. All those different shapes. Do you dot the *e . . . t* and cross the *i*? And where do you put the loop on the *b* and the *d* and the *p*? And how many humps on the letter *m*? It certainly seemed like an impossible task to make sense out of all that.

3. Bring about the conscious/unconscious dissociation. Erickson's concept of consciousness was closely linked to the idea of hemispheric dominance, with the classic distinction of the left hemisphere (awake/conscious) being responsible for language and the right hemisphere (trance/unconscious) being responsible for visuospatial understanding. Erickson often embedded suggestions in his inductions that instructed the client to change focus from the customary left hemispheric patterns of thinking. Generally Erickson regarded the conscious mind as the weaker, less intelligent, less reliable, and more easily duped. His consistent refrain, "you know more than you think you know," demonstrates his belief in the superiority of the unconscious. The following continuation of the induction focuses on the contrast between the conscious mind (that know letters and numbers) and unconscious mind (that forms images), leading to the conclusion that the work of the unconscious mind goes on outside of awareness.

Therapist: Gradually you formed a mental image of each letter, many mental images because letters are in script and in print, various shapes and sizes. And finally you had mental images located somewhere in your brain and you added mental images of persons and words and numbers and objects and even ideas. Not knowing at the time you were forming mental images.

4. Consolidate and deepen the trance. Erickson asks the client to focus on the alterations that have occurred from attention and dissociation, referred to as ratifying; letting the client know of his or her potential for trance phenomena is known as deepening, which validates that something unusual has indeed occurred. In this stage, the Ericksonian concept of utilization is important. This concept states that the therapist should take advantage of any of the client's own idiosyncratic responses. An example might be when the therapist gives the suggestion to the client:

Therapist: And as you become aware of the deepening of your state of relaxation, you will notice that somewhere in your body, there will be a signal that lets you know that you are relaxed. It may be your hands or your arms. You may feel a muscle relax or tense. Only you will know, and you may be surprised by the realization that your body speaks to you.

The concept of utilization is used when the therapist suggests that the client will have a response of some sort rather than prescribing what that response will be.

Therapist: While I've been talking to you, your respiration has changed, your blood pressure has changed. Your muscle tone has changed. And muscle reflexes have changed. You may feel the changes in a number of ways. Close your eyes now and feel the sense of comfort. And the more comfortable you feel the deeper into trance you'll go.

5. Set the stage for learning. Learning is an important aspect of Ericksonian hypnosis. He offers the suggestion that, in contrast to traditional psychotherapeutic concepts of "working through" or "dealing with," the client will learn, or more specifically the unconscious will learn or will be able to impart learned material to the conscious mind.

Therapist: And in the trance state you can let your unconscious mind survey that vast array of learnings that you achieve, that you have achieved during your lifetime. There are many learnings that you've made without knowing it. And many of the learnings that were important to you consciously have slipped into your unconscious mind and have become automatically useful to you. Sometimes you will allow them back into your conscious mind, when you are ready to have them help you that way. And they are used only at the right time, in the right situation.

6. Use the trance therapeutically. In this area there are three major approaches or types of interventions used: indirect suggestions, use of metaphors or short anecdotes, and giving explanations, or prescriptions for utilizing client resources.

7. Conclude the trance state. The therapist concludes the therapeutic work of trance and offers suggestions for continued learning or posthypnotic behavior. It is important to recap any themes used throughout the trance in the conclusion. For instance, if the client wondered about his ability to go into trance, the following conclusion might be appropriate:

Therapist: Just as you wondered earlier about your ability to go into a trance and about the ability of the trance to be effective, your conscious mind will wonder about the information it learned from your unconscious mind. And as you open your eyes, you will continue to wonder about what wonderful things are capable of being learned from your unconscious.

Ericksonian Hypnotherapeutic Techniques

Several broad categories of techniques are used in the trance portion of Ericksonian hypnotherapy. Since Ericksonian therapy is not centered exclusively around hypnotherapeutic techniques, these interventions may also be used in other nonhypnotic circumstances. They include metaphors and indirect suggestion, among others.

Metaphors

The utilization of metaphors in therapy is not restricted to Ericksonian frameworks; it has long been a standard tool in psychoanalytic work and is used by a wide array of therapists. In the traditional use, the metaphor comes from the client's life, and the therapist uses it to assist the client in gaining insight into the unconscious processes. Ericksonians are more likely to use metaphors created to teach a client a specific lesson. In fact, Erickson referred to his metaphors as "teaching tales" for the unconscious. His metaphoric tales were designed to circumvent the conscious mind and avoid the development of insight, which Erickson felt was counterproductive to the process of changing behavior (Erickson and Rossi, 1979). Among the benefits of using metaphors in therapy, they are nonthreatening and interesting, promote a sense of autonomy in that the client struggles to intrepret them and thus reaches individual conclusions, bypass resistance to changing, help structure the therapeutic relationship, model a sense of flexibility, foster a sense of confusion, which heightens the susceptibility to trance, and present the unconscious with a handle by which to remember the intended lesson (Zeig, 1982).

The following example, originally used by Erickson, has as its purpose the lesson that the unconscious mind can be trusted to communicate appropriately if given time. This metaphor, if used at the beginning of a trance, may suggest to the client that she wait until she desires to talk or her body communicates in some other nonverbal manner:

> A lot of people were worried about a friend of mine because he was already four years old and he didn't talk. He had a sister two years younger than him who talked, and she is still talking but she hasn't said anything that's had any impact on people, while my friend, her brother, is a superb therapist and author. But, back then many people got distressed because here was a four-year-old boy who couldn't talk. But, his mother said, comfortably, "When the time arrives, then he will talk." (Rosen, 1982).

The next example points out both the variety of experiences available and that dreaming is included in the collection of experiences. Erickson suggests in this story that therapy might be beneficial even if hypnosis is not. The client may complete his work in a dream.

When you go to bed at night you go to bed to sleep, and you always dream, even when you don't recall your dreams. And in your dream, you do not intellectualize, you experience. I refused to give some candy to my son, Lance. I told him that he had already had enough. The next morning he awakened, very happy. He told me, "I ate the whole sack full."

And when I showed him that the sack still contained candy he thought that I must have gone out and bought some more because he knew that he had eaten it. And he had eaten it—in his dream.

Another time, Bert teased Lance and Lance wanted me to punish Bert. I refused. The next morning Lance said, "I am glad you gave Bert a licking—but you did not have to use such a big baseball bat." He knew I had punished Bert severely. He turned his guilt over wishing that his father would punish Bert into criticism of the severity of my punishment. So, something had happened to him.

Many subjects who tend to intellectualize, instead of going into a trance, will, some night, when they are thinking about other matters, dream that they are in a trance. And, in that trance state of the dream they will do certain things. They will come and tell you the next day, "I dreamed a solution to that problem." Therapy is primarily a motivation of the unconscious to make use of all its many and varied learnings. (Rosen, 1982)

To be effective, metaphors must be structured to meet the specific and idiosyncratic needs of a client. The most elaborate and well-constructed metaphor will be of no use if it does not communicate with the client.

Treatment Planning With Metaphors. The following method for treatment planning, based upon Ericksonian approaches, can guide the development of metaphors (Lankton and Lankton, 1983; Otani, 1990). There are six areas in which one can expect behavior change:

1. Bonding and stabilizing age-appropriate intimacy.
2. Self-image enhancement.
3. Attitude changes.
4. Change in social roles.
5. Changes in family structure.
6. Enjoyment of life.

After assessing the client's needs through taking a history, the problems are framed for these six different areas, as this example shows:

1. Bonding and stabilizing age-appropriate intimacy. A client has difficulty with separating herself from abusive family relationships and establishing more supportive ones.
2. Self-image enhancement. The client must feel secure in her ability to be autonomous and self-caring.

3. Attitude changes. The client expects relationships to be coercive and/or manipulative and needs to see the potential for intimacy.
4. Changes in social roles. The client has to learn to act in a more assertive style.
5. Changes in family structure. The client must separate from family and form new and more intimate relationships.
6. Enjoyment of life. The client needs to break out of self-defeating patterns and seek satisfaction from life and accept the possibility of a positive future.

These major themes address change on cognitive, emotional, and experiential continua. Although each of these areas of concern could be addressed directly and suggestions could be offered that might remediate the area, Erickson would caution that the therapist is likely to meet with resistance or that the person will be acting out of a conscious awareness of the dilemma and therefore no real change will be effected. The use of metaphor will evoke images that are more powerful to the unconscious mind.

The next step in this process is to think of appropriate metaphors by examining each dilemma and therapeutic outcome in the light of the question, "What is this situation similar to?" With creativity, these parallels lead to the development and embellishment of a story or metaphor that will address, indirectly, the therapeutic issue. Following is an example of possible skeletal dramatic plots for each issue.

1. Difficulty separating from family. A Dutch girl has a garden that is periodically flooded by seawater. She knows that water is the origin of life and sustains her in certain ways, but she needs to build a dike that will protect herself and allow her garden to flourish.
2. Feeling secure in the ability to function autonomously. A young owl is forced from the nest, feels alone, and senses that he must now learn to fend for himself.
3. Seeing relationships in a positive light. A person begins a new job and because of fear sees all co-workers as cold and indifferent. The person opens herself up to new relationships and stays at the job.
4. Acting in a more assertive fashion. A child is given the job as a street-crossing guard at his school. The job requires assertiveness without aggression. Passivity may result in injury.
5. Separating and forming new relationships. A bee finds her hive to be too full, without enough available food. She flies off and is at first frightened and feels alone. But she persists and eventually meets an attractive drone. Love ensues.
6. Enjoying life. The garden is pollinated by the bee, and new and exotic types of flowers grow.

Following the construction of the beginning of the metaphors, endings are chosen that will indicate success:

1. The girl builds a dike and successfully keeps the damaging seawater from ruining her garden.
2. In his developing wisdom, the owl finds a way for himself and learns to depend on his own innate knowledge.
3. The person finds that the new co-workers are accepting and the job is the most rewarding so far.
4. The child masters assertiveness, learns to help others, and earns respect for his levelheadedness.
5. The bee becomes a queen, begins a new hive, and finds herself a productive life full of honey.
6. The garden blooms year round, filling the person's life with sweetness and happiness. The flowers are not only interesting and appealing aesthetically but also useful as herbs and medicines.

This process can be summarized thusly:

1. Listen to the client's problem.
2. By focusing on the six areas of outcome, generate a list of themes that are part of the existing situation and the proposed solution.
3. Construct appropriate metaphors that parallel those themes.
4. Formulate appropriate outcomes.
5. Deliver the metaphor in such a manner as to create suspense or tension.

The use of these metaphors may serve as the basis of several hypnotherapy sessions or a single session. Over time, they can lead to a major character revision. Although these may be used singly, more often Ericksonian hypnotherapists utilize metaphors in a fashion known as multiple embedded metaphors.

Multiple Embedded Metaphors. Multiple embedded metaphors are based on the assumption that if a series of stories based on metaphors is presented in an embedded fashion, the conscious mind is foiled in its attempts to make sense of the messages. Thus, it is more likely to be "understood" by the unconscious mind. Indeed, the experience of Ericksonian therapists supports the notion that clients will be amnestic for the most deeply embedded stories, although research has not yet provided empirical support for this claim. Lankton and Lankton (1983) have developed a model of utilizing multiple embedded metaphors:

1. Induce hypnotic trance.
2. Start but do not finish metaphor 1, which focuses on a specific aspect of the client's problem. This is often called the matching metaphor and is designed to focus the client's attention. Knowledge of the client's attitudes toward the hypnotic process is essential.
3. Start but do not finish story 2, which centers on retrieving the appropriate internal resources that will assist in solving the problem. A resource may be a memory or an experience. The point here is to find and retrieve small pieces of images, experiences, motor responses, and mechanisms that will benefit in assisting the client. A thorough knowledge of the client's worldview and his or her developmental attainments helps to formulate appropriate metaphors.
4. Start and finish story 3, which focuses explicitly on the problem and any accompanying limiting thoughts. This is the direct work on the "core of the neurosis." There are several techniques that can be used in this phase, and they will be discussed later in this chapter.
5. Finish story 2. This process is also referred to as linking resources to the client's social network. Combining the attained resources with the new realizations gained during the direct work phase allows for reworking of the client's worldview.
6. Finish story 1. There may be several possible endings for this matching metaphor: a good ending, no ending (one where the client must finish the story, possibly by a dream), a surprise ending, or a tragic ending (which may serve to motivate the client to make wise use of time).
7. Bring the client out of trance and reorient him or her.

Indirect Suggestion

Erickson favored change over understanding and felt that insight could be counterproductive to bringing about change. Although direct suggestion is associated with classic hypnosis, Ericksonian hypnotic techniques focus on indirectness: "Sooner or later you'll be wondering about going into a very deep trance. And you may do that suddenly or gradually." Whereas it is felt indirect suggestion can bypass conscious criticism and thus be more effective than direct suggestion (Erickson and Rossi, 1980), direct suggestion is seen by Ericksonians as useful when the client knows what change he or she wants to make, is highly motivated to make it, and has all the necessary resources to effect the change. This latter situation, although welcome, rarely describes many of the clients who present themselves for hypnotherapy. Ericksonians believe indirect suggestion is superior to direct suggestion for three reasons: (1) the client, because of the ambiguity, is allowed to display idiosyncratic and thus powerful responses; (2) there is the potential to draw upon previous learnings from the client's past; and (3) indirect suggestions are not as likely to evoke resistance. Erickson enumerated at least twenty-three techniques of indirect suggestion (Erickson and Rossi, 1980); here we examine the primary techniques.

Open-ended Suggestions. These statements are designed to be interpreted in the broadest manner possible as a means of enhancing the utility of the trance at any stage. In the initial stages of the trance, the suggestion that "there are many ways of finding the most comfortable position conducive to trance" can be given to encourage the client to seek out the optimal way to enter trance. In the concluding portions of the trance, suggestions such as, "You may find yourself reviewing and remembering these learnings for some time to come," allow the client to focus on what important information was gained from the trance and how to focus on it.

Truisms. These are statements regarding the state of the world that are undeniably true and are useful primarily in developing an attitude of acquiescence prior to therapy. The rationale is that a client who agrees to these basic statements will be more likely to agree with the therapeutic interventions. An example of use of truisms at the beginning of hypnotherapy is the statement, "Everyone finds it useful and important to relax sometimes." At the later development of the trance, the following statement is used: "Just as each individual is different, each person experiences the trance in a different manner." Truisms can also be used in the middle stages of the trance to remind clients of skills that everyone possesses, such as the ability to signal to the therapist by nodding the head or signaling nonverbally.

Suggestions Covering All Possible Alternatives. One of the hallmarks of Ericksonian approaches is the use of the client's idiosyncratic approach to the world. Therefore, there is a prohibition on prescribing specific behavioral or attitudinal changes such as, "Your hand will feel heavier." To do this may only heighten any sense of resistance on the client's part. Failsafe statements such as, "You may notice a change in your hands. They may get heavier or lighter, they may want to stay where they are or they may want to rise up toward your face," are a way of ensuring the therapeutic alliance. At the stage of developing the trance, statements such as the following are useful: "You may find yourself going into the trance slowly, quickly, or not at all." The main rationale is to offer the client the option to determine his or her own responses to the therapeutic intervention.

Apposition of Opposites. This technique involves the juxtaposition of opposing behaviors or states—for example, "You may find yourself feeling lighter the deeper you go into the trance," or, in age regression, "The older you become, the younger your memories may be." Erickson believed that using contradicting messages is more likely to promote the confusion that he saw as a part of the hypnotic process.

Binds of Comparable Alternatives. Binds are statements that offer the client a free choice of two or more comparable alternatives that may lead the client into alternative forms of constructive behavior. Although the patient is given a choice, he or she feels compelled to choose one of the alternatives. In the use of binds of comparable value, suggestions such as, "Would you prefer to use your left hand or your right hand to respond?" could be utilized at the outset of the trance. When offering suggestions after the trance statements, such as, "You can choose how you will use this trance or you may simply discover its use," can provide the client with direction but still offer choice.

Conscious/Unconscious Double Binds. The duality of the unconscious and conscious minds is an essential concept in Ericksonian hypnosis. Erickson believed that the presentation of a double bind at the conscious level will effect change in the unconscious, as in statements such as this one: "You think you know the real reasons behind your problems but maybe your unconscious sees things differently. Maybe your conscious understands imperfectly what your unconscious understands perfectly. Whereas your conscious mind may be confused, your unconscious mind moves forward with clarity" (Erickson and Rossi, 1980, p. 424).

Double Dissociative Conscious/Unconscious Double Binds. This can be accomplished by taking a compound sentence and reversing the assignment given to the conscious and unconscious mind in the first part of the sentence. This can be reduced to the following formula: "Your conscious mind can do A while your unconscious mind does B, or your unconscious mind can do A while your conscious mind can do B." A concrete example is, "Maybe your conscious mind can give you permission to go into a trance while your unconscious mind prepares for change, or maybe your unconscious mind will trigger your willingness to enter a trance while your conscious mind gets ready to receive new information."

Reverse Conscious/Unconscious Double Binds. This intervention is used with clients who present as oppositional or skeptical. Erickson stated that before using this type of intervention, it may be necessary to define the relationship with the client as adversarial with a comment such as, "There are many things that I think are in your best interest, and I intend to bring these things to pass because it is my job." This reinforces the client's desire to resist any future intervention. This can be followed by interventions such as, "I don't want you to listen to me even if you feel like you want to relax and pay attention. I am positive that there is nothing that I will say that will be of any use to you, so don't even try to absorb any of this information." These paradoxical techniques often have the intended effect of riveting the client's attention.

Non Sequitur Double Bind. This indirect method is based on the premise of offering the client two alternatives, both of them beneficial. As Erickson and Rossi stated (1980, p. 426), "In the non sequitur double bind, there is a similarity in the content of the alternatives offered even though there is no logical connection. Thus one cannot figure it out, one cannot refute it, so one tends to go along with it." An example in the earlier stages of the trance might be, "Let's start our work now or else use the time effectively." A use later in the trance might be, "You will either go into a trance as we speak, or you will notice a subtle change in your consciousness and experience." As in all other binds, the client has a choice, and both choices are beneficial to the client.

Techniques for Direct Work

From an Ericksonian perspective, the work of character change occurs in the deepest and often an amnestic part of the trance. Following are examples of the techniques that can be used in this phase of the trance. This does not represent an exhaustive listing but is suggestive of the kinds of techniques that are useful.

Punch Lines. This technique refers to the embedding of directives within metaphors. Often these directives are couched in terms of quotes so that a client may choose to hear or ignore them. The use of punch lines is a way to minimize client defensiveness that might otherwise be encountered if a direct statement were made. The use of punch lines may be effective with sensitive issues such as sexuality, admonishment, or any other issue with which the client's conscious mind is likely to take exception. For example, a statement such as, "You'd be far better by doing those things that you know will help you," can be embedded in a metaphor and addressed as if to a character in the metaphor. Often Erickson based his metaphors on his own experiences. One of these involved the time when he helped his mother say "good-bye" to her home in preparation for moving. The metaphor stressed repeated "good-byes" and is useful when working with clients who have grief or loss issues. Punch line metaphors are usually based on universal themes, such as rites of passage or the intrinsic worth of the individual, and then they allow other common issues to be developed. Therapists will probably be more effective to the degree they start basing punch lines and metaphors in terms of their own experience rather than always using those of Erickson.

Scramble. This technique essentially involves confusing the client on the sequence of the indicators that he or she may use as a reminder of the problem or to help him or her gauge the severity of the problem. This distracts the client from the focus on the repetitive and reinforced pattern of problem definition and assists the client in associating the sequence of events of the problem with relaxation or perhaps another positive experience.

Reframing. By breaking out of a limiting pattern of preconceptions, clients can often develop a broader understanding of the possibilities of their behavior. This reframing can be useful from the outset of the hypnosis when, by relabeling motives and needs in a positive light, a reduction of resistance can occur. Later, the use of restructuring the client's experience can facilitate a set of new learnings and desirable experiences.

Dissociative Reviewing. The purpose of this technique is to allow the client to remain comfortable while examining painful historical material. These directives are usually aimed at helping the client to establish physical and emotional distance from the painful material. An example similar to one used by Erickson follows: "So, would you like to see your adult body sitting in that chair over there? And your unconscious mind over here, but your body's over there? Explain to me the position in which you're sitting now." This exemplifies the goal of allowing the client to observe himself or herself from a distance while working through painful material.

Reciprocal Inhibition. This technique allows for the immediate modification of the painful sensory components that lead to dysphoria. It is accomplished by establishing the negative image and then asking the client to imagine an incompatible positive image. The therapist guides the client into superimposing the incompatible positive image on the negative image. An example might be of a woman who suffered from incapacitating gastrointestinal pain. Through discussion, it was discovered that the precipitant for this pain was a previously unconscious image of a photograph showing her mother and aunt, both of whom had died of colon cancer. Quite likely, the photograph had been incorporated years ago as a core memory and precipitated the pain. When the woman could associate the memory of the photograph with an incompatibly positive image, the photograph lost its ability to elicit the pain.

Life Mazes. The use of life mazes during trance involves giving the client a purposefully confusing set of instructions designed to send him or her on an imaginary journey to both the past and the future. During this journey, the client is asked to imagine different versions of the past and future—both much worse and much better than he or she perceives it to be. The transitions between these different reality states are relatively rapid, resulting in a blurred sense of reality. Ideally, the client begins to have difficulty telling the past from the present or the future and may lose any sense of a rationale for doing so. As a result, energy bound to unpleasant historical events can be released or at least decathected, and the client can be guided into choosing a set of future schemas and goals.

Specific Uses of Ericksonian Hypnotherapeutic Techniques

Possibly one of the most useful applications of the Ericksonian model is in the strategic treatment of specific needs. Ericksonians assert that the true value of their approach lies in the imminent applicability to any particular symptom cluster, whether situational or more long standing and pervasive (Otani, 1990; Lankton and Zeig, 1988). It is important to be aware of the idiosyncratic worldviews of the client and to construct appropriately corresponding inductions and metaphors. This section discusses the utilization of Ericksonian techniques with specific presenting problems or therapeutic needs.

Pain Control Techniques

As a result of his lifelong battle with postpolio syndrome, Erickson was intimately acquainted with chronic pain and developed several relevant techniques to control it following upon a basic postulate that hypnosis requires the exercise of judgment and choice of specific techniques on the part of the practitioner. An initial goal when working with patients who are in chronic pain is to understand the physiological components of that pain, the specific medical ramifications, and the impact of medication. It must be remembered that pain is a natural signal; hence, utility must be evaluated before wantonly attempting to alleviate it. A major responsibility on the part of the practitioner is to teach the patient to recognize and attend to pain as a warning signal (Klein, 1990). Erickson (1967) and Lamkton and Zeig (1988) developed several applications for the alleviation of pain.

Direct Suggestions for the Total Alleviation of Pain. Although not appropriate or useful with many clients, Erickson found that with patients who had a strong sense of internal discipline, the suggestion, "You have found that you no longer need to feel the pain. You can now let it go when you are ready," may be enough to result in temporary relief of pain.

Permissive Indirect Prohibition of Pain. These statements are suggestions couched in more indirect, and therefore receptive, language. Statements such as, "Wouldn't it feel nice if your leg were resting on a warm, fluffy cloud of comfort, and to be able to go to that place when you want to?" may be enough to mobilize the unconscious toward the cessation of the pain.

Amnesia. Total or partial amnesia may be used and may be explained as a natural phenomenon, as when a client chooses to become engrossed in an external activity, such as a book, movie, or sport event.

Hypnotic Analgesia. Through the use of indirect suggestion, such as experiencing a cool breeze or a soothing ointment, a reduction in the severity of pain may be accomplished.

Hypnotic Anesthesia. This can be explained as building up emotional or psychological situations that are contrary to the experience of pain. For example, if a client accepts the notion that a particular part of one's body is so damaged that the nerve must also be damaged, then there would logically be a reduction of the sensation of pain.

Hypnotic Replacement or Substitution. This calls for a modification or substitution of the sensation of pain with another physical sensation. An example might be to replace pain with a sense of tingling.

Hypnotic Displacement of Pain. Causing the focus of discomfort to move from a central to a peripheral part of the body may bring about both a sense of control and a sense of decreased distress.

Hypnotic Dissociation. This technique involves the disorientation of time or body as a means of removing oneself from a sense of pain. For example, while undergoing a minor dental procedure, a patient might be encouraged to remove himself or herself from the situation figuratively and go to a more pleasant place to enjoy the scenery or some specific experience.

Hypnotic Reinterpretation of the Pain Experience. Reframing pain as another less noxious sensation can be accomplished in a series of steps. An example might be helping a client gradually to reinterpret a throbbing pain as a slightly unpleasant but mild muscle cramp.

Hypnotic Time Distortion. In this variation of the dissociation technique, the client is encouraged to extend the time when he or she is pain free and to condense the periods of pain.

Hypnotic Suggestions to Lessen Pain Progressively. This is a technique in which clients are asked to imagine a slight diminution in the pain that they are experiencing. This is increased gradually until the pain has significantly decreased.

Each of these techniques can be used either singly or in combination to effect a reduction in pain. Klein (1990) has developed a five-category classification of these pain techniques, depending on the needs of the clients:

1. *Acceptance.* The techniques in this category are focused on the accommodation of pain in one's life. Erickson believed that if individuals stopped running from the fear and pain and squarely faced it, it would lessen and be more manageable. Pain control measures may focus on the acceptance of any part of the phenomenon in its real or altered form. Rather than measuring the utility of the intervention by rating the diminution of pain, acceptance focuses on the increased productivity of the person's life.

2. *Division into Parts.* A frequently frightening and overwhelming part of pain is both its history and its future. Patients who find themselves faced with a history of chronic pain with no real prospect for relief in the future are likely to be distressed. In addition, pain may be associated with a particular loss or grief issue that compounds the severity of the pain. Finally, the spatial qualities of the pain can affect its manageability; small areas of pain are easier to control and manage than larger ones.

3. *Dissociation.* Rather than experiencing the pain at the site of its origin, removing the focus of the pain to another part of the body or to remove oneself from the body and to view it from across the room may prove beneficial in dealing with pain. For example, during minor surgery performed on a client's left hand, the client may be instructed to focus all pain receptors on the right hand, making it hypersensitive. Another option during a painful procedure is to have the client remove himself from the room, go to another place, or simply observe the procedure from a distance.

4. *Transformation.* Frequently it is the intensity of the pain that is most unmanageable. To alter the parameters of the pain by enlarging its area and thus diffusing it may increase the sense of control that the client has over the pain. As an example of a paradoxical pain technique, to ask the client to expand the sense of pain may also give him or her the ability to contract or diminish the quality of the pain.

5. *Resolution.* One of the most depressing aspects of chronic pain is the sense of diminished focus that it brings to life; people find that they can focus on little else but the pain. Resolution techniques offer the client the chance to look at the world beyond the pain in the hope that the expanded sense of vista will bring about a sense of perspective to the pain. An example Erickson used while working with an elderly woman who had seemingly lost her will to live was to focus her continually on the grandeur of her environment, even including having her research natural landmarks.

These are some major tasks in pain control into which the pain control techniques can be fitted. These are probably most useful within a deep trance. The caveats about the need for the presence of pain as an indicator of danger should be heeded. As with all other Ericksonian techniques, the interventions should be both tailor-made for the client and relatively simplistic. Despite this appearance, however, they require a preparation by the therapist as well as thought on the part of the client to effect these changes.

Mind-Body Healing Techniques

A rather innovative use of Ericksonian hypnotherapeutic approaches is in the ara of mind-body healing (Rossi, 1986). As early as 1943, Erickson explored the connection between somatic symptoms and early experiential learning. He believed that early experiences could become encoded in the limbic system or other physiological structures, eventually producing illness or physical distress. Erickson (Erickson and Zeig, 1948/1980) felt that the use of trance provided a unique psychological state in which the client could reassociate or resynthesize information, thus utilizing his or her own capacities to effect physical healing. An important concept in this area is that of state dependent learning, which holds that the learning people undergo is affected by their situation and environment. Following from this is the notion that a person who is placed in that situation or state again will reexperience what he or she learned originally.

An example might be helpful. For many of us, the dentist is not one of our most loved professionals. We associate the dentist's office with many unpleasant memories that usually involve both fear and pain. As a result, it is often the case that people may feel slightly queasy even if going to the dentist for a rather benign purpose, such as a routine cleaning. We have learned that in this situation, pain is a real possibility. So, when faced with that situation again, even if we consciously know that there is likely to be little discomfort, we nonetheless feel frightened—a simple example of how we learn physiological responses that seemingly defy our conscious minds.

Erickson and Rossi (1976) developed a basic formula for accessing the connection between symptoms and state dependent learning. Typical of Ericksonian techniques, this does not suggest how healing will progress but rather puts clients in touch with their own encoding of the problem and allows for the communication of this information in a manner that will facilitate healing. This formula has three basic steps:

1. A time-binding introduction that signals the beginning of an internal search for the source of the memory or previous learnings. As is typical of other Ericksonian approaches, this signals the unconscious mind or creative side of the individual to become active—for example, "As soon as your inner mind knows . . ." or "When your unconscious knows that it can resolve that difficulty, then you will find yourself becoming relaxed and your eyes will close." Focusing on the expectancy for solution

and the method by which this solution will come is important at this stage.

2. Accessing state-bound sources of the problem. The purpose is to begin a review of memories associated with the problem. As a natural part of this process, reframing of the problem will likely occur, which can result in new learnings about the nature of the problem—for example, "As you are there, now you can review some important memories related to the source of that problem . . ." or "Your inner mind or unconscious knows all it needs to know to solve this problem, and it will continue to work by itself to solve the problem in a fashion that will fully meet your needs." The purpose of this phase, in addition to prompting the review of memories, is to focus on the more creative and powerful unconscious.

3. Ratifying the problem solving. This stage is dependent on the client's responsiveness to the previous stages of hypnosis. At this particular stage, as in other ratification stages, the display of some sort of ideo-motor signaling is indicated—for example, "When your mind knows that it has worked enough on this problem for now, you will find yourself moving slightly and wanting to open your eyes" or, "When your unconscious knows that it can continue to work effectively on this problem, you may find some part of your body wanting to move and you will feel your eyes wanting to open." The purpose of this stage is to signal the end of the formal phase of hypnotherapy and to indicate to the client that the therapeutic work will continue even though he or she is conscious.

Incubating Mind-Body Healing. This is based on the notion that we can create our own reality and that we have some control over our unconscious. Erickson suggested that clients could generate their own futures by accessing inner possibilities. Once again, this is composed of three stages.

1. Readiness signal for reviewing the present problem: "When your unconscious mind is prepared to consider and review all aspects of this problem, then you will find yourself becoming more relaxed and your eyes may close."

2. Incubating the potential for future healing: "Now explore and consider in the depths of your mind the possibilities for healing and cure. See yourself as healed. How would you feel if you were healed? How would your life be different if you were completely healed? Now let your mind trace for you the steps you will need to make to get from where you are to your healing. What steps will you need to make to help you heal yourself?"

3. Ratifying the mind-body healing: "When your unconscious mind knows that it has found the way to healing and can continue the process on its

own and when your conscious mind knows that it can cooperate with your unconscious mind, then you will find yourself feeling relaxed, alert, and refreshed."

Symptom Scaling and Prescription. Asking the clients to experience the problem focuses on more unconscious aspects of the problem. Asking them to scale the problem quantitatively involves the use of the conscious mind and yet simultaneously coordinates the conscious and the unconscious minds. It also gives clients more experience in controlling the problem's experiential and behavioral manifestations. The ultimate goal is to assist clients in "turning off" the problem. Following on the model of the basic accessing formula, this technique also has three steps:

1. Symptom scaling and prescription: "On a scale from one to one hundred where one hundred is the worst, assign a number that describes the degree to which you are experiencing the problem at this point."
2. Problem prescription: "Now let the problem get worse. What number would you assign to it then? Now let it get better. What number would you assign to it now?"
3. Ratifying the therapeutic response: This ends when the client indicates that he or she has been able to lower the original scaling of the problem and feels confident in the ability to continue this work.

Ultradian Accessing Formula. Rossi (1986) has explored the use of what he terms ultradian healing responses, which he asserts occur every ninety minutes or so. At this point, the individual is psychobiologically prepared to experience healing. Rossi also states that if these periods are not addressed during the course of therapy, they will usually result in therapeutic resistance. This is also a technique that can be taught by the therapist and utilized at the client's discretion. It has three steps:

1. Recognizing and using natural ultradian rhythms. The point at which the client appears to become distracted or quiet or some other withdrawal behavior occurs may be an appropriate time to introduce this therapeutic approach: "I notice that you have become quiet [or whatever withdrawal behavior is being exhibited]. I wonder if your unconscious is signaling that it is ready to enter into a period of healing? If that is the case, you will find yourself becoming comfortble [or even more comfortable]."
2. Accessing and utilizing ultradian healing: "You can continue to become more and more comfortable just as you do when you take a break or a nap, so that your unconscious can do the healing it needs. You may or may not be aware of what your unconscious is doing to bring about

healing or resolution of these difficult issues. [Pause and remain quiet to allow five to twenty minutes of work.]"

3. Ratifying the continuation of ultradian healing: "When your unconscious knows it has dealt with this issue sufficiently for now and when your conscious mind knows that the healing will continue and that you can choose these moments when you need to, you will become alert, refreshed, and open your eyes."

Although these techniques are utilized to facilitate physical healing, many of these techniques can also be used to access painful memories or to assist in the exploration of painful affect for which the client is unable to retrieve the cause.

Conclusion

The work of Milton Erickson was seminal, and his disciples have made significant advances using his basic philosophies. The Ericksonians pride themselves not for adhering strictly to the principles laid down by Milton Erickson but for capitalizing upon his knowledge in ways that are creative and specific to each client. In their best work, this seems to be the case, though at times some become enmeshed in jargon that leads to little that is productive, and at other times some simply seem to be worshipping at the words of the guru. At the same time, the material in this chapter represents only a portion of an innovative approach. The Ericksonian approach will no doubt be quite influential for many years to come.

6

Direct Suggestion and Posthypnotic Techniques

> Let us begin by committing ourselves to the truth—to see it like it
> is, and to tell it like it is—to find the truth, to speak the truth, and
> to live the truth.
> —Richard M. Nixon

This chapter discusses specific forms of suggestion that are designed to accomplish specific goals. Direct and posthypnotic suggestions are used as an adjunct to traditional psychotherapy, as well as in medical and dental applications in order to alter behaviors in such a way as to improve psychological functioning, control unwanted habits, and develop coping strategies for pain management. Consider a behavioral treatment strategy for a phobia that utilizes hypnosis. The hypnotic component may contain a direct suggestion that anxiety related to the phobic object will diminish over time, guided imagery of experiencing the feared object in pleasant surroundings, and posthypnotic suggestions that the client will feel a heightened sense of self-esteem whenever the feared object is confronted and tolerated. This chapter presents an overall description of suggestions, with particular attention to direct (as contrasted to indirect) methods, as well as posthypnotic techniques. Strategies for the use of these methods are offered, and case studies are presented.

Suggestions

Basic Definitions

A suggestion is a communication that begins a series of ideas or behaviors. When we suggest an idea or course of action to another individual in a normal day-to-day interaction, we anticipate that the suggestion will be followed, ignored, or partially implemented (possibly depending on if it is a friend, foe, or family member). When we make a direct suggestion to the conscious mind in the waking state, the individual makes a conscious decision about it. The decision may be influenced by personality or situational variables. The stimulus (suggestion) and response are intrinsically different from the transaction that transpires in a hypnotic trance.

92

There are as many views of what a hypnotic suggestion is as there are theories of behavior. Most are, in one way or another, conceptualizations of a stimulus-response connection or a method of therapeutic maneuvering in behavioral terms, although Freudian concepts propose that suggestions have power in their ability to stimulate transference; another Freudian view is that a response to a suggestion is an expression of submission arising from a parent-child relationship between the therapist and subject.

Any definitive explanation of suggestion should include the following:

1. When a normal individual is placed in a specific situation and is confronted with a specific stimulus, a response that is appropriate to the stimulus in that situation is elicited.
2. The response should be elicited under identical situations.
3. The response should be available for replication.

Obviously hypnosis is not a normal situation that most individuals find themselves in, and the trance state is idiosyncratic. It is also true that the stimulus is not normal in the sense of being a directive given in a waking situation. That is, to an observer, a direct hypnotic suggestion or posthypnotic suggestion would not be viewed as appropriate to the situation. For example, if the hypnotist suggested that a force was pulling the subject's arm upward when there obviously was not a force pulling the arm, for an observer, or indeed a subject who was in a waking state, this would be a preposterous proposition.

Therefore, a suggestion when proposed in this unique situation (hypnosis) becomes a surrogate for another nonpresent stimulus. Suggestions are merely a form of communication, and if it were true that all communications had the same power to influence as do direct and posthypnotic suggestions, then it could be accurately stated that the content and the meaning of the communication were synonymous—or, as Weitzenhoffer (1953) writes, "Content and meaning are essentially the same thing; hence, if content were the dominant factor in making a suggestion out of a stimulus, all meaningful stimuli would automatically have the power to evoke suggestibility phenomena at all times. This is not the case." This essentially means that the different structure of suggestion makes for different response strength in the subject; differences in the structure of suggestions that may appear on the surface to be minor may indeed be significantly different in meaning to the subject (Edmonston, 1986; Goodwin, Hill, and Attias, 1990).

These basic definitions of suggestive processes lead to a more formal definition of a suggestion as an idea, or group of ideas, proposed by the hypnotist to the subject and that cause the subject to act as if the phenomenon for which the ideas stand actually exists. Thus, there are two basic sources of suggestions: from the subject and from the hypnotist. Auto- or self-suggestions come from the subject, and heterosuggestions come from the hypnotist. While it is true that any and all communications may constitute a suggestion, they obviously do not always function in this capacity. And although this chapter will generally devote itself to describing specific forms of communications that occur under the influence of hypnosis, direct suggestions can also be understood as occurring in the waking state.

Cautions in the Use of Direct Suggestions

Hypnosis can be thought of as a role-playing phenomenon in which the subject assumes a role under the "direction" of the hypnotist. Hypnosis is a technique that allows the therapist to speak directly to the emotionality of the subject, and even to touch him or her, a normally taboo intervention. The relaxation and emotional vulnerability of trance suggest that a substantial trust exists between therapist and subject, in which the therapist is given control not usually accorded during the regular portions of the session.

Because symptoms often mask deeper psychological disturbance, care should be taken when working toward symptom removal through direct hypnotic suggestion. In structuring any hypnotic therapy, it is important to understand the individual and that person's unique methods of problem solving. Erickson, Hershman, and Sector (1961) put it succinctly:

> In giving suggestions, the real question should be: How much of the symptomology does the patient really need? Does he need all of it? A part of it? One raises the questions in the trance state; then one might suggest that it be cut down until he has only the amount of symptomology that is useful to him. It is a way of winning a patient's cooperation. The therapist is not asking him to transform himself completely as a person. He is merely trying to help the patient keep what he needs, whatever truly belongs to him. (p. 355)

The use of direct suggestions is not advised when treating certain emotional disorders where symptom substitution, rather than amelioration or elimination of symptoms, is likely to result.

Several factors appear to determine the extent to which direct suggestions may be used during a therapeutic regimen. First, a deeper hypnotic trance must be achieved for a direct approach as compared to an indirect approach (Berrigan et al., 1991). This is due to the fact that the suggestions are overt and may be resisted by the subject's natural defenses.

Next, the extent to which posthypnotic activity, as well as further hypnosis, is necessary to maintain progress in the therapy is related to the use of direct techniques. Because indirect suggestions theoretically allow the unconscious to affect change, they appear to have greater prophylactic effect than direct suggestions. Therefore, symptom relief more than personality change is affected through direct suggestions, and repetitions become important, as in any other form of behavior therapy. With directive methods, the work of change is accomplished by the overt actions of the client rather than through unconscious processes. To this end, the use of posthypnotic suggestions and repetition of direct suggestions is needed to reinforce the desired behavior; hypnosis is an adjunct to a comprehensive treatment program when it is used in psychotherapy.

The character structure of the client is important in determining if direct suggestions should be used in the therapy; prescription of direct suggestions is made in inverse proportion to the level of diagnosed personality disorder pathology. That is, while direct suggestions can be most helpful with habit disorders, neuroses, and similar problems, it is unlikely that a direct hypnotic technique will be useful in treating a borderline or an antisocial personality disorder. Additionally, conversion symptoms appear extremely resistant to direct suggestions, and if symptom relief is obtained, it is usually likely that symptom substitution will occur.

The use of direct suggestion implies that the hypnotist is more interested in amelioration of symptomology and the control of distress than in the etiology of the disorder. In this respect, it is kin to behavioral and cognitive-behavioral therapies. As in diagnostics that lead to behavioral therapies, it is essential that the client be well understood by the clinician; the meaning of the disorder or symptom should be understood within the framework of the total person before proceeding in any technique, even with a strictly behavioral approach.

Directives: Direct Suggestions in the Waking State

There are different types of direct suggestions, used in different therapy situations. Critenbaum, King, and Cohen (1985) describe a type of direct suggestion called a directive. Directives are given when the subject is in a waking state, and they are believed to be akin to "therapy without trance" (p. 97). Directives are an injunctive form of language that carry weight in proportion to the prestige of the therapist. Directives are a form of communication used often by orators, preachers, and politicians, as well as therapists. They are important because they delineate the purpose of direct suggestions and indicate the context for their use. Each of these directives, while offered as examples of suggestions given in the waking state, may also be understood as a form of suggestion to be used with a client in trance.

An *information-providing directive* provides data that the client may use to solve a problem. For example, an individual presents with overeating problems. This individual may not be aware of how daily behavior patterns lead to overeating. Many people who overeat often do so when they are not hungry, when they watch television, or when they are bored; they may eat everything on their plate regardless of how full they become. Directives would take the form of didactics regarding this information and encourage the individual to consider which of these behavioral patterns he or she engages in and which he or she would be willing to change. These directives could be given during a trance as direct suggestions or during the waking part of the therapy session.

Directives that evaluate a client's motivation for change are used to ascertain the degree to which a client will comply with overt behavioral therapy approaches and screen for areas of conflict that may arise in the therapy. A man came into therapy complaining of a myriad of depressive and anxiety-related symptoms. He had been in therapy many times previously and appeared to take some delight in describing how little the other therapists had done for him; there always seemed to be a "problem" with the previous therapist. On the other hand, this man was intelligent, articulate, and appeared to have good insight into his problems.

He said he wanted to have cognitive-behavioral therapy. To get an idea of how appropriate he would be for that kind of approach, he was given a directive to go home and keep a journal for ten consecutive days; when he had accomplished that, he could call in for another appointment. This client was unable even to start a journal or to keep any kind of written or recorded record of his symptoms. By using this type of directive, we were able to identify that resistance would be a major problem and structure the treatment accordingly. This was essentially a technique to gain control over the therapy. The client had failed in previous treatments because he had manipulated the therapists into a one-down position, and when the program did not work, the client blamed the therapist for the failure because of the therapist's ineffectiveness. This type of directive places the responsibility for therapeutic progress squarely on the shoulders of the client and does not allow the client to manipulate the therapist into a pathological relationship.

Metaphorical directives are not so direct. They are used extensively by therapists of all persuasions and encourage the client to see problems and solutions from another perspective. Their purpose is to get the client to do something that will move him or her toward a goal in a manner that uses the client's own problem-solving capacity instead of the therapist's providing a solution or concrete information. For example, a metaphor that is helpful when a client feels stuck and fearful about proceeding is the story about a young girl (or boy) who had a terrifying accident as a child. This accident occurred when she was swimming, and although she was not hurt, she came to associate going into the water with dread and foreboding. Later in life, it became necessary for this girl, now a woman, to travel across the country to achieve a goal. In doing so, she came to a river, which she was terrified to cross. This presented the dilemma that a client may face in making progress in therapy: giving up the symptom will entail confronting a terrifying issue.

This particular metaphor concludes with the woman realizing that her journey can proceed only when she crosses the river.

Self-hypnotic directives work insofar as they can provide the client with a method of circumventing their irrational beliefs. Clearly, we all attempt to solve problems using cognitive processes. All is well and good when thinking about a problem leads to a solution, but experience tells us that many problems cannot be solved simply by thinking. If that were possible, obsessive individuals would rule the world (on second thought, some do). Self-hypnosis allows the subject to enter a trance state in order to consider issues in an alternative cognitive state. This is done by making a direct suggestion during trance that the individual will find it possible to enter trance by repeating to himself or herself the steps that comprised the induction process (this induction should be one that the client has identified as being comfortable). The suggestions given under trance will be that entering into self-hypnosis will allow the subject to work on problems in a new way—that is, by allowing the unconscious mind to work on the problem, even while the conscious mind is involved in another activity. The suggestion could be that the unconscious mind will challenge the automatic thoughts of the conscious mind, which are self-defeating and negative and work to prevent the positive steps required for symptom relief.

Directives that block attempted solutions utilize studies that have indicated that the right and left hemispheres of the brain use language differently. Trance is basically a right hemisphere experience, and it has been theorized that the right hemisphere is more primitive in its use of language and is reflective of primary process thinking (Critenbaum, King, and Cohen, 1985). The right hemisphere represents ideas metaphorically and pictorially and as such cannot depict a nonoccurrence. This may appear confusing, but it makes intuitive sense. For example, if someone tells you, "Don't draw that picture," you will imagine yourself drawing a picture since your right brain cannot deal with negatives. It cannot imagine a nonoccurrence—your not drawing the picture. If a therapist directs a subject not to do something, the negative will drop out through right-brain processing, and the person will think of nothing but doing that thing. In other words, many clients obsess about their symptom, and telling them not to think about it only increases the thinking. Therefore, to begin the therapeutic process it is often necessary to use a directive to block an attempted solution that is being tried by the client.

Direct Suggestions

The use of direct suggestions is indicated when it appears to the therapist that the client can benefit from techniques that remove, ameliorate, replace, or intervene in distressing symptom patterns (Brown and Fromm, 1987; Dorcus, 1956). Several different techniques are commonly used.

Symptom removal techniques involve directions that the symptom will disappear or be less anxiety provoking within a general or distinct time frame. For example, a suggestion might be made that the fear response in an anxiety disorder will dissipate gradually throughout a time-limited treatment program.

> *Direct suggestion:* "As we proceed through the treatment process, you will feel a reduction of anxiety and a reduction in the symptom(s) you feel. You will feel a reduction in your symptom(s) with each step of the process, and by the end of the six weeks you will feel no anxiety whatsoever when thinking about or encountering the [feared object or situation]."

Amelioration techniques involve secondary processes that work to change the client's perception of the symptom by altering the sensation, perception, and stimulus reception process through general relaxation techniques that target anxiety and somatic symptoms. This is analogous to cognitive restructuring and is often used in medical and dental applications.

> *Direct suggestion:* "During the drilling you will not be bothered by the sound of the drill at all. Instead, it will remind you of the sound of the wind blowing through the trees, and you will be relaxed and comfortable. The sound and feel of the procedure will not make you feel anxious or uncomfortable but instead will be a cue to return to the 'safe place' that we talked about earlier."

Symptom replacement and symptom substitution are essentially equivalent approaches to symptom relief. The basic idea is that there is a neurotic need addressed by the symptom and that the client may be able to replace a very anxiety-provoking symptom with a more benign one. Symptom substitution is a serious problem when working with neurotic clients. Symptom-replacement techniques are attempts by the therapist to control the process in a positive manner, which gives the client self-esteem in gaining power over the symptom. For example, irritable bowel syndrome (IBS) is often one symptom of stress, and direct suggestions and/or substituting through hypnosis a more benign symptom such as nausea (to be replaced with an even more benign symptom later in the treatment) would be positive due to the seriousness of IBS (Prior, Colgan, and Wherwell, 1990). A less serious example might be substituting restlessness and the need for exercise when hunger strikes a client presenting with weight-control issues.

> *Direct suggestion:* "You have come to associate eating with many of your favorite daily activities, such as watching television or reading the newspaper. You feel hungry even though you have recently eaten, because you have come to associate these activities with eating. But you want to lose weight, not gain weight, so instead of eating when you feel hungry, your hunger will be a cue to you to exercise. When you feel hungry, you will feel a sense of restlessness, feel that you must get up and go for a walk or do simple calisthenics; you will decide which is more appropriate for the situation you are in. You will feel good about your decision, because it will move you closer to your goal of losing weight."

Intervention strategies are those that add characteristics in the way of sensations or perceptions to the symptom pattern. This is a systems perspective, whereby a change in the symptom process will lead retroactively to symptom removal without utilizing any of the other techniques. Intervention strategies use such techniques as age regression, hallucinations, sensory alterations, and time alterations. Often a client has trouble imagining what he or she would be like without the symptom; using direct suggestions to facilitate self-awareness through time alterations may enable the client to perceive himself or herself in a new light.

> *Direct suggestion:* "I want you to imagine yourself, how you will be, one year [or any other time span] from now. You will not have your symptom. You will be a different person in that regard, but otherwise you will retain the same positive qualities that make you who you are. Your uniqueness will remain. You will feel comfortable and secure, knowing that you have made this positive change in your life." [Under these conditions and still in trance, the client is then asked to describe how he or she would be different or the same without the symptoms and describe the steps he or she has taken and will take to get rid of it.]

Beyond the strategies for direct suggestions, the following qualities of direct suggestions make them more likely to be successful:

Repetition: Repetition is important in making direct suggestions (Cheek and LeCron, 1968). As in advertising, ideas should be rubbed in—but only to a point, because there are diminishing returns with greater repetition. Three or four repetitions, ideally interspersed with other hypnotic commentary, is usually adequate.

Time frame: Suggestions should be worded so that they are set in the immediate future rather than in the present. An example for a dog phobia would be, "You will begin to feel less and less anxiety when you think about dogs."

Motivation: Establishing motivation through direct suggestions or directives will make it more likely that the suggestions will carry enough force to work real change in the subject. One method is to suggest directly that the client will feel positive benefits from the therapy, that the future will appear brighter, and that self-esteem will improve as a result of following the suggestions.

Hypnotherapy using direct suggestions is often a major part of a behavioral or cognitive-behavioral treatment procedures, used in both psychotherapy and medical and dental applications (Hilgard and Hilgard, 1975; Edmonston, 1986; Brown and Fromm, 1987). For example, in a text on the management of pain through hypnosis, Hilgard and Hilgard (1975) describe three classes of procedures: one involves the direct suggestion of pain reduction, the second technique works to alter the experience of pain in some way, and the third works to direct attention away from the pain.

There are primary and secondary factors associated with pain management. A primary factor is the pain itself; secondary to the pain is the anxiety and social factors that accompany it. In treating subjects who have severe but intermittent pain, Hilgard and Hilgard report that amnesia can be an important tool. The reason is that when individuals have chronic spells of intense pain, they come to have great anticipatory anxiety associated with the pain, and often this secondary symptom becomes as important in treatment as the pain itself. To alleviate the anticipatory anxiety, a direct suggestion can be made designed to induce an amnesia in the subject such that previous memories of the painful experiences may be forgotten. It can also be suggested that each subsequent episode of pain will be a transitory experience. In this way, the pain may be experienced as a momentary inconvenience and not remembered or anticipated as an excruciating experience.

Another method is to use direct suggestions to deny the existence of the painful body part. Hilgard and Hilgard (1975) offer the following script: "Think that you have no left arm. Look down and see that there is no left arm there, only an empty sleeve. An arm that does not exist does not feel anything. Your arm is gone only temporarily; you will find it amusing, not alarming, that for awhile you have no left arm" (p. 66).

In psychotherapy, use of direct suggestions is recommended when the client and therapist have a good working relationship and when the client appears motivated to make the behavioral changes that may lead to therapeutic change—for example, to approach the feared object that is the basis of a phobia. Additionally, it is believed that for direct suggestions to be successful, it is usually required that a deep trance be accomplished, and it does appear to be a consistent factor (Berrigan et al., 1991). If these conditions are met, direct suggestions can be a successful part of hypnotherapy. The following case example is illustrative.

Sandy, a thirty-four-year-old woman, came into our office seeking treatment for a dog phobia. Historically, she had experienced a trauma involving a neighbor's dog when she was seven years old. The dog, a pit bull terrier, got loose in her neighborhood and attacked a boy who lived across the street from her, severely mauling him. The police had to shoot the dog to get its jaws unlocked from the boy's leg. Sandy witnessed this event and developed a generalized phobic response to dogs. Even viewing dogs on television disturbed her until she was a teenager. Until the time she came into our office for treatment, she had never directly approached a dog or stayed in the same room with a dog since witnessing the accident. Her life revolved around her phobia, and she picked friends and activities on the basis of the proximity to dogs.

Sandy became ready to face her fear and entered into therapy when the man she had fallen in love with was a dog lover and had a show-quality weimaraner that he wanted to keep. The treatment plan consisted of cognitive-behavioral psychotherapy to deal with the intense anxiety and irrational fear our client had about dogs, and hypnosis, used both to boost her self-esteem and also to allow her to move quickly into proximity with the feared canine.

She was an excellent hypnotic subject. After only three sessions, she was able to move quickly into deep trance, the most suitable state for direct suggestions. Once the deep trance was established and confirmed by glove anesthesia, direct suggestions were given that followed this course:

1. *Guided imagery:* "You are in your special place of comfort [a previously agreed-upon location and atmosphere—in her case, working in her backyard garden] and you feel relaxed and at peace with yourself. The sun is shining upon you, and the warmth is very comforting. Music that you love is playing in the background, and there is nothing else that you are required to be doing at this time."
2. *Progressive relaxation:* "At peace in your garden, in the distance you hear a sound that you think may be a dog barking. You do not feel

anxious. The sun is upon your face, and the music is sweet. You see something out of the corner of your eye, across the field in the distance. It is an animal. You consider that it may be a dog. You do not feel anxious. Feel the sun shining on your face. Hear the music you enjoy." These direct suggestions proceed through a hierarchy until she is able to tolerate imagining a dog coming into the garden, approaching her, and licking her face, and she is able to do so without anxiety.

3. *Posthypnotic suggestions:* These followed two courses: confiding in her fiancé her fear of dogs, which was intensely embarrassing to her, and building self-esteem and confidence in her ability to overcome this fear prior to the wedding. The first course followed these lines: "When you decide to tell Dan, you will feel relieved and good about yourself at having come to such an important conclusion. You will be comfortable with the decision. You will feel pride in your accomplishment and re-ward yourself in some way—perhaps by purchasing something you have wanted or by having a long, expensive, and enjoyable lunch with a friend. When you prepare to tell Dan you will remember what has been discussed in therapy about how common your fear is, and even if he acts surprised or amused you will not feel embarrassed or silly, but will feel proud of the courage you have shown in confronting this fear."

The second part of the posthypnotic suggestions followed these lines: "You will find an appropriate time and place prior to your wedding to begin the exercises we have agreed on in your therapy. You will feel proud of having finally decided to confront your fear and confident in your ability to overcome it. The time and place you choose will be appropriate and will give you plenty of time to work on your fear prior to the wedding, but you will not feel anxiety or pressure about making this decision. You are able to retreat to your special place whenever you need relief from your fear or are experiencing anxiety that you need relief from."

As is evident from this example, direct suggestions enjoy an evident relationship between the presenting problem and the treatment plan. This is the major benefit from our perspective: the treatment becomes a joint effort between the therapist and client, and the client learns how to solve problems rather than just solving them. This may not appear to be much of a dis-tinction, but indirect methods are thought to utilize unconscious mecha-nisms, which are appropriate in many, perhaps the majority of, cases. When the factors that indicate a didactic treatment approach are positive, the direct method has some distinct advantages.

Perhaps it would be best to envision using direct suggestions when a clear relationship exists between the presenting problem and the treatment plan (Yapko, 1983), as in the previous example where there were no com-plications from a coexistent personality disorder. The client was intelligent and motivated, and it was easy to establish a therapeutic relationship. The didactic approach appealed to her; she wanted to learn how to solve her problem as well as alleviate her symptom. It was clear from the initial sessions that she was psychologically minded even though she had not had previous psychotherapy. She understood that her experience as a child had led to her phobia and that some measure of discomfort would be required to challenge the fear.

In fact, many clients have a good idea what they do not want from therapy: a detached professional who does not seem to respond to them on an emotional level. Many clients fear that the therapist will ask them to "assume the couch" and sit impassively while they reveal their deepest secrets. These clients may leave a session of psychodynamic therapy wondering what they are paying for. The direct approach is for them, at least as an introduction to the therapy process.

But lest readers assume that directive methods are reserved solely for more sophisticated clients, we present two case studies in which hypnosis was used with prison inmates:

Meyer and Tilker (1976) were confronted with a difficult case while employed as therapists at the Psychiatric Clinic of the State Prison of Southern Michigan. The client was a twenty-six-year-old male, Mr. A, who had been incarcerated for his second narcotics offense. He had an extensive psychiatric history and had been in individual therapy twice while outside of prison. The working diagnosis, although he had never had formal psychological testing, had always been sociopathic personality, antisocial type (in DSM-II-R, an antisocial personality disorder). Mr. A had received parole, effective in six weeks. Because no progress had been made with him in any previous therapy, an attempt was made to implement direct suggestions through hypnotherapy. He proved to be an excellent hypnosis subject and was able to attain both glove anesthesia and amnesia for posthypnotic suggestions in the first one-hour session. Over the next four weeks, he was seen for seven more fifteen-minute session and always went into a deep state of hypnosis in response to a rapid induction technique.

During those sessions, only direct suggestions were given for the full fifteen minutes—in this case, that he would stop craving drugs or alcohol. A posthypnotic suggestion was used to emphasize that every time he was able to resist or complete another activity that he saw as an indication he was developing a healthier personality, he would think for a few minutes how well he had done and how easily he could repeat the event.

He reportedly took no drugs in the first three weeks after parole but did drink himself into a stupor three times. Three months later, he said that he had not used drugs or alcohol since his discharge, and the interview indicated that most areas of his life had dramatically improved. He was holding a job and had plans to get married. Contacted by mail six months later, he reported that these trends were continuing.

The self-reports of a chronic drug and alcohol abuser are not the best empirical evidence of a therapeutic technique's efficacy. To test the procedure under more rigorous controls, a second inmate, Mr. C, was selected.

Mr. C was less verbal, appeared less intelligent (tested IQ of 85 to 90), had chronic low-grade anxiety as well as a weight problem, and was not self-referred for treatment, all factors that markedly contrast with Mr. A. Mr. C, a thirty-four-year-old white male who was serving his third term for larceny, admitted to strong feelings of inferiority in situations he construed as competitive. He was in chronic trouble while in prison; his problems appeared to be due to passive resistance to security officers or the stealing and selling of illegal contraband. On the two previous convictions, Mr. C had violated his parole on both occasions. His first parole lasted only two months before he was apprehended and returned to prison. He stated that he had never interrupted his pattern of stealing at any time from the age of sixteen. He did not view his problems as psychological but rather assumed naively that he would be given pills that would cause him to lose weight and lower his anxiety.

The first several sessions were directed toward the patient's rapidly attaining a hypnotic trance marked by both glove anesthesia and amnesia for posthypnotic suggestions. After three twenty-minute sessions, Mr. C could do both. Utilizing a strict time constraint developed a priori, the therapy lasted for twenty-three weeks, which included fourteen sessions, totaling 210 minutes of hypnotic therapy.

In each session after rapid induction, direct suggestions were repeated and elaborated to the effect that Mr. C would find himself gradually able to resist eating extra helpings of food and on occasion would be able to resist a first helping of starchy foods. It was emphasized that each time he was able to do so, Mr. C would feel very proud of himself for having succeeded in spite of his tendencies to do otherwise. He was directed that on these occasions, he would immediately reflect on the fact that he had been able to make some changes by himself and be justly proud of these changes. It was also directly suggested to him that he would find himself making changes in other areas that were meaningful to him and at a pace comfortable to him. Areas directly suggested were the handling of situations involving competition with others and decisions about whether to steal various items and whether he should get into arguments. Again it was emphasized that every time he did something positive, he would feel good about himself. It was emphasized that if he failed in particular instances, he would not feel guilty but would realize that steps toward improvement are gradual and would simply wait for a later time, when he would succeed. These direct suggestions were the entire content of all sessions.

At the end of these sessions, Mr. C had lost thirty-five pounds. He reported that he was free of the anxiety that had plagued him most of his life. He spontaneously verbalized that he felt good about himself and was optimistic about his life. He said he realized that there were things about himself he should be proud of and that he was not particularly bothered about what others may think. After the therapy was terminated, the authors received reports from prison staff that Mr. C's attitude had markedly improved, as evidenced by both his work and recreational involvement.

An interview with Mr. C held a month after release indicated that his improvement was continuing: he had held a steady job, was preparing to marry, and had no desire to be involved in any criminal activities. Checks at both nine and fifteen months after parole indicated his situation was stable and positive; interviews at the fifteen-month mark indicated he was still free from anxiety and happy in his marriage, and he had maintained his weight loss.

Two techniques were used in these cases to elicit behavioral response and positive self-reinforcement to maintain the behaviors until the environment could act as a positive reinforcer. The behaviors that were causing difficulty were effectively attacked through direct suggestion; secondary processes, such as anxiety and self-image, were also treated through posthypnotic suggestions, supporting the behavior change. These two cases were of a type that therapists often consider to be not amenable to psychotherapeutic intervention of any sort, especially in regard to long-term or substantial change.

An important consideration with such clients as Mr. A and Mr. C, who may not have had much experience accepting responsibility for their actions, is to try to instill in them a sense of personal and social responsibility. One of the benefits of the direct approach, then, is that it leads to a therapeutic alliance that is a shared approach to treatment: the therapist offers direction in problem solving or helps the client to come up with solutions, which will then become the suggestions themselves; the client is ultimately responsible for carrying out the directives and for taking responsibility for the progress of the therapy.

The main disadvantage to the direct approach may be that a useful tool, the unconscious (or at least subconscious) mind, is largely circumvented. For clients who are experiencing psychological distress, the symptoms are the client's idiosyncratic methods of problem solving. Not being aware that symptoms may mask deeper emotional conflicts is a disservice to the client, because the emotional need will be addressed, usually through another symptom at another time.

Another disadvantage to direct suggestions is that it may increase the tendency of clients to intellectualize and further the distance between their emotional and intellectual selves, when one goal of therapy for them may be integration. A failure of the client to make progress under these conditions may be interpreted by the therapist as resistance, leading to an excerbation of the problem.

Clients who have problems with authority figures may not do well in directive hypnotherapy. Because direct suggestions involve telling the client what to do, feel, and experience, a client with authority figure problems will probably not respond well to them. This should become evident in the assessment sessions as resistance rears its head and the therapist feels distance. Issues regarding problems with authority figures in the past should be addressed; resistance to discussion of these issues should alert the clinician to the possibility of this type of problem.

Posthypnotic Technique

Posthypnotic suggestions direct the client's behavior in some fashion after the session. When successful, posthypnotic suggestions are acted upon compulsively and in this manner are similar in nature to conditioned reflexes (Cheek and LeCron, 1968). Yet they are complex tasks that are more resistant to extinction than conditioned reflexes and are probably mini reenactments of the original trance. If there is a difference in the actual trance and the psychic state during the behavior precipitated by the posthypnotic suggestion, it may be in degree rather than type, unless the posthypnotic suggestion is to enter a deep trance upon some cue (these suggestions are often planted to save time in future sessions). Erickson, Hershman, and Sector (1961) report that posthypnotic suggestions are "essentially identical to the trance in which the posthypnotic suggestion was given. It is another sign that the subject is responding to posthypnotic suggestion" (p. 347).

Posthypnotic suggestions may last from months to years and can be reinforced through subsequent suggestions. They are usually followed, regardless of the depth of the original trance; nevertheless, the greater is the depth, the more likely the suggestions are to have an effect (Berrigan et al., 1991; Meyer and Tilker, 1976). The nature of the suggestions is a major factor in whether they are carried out. As in all other hypnotic suggestions, it appears reasonable to assume that a client cannot be made to do what he or she would not otherwise do. The suggestions should be of desired behaviors, whether unconsciously or consciously. Amnesia for the suggestions may be given during hypnosis; otherwise, the subject may or may not remember the suggestion at the time of the posthypnotic act. When amnesia is suggested, the subject knows what he or she is doing but not why.

The content of the posthypnotic suggestion determines whether it is carried out. Ridiculous suggestions are usually rejected, unless done as part of a stage routine, in which case the subjects are usually selected carefully for a proneness to exhibitionism. A client who carries out a posthypnotic suggestion and is told that he or she has done so will often rationalize this behavior. For example, a client was given a posthypnotic suggestion to take off her shoes upon emerging from hypnosis. As she came out of the trance, she rubbed her feet for a few seconds and then removed her shoes, commenting on how sore and itchy her toes were.

The strength and durability of posthypnotic suggestions is directly related to the hypnotic trance, trust in the therapist-hypnotist, and the quality of belief in hypnosis that the subject has accrued. If a subject carefully follows complex suggestions made during the trance, the likelihood of posthypnotic response should be good to excellent.

Posthypnotic suggestions are used for many reasons. We will examine some of the most common uses, but these should by no means be considered inclusive, for there are as many reasons for and permutations of these techniques as there are clients. Each situation will be different, each case unique.

1. *To assess the depth of the trance and suggestibilty of the client.* For example, a posthypnotic suggestion might direct the client to sleep deeply immediately after coming out of trance or to look out the window. The extent to which these suggestions are followed gives the therapist an idea about the depth of trance and suggestibility of the client. This kind of posthypnotic suggestion may also be used to ascertain whether other direct suggestions are having an effect. Trenerry and Jackson (1983), in treating a client with hysterical dystonia, gave a posthypnotic suggestion that symptoms would be gone for two days and then would return. This was done both to demonstrate to the client that she had control over the symptoms and to demonstrate to the therapist that the direct suggestions were working.

2. *To achieve a psychological or physiological state prior to stressors.* Many clients know all too well which objects or situations cause them anxiety. Posthypnotic suggestions may work well as inoculations. For example, a client who has performance anxiety may be inoculated by suggestions of relaxation if aware of impending public performance. These suggestions could be of symptoms incompatible with anxiety, such as normal heartbeat and breathing or of guided imagery of safe, comfortable

places. Brown and Fromm (1987) report that this type of posthypnotic suggestion is used in a variety of clinical ways. One use was in the case of a man who suffered from premature ejaculation. For this client, sexual performance was very anxiety provoking, so posthypnotic suggestions were given that allowed him to achieve anxiety reduction far in advance of having sex. Reduction of anxiety made it possible for him to carry out the other behaviors (pause and squeeze techniques) that ultimately led to successful outcome.

3. *To install behaviors and techniques that will allow clients to achieve trance state.* Giving a posthypnotic suggestion that will allow the client to achieve trance at an appropriate time is common in medical and dental applications. Patterson, Questad, and de Lateur (1989) gave posthypnotic suggestions to clients in burn wards that allowed nurses and other staff to bring the client into trance when painful procedures were to begin.

4. *To set the unconscious working to solve a problem.* This is common in hypnotherapy and is used in both direct and indirect approaches. Suggestions are made that the client has the psychological tools to solve the presenting problems and that these tools will be used in an effective way when the client is ready. A direct suggestion approach in treatment of a phobia, for instance, may be that the feared object will be encountered in a way that minimizes initial anxiety. Indirect suggestions are more likely to be vague about how the problem will be solved and in this way allow the unconscious to find the best problem-solving method.

5. *To give the client control over anesthesias.* Once glove anesthesia is achieved, another suggestion can be made directing the anesthesia to another spot on the body or to a body organ. Brown and Fromm (1987) report that this technique may be an aspect of weight reduction therapy or of sex therapy. In weight reduction therapy, the anesthesia is transferred to the pit of the stomach to suppress hunger by posthypnotic suggestion; in sex therapy, premature ejaculation may be treated with a posthypnotic suggestion that the anesthesia be transferred to the glans of the penis. Both of these would be under the voluntary control of the client. Another use of this type of posthypnotic suggestion is in pain management. If a client has control over pain reduction by way of locating an anesthesia, anxiety over painful procedures can be reduced. In Patterson, Questad, and de Lateur's (1989) study, patients who had been hypnotized and given posthypnotic suggestions allowing them to focus glove anesthesia on the area that was to be debrided or have a dressing changed were able to tolerate the treatment better.

6. *To induce amnesias.* There are many reasons why the clinician might want to create an amnesia. It could be that age regression has led to recall of long-suppressed memories and that the therapist has determined that it would be best if the knowledge of these experiences remain suppressed until the client can gain some coping resources to deal with them. These could be

memories of abuse or other trauma. MacHovec (1985) has treated post-traumatic stress disorder clients using hypnosis and has found it useful to reintegrate clients' memories of traumatic events gradually with the other aspects of the therapy—for example, grief processes over the repressed memories of a loved one's death.

Another reason for instilling an amnesia is to reduce anxiety after a painful medical or dental procedure. Anxiety over dental visits could be reduced if the client were given the suggestion that he or she would forget the painful unpleasantness of the root canal; it could be directly suggested (after prior approval by the client) that the memory of the procedure be forgotten.

7. *To recreate pleasurable psychological or physiological states.* Brown and Fromm (1987) report that in treatment of addictive disorders, it is essential to plan for relapse. One method is to use a posthypnotic suggestion that the client will be able to achieve through imagination the psychological benefits previously received from the substances he or she abused. This type of posthypnotic suggestion may also be used in sex therapy—for example, when a wife or husband has lowered sexual desire and/or response after surgery or trauma. A suggestion is made that the client will recall past pleasurable sexual experiences to aid in gaining sensations during actual intercourse.

8. *To reinforce other behaviors.* This is probably the most common use of posthypnotic suggestions. Any desired behavior, whether it is directly or indirectly related to the presenting problem, may be reinforced through the use of posthypnotic suggestions. For a client who wants to learn new skills for weight reduction, suggestions may be made that normally bland (but healthy) foods taste good, that self-esteem will improve through periodic fasting, that a feeling of being full will be achieved after only a few bites of food, or that after an agreed-upon number of calories is consumed, the client will no longer be hungry. Posthypnotic suggestions of this kind may be constructed for any habit control problem—for example, that apples are more satisfying than cigarettes.

9. *To promote the use of skills learned in therapy.* Since hypnosis is only a minor part of therapy in numerous cases, posthypnotic suggestions can be used to move the treatment along. Any kind of coping behavior, from improved self-esteem to ways of dealing with depression and anxiety, may be encouraged through the use of posthypnotic suggestions. Marital therapy cases with communication problems can be encouraged in individual sessions to take chances toward intimacy with their partners; borderline clients can be encouraged to monitor their behaviors; depressed clients can be encouraged to monitor their thoughts. Coping resources may be called upon at any time or at times of stress; posthypnotic suggestions can leave the timing up to the needs of the client.

10. *To reduce awareness of stimuli.* Koe (1989) presents a case of sleep

terror successfully treated with hypnosis. One aspect of the disorder was that the onset of the terrors was related to sensitivity to environmental stimuli; sounds during the night precipitated the sleep disorder. Posthypnotic suggestions given that awareness of stimuli would be reduced during sleep and uncovering therapy were successful in eliminating the sleep disturbance. There are many other uses of this technique, including reducing attention of distracting stimuli in performance anxiety or medical or dental procedures.

Posthypnotic suggestions constitute an important factor in successful hypnotherapy. They can be used in a myriad of situations. As with all other suggestions, clinicians should be aware of the consequences of their use and should thoroughly assess what behaviors are likely as a result of the suggestion. Clinicians should heed these points:

Hypnotic subjects are literal minded. If you encourage behaviors, be sure that part of your suggestion contains a caveat that the client will follow the instructions only in a positive manner and at the appropriate time. It is also a good idea to include a beginning and ending point for the behavior, unless the suggestion is that the unconscious work to improve psychological functioning. For example, you would not want a weight control client to have anesthesia in the pit of the stomach for days on end.

Know your client. Be sure you know what the client will do with the suggestion. There is no substitute for a good historical and diagnostic workup, even in cases where the presenting problem appears relatively circumspect and straightforward, such as in habit control treatment.

Consider carefully the positive and negative effects of the suggestion. All suggestions affect the unconscious. Therefore, thoroughly consider what a client is likely to do under the influence of suggestion(s). Suggestions for weight reduction, for example, must include directions for adequate nutrition. Those for inducing anesthesia must include sufficient controls so that the numbness can be eliminated. Ensure that suggestions to induce relaxation are situation specific. Anxiety is a useful defense mechanism; for example, a client should not be in a state of significant relaxation while driving in rush hour traffic.

Clinical Applications

We had occasion recently to treat a woman who had lost her left leg in an automobile accident. Julie, a twenty-seven-year-old nurse, came seeking hypnotherapy to deal with a condition referred to as phantom limb. This often occurs when a limb is amputated and is due to the brain's attempting to seek the stimulation of the (now-departed) nerves that had been sending information from the limb. This condition can last for some time, even years, and it can be uncomfortable or even painful. Julie had been without her leg for almost nine months at the time she presented for her first session.

We first got a history of her symptom and the factors surrounding it. She was experiencing a lot of anticipatory anxiety because she did not know when the pain would begin, but she usually felt it each day for a few hours. If it happened at work, it could be incapacitating. In the middle of the night, it was simply painful and frightening. There was also the issue of Julie's self-esteem and self-image, which were severely damaged by her accident. She had lost confidence in her ability to do the things she had loved to do, although her doctors assured her that with the new prosthetics available, she could jog, ride a bicycle, and even play tennis. Depression was thus part of the picture.

We decided together that we would work on the anxiety and pain first and then deal with the depression, trying to get Julie back into the swing of her life. Julie was an excellent hypnotic subject, as is often the case with pain clients. She achieved a deep trance during our first session, using the eye fixation method and testing the depth via glove anesthesia.

We had agreed that she should have an imaginal refuge she could retreat to when she was feeling anxious or if the pain was beginning. Julie would use this "safe place" only when she was not at work, not driving, and not in other situations where she needed to be alert. The safe place served two functions. First, she had an autohypnotic technique she could use to relax and avoid pain, and second, it gave her confidence in her ability to cope with her condition.

Julie had grown up in the state of Washington and fondly recalled walks on the beach as a youngster. Therefore, we set her safe place on a beach she loved, on a warm, summer day, with a cool breeze blowing the salt smell of the ocean on her face. Direct suggestions were used to set the imagery.

Guided imagery: "Julie, you are feeling warm and comfortable. It is a summer day, and you can feel the sun on your face. You are sitting on a picnic table near the sandy beach, and you decide you want to go for a walk down that favorite path. You stand up, and as you do, you feel the breeze blowing across your face; you smell the salt spray from the sea, the scent of the kelp, and the mustiness of the warm sand. What do you smell?" [At this point, it is a good idea to check for the sensory hallucinations. If the client is not smelling and experiencing the hallucination, deepening through more progressive relaxation or another technique will help.]

"Good. Now you are proceeding down the beach to your safe place, the cove on the west side of the inlet. You see the cove. You feel relaxed and comfortable. Proceed to your favorite spot, and indicate to me when you are there by raising your finger. [Once we established that she was there, we could proceed with one of the pain reduction techniques we used.]

"Julie, I want you to look around you on the beach. You will see a bottle half buried in the sand. Pick it up. There is a piece of paper in your pocket, as well as a pencil. Take them out. Write 'my pain' on the paper. Now roll the paper up and put it in the bottle. Now stand up and throw the bottle as far out to sea as you can. You will count to ten as you see the bottle get farther and farther away. With each count, your pain becomes less and less, until at the count of ten you feel no pain from your leg. You will realize that the bottle is likely to come back in. The tide and waves will bring it back. All you have to do is pick up the bottle and throw it back out to sea, and count from one to ten."

It is important to note that the dialogue did not follow this straight-through pace. Throughout the process, we were making sure she was experiencing the imagery and feeling the sensation by asking simple questions and looking for a finger movement in response.

This technique was very successful for Julie; however, we needed to deal with her pain in a less complex manner for those times when she could not go into autohypnosis and retreat to her safe place, where she could throw the pain away. We did this by transferring a glove anesthesia to her missing leg—not to the missing leg, obviously, but to a spot on her thigh that, when numb, would not allow any pain messages from the phantom limb. This was the suggestion we gave:

Direct suggestion: "Julie, I want you to notice that your hand is getting numb. As I touch it, you notice that you are feeling less and less sensation from it, as though it is covered in a protective covering. I could be touching the chair, and you would not know the difference. I want you to be aware of the fact that you are controlling the feeling in this hand. You are making it numb. Now I want you to use that power to make another spot numb. I am going to touch you on the left thigh, and on that spot you will notice you will lose sensation. I am touching your thigh with one finger, and I want you to take that numbness and extend it around your thigh in a band, just as if you have a tourniquet around your thigh that is cutting off the feeling instead of the blood supply. Now that loss of feeling means that no sensation below it will get by; no loss of sensation will occur above the ring of numbness."

Two approaches were used in posthypnotic suggestions. To alleviate the pain directly and indirectly, Julie was given posthypnotic suggestions that she would be able to control the pain and that if she experienced pain it would be tolerable.

Therapist: Julie, you have indicated to me that you experience pain at certain times during the day, such as in the morning, late in the afternoon, and in the evening just before you retire. In the morning after you rise, you will feel refreshed and invigorated. You will be aware of the fact that you often have felt the pain of your leg at these times, but you will feel no apprehension about it. If you begin to feel pain, you will use the anesthetic technique you have learned to eliminate the pain. You will feel the pain and make it go away by using the band of numbness you have control over. The pain will never be so severe that you will not be able to tolerate it.

The direct techniques that we used with Julie were successful in helping her to deal with her loss. In addition to hypnosis, we used interpersonal process techniques to help Julie regain her lost self-esteem and deal with her depression. But direct suggestions were used throughout the therapy to reinforce and enhance the psychotherapy.

Conclusion

Direct suggestions have an important place in hypnotherapy, especially since cognitive-behavioral and behavioral therapies have been shown to be so effective in treatment of specific disorders. The extent to which direct suggestions and posthypnotic techniques may be used in hypnotherapy is bounded only by the imagination of the therapist. Entering into a therapeutic alliance in which the input and motivation of the client is encouraged and supported is fertile ground for a direct approach. Direct suggestions and posthypnotic techniques benefit motivated clients by giving them the tools they need to change and by showing them that change occurs through efforts they ultimately have control over. In medical and dental applications, direct suggestions and posthypnotic techniques work not only to alleviate the pain of the procedures but also to reduce the associated anxiety, and thus they may make it more likely that the patient will comply with the treatment.

7
Hypnotic Age Regression

> Life can be understood looking backward,
> but must be lived forward.
> —Soren Kierkegaard

Age regression, a method of recovering reflections from another time, has long been a favorite tool of dynamic therapists, though often not more than a curiosity for cognitive psychologists (Nash, 1988; Bodden, 1991). Freud, citing Breuer and Jackson, traditionally invoked the concept of psychological regression to explain changes evident during special states. From his work, many dynamic therapists embraced the notion that revisiting the past promised an antidote for the future. They maintained that once a person gains awareness from retrospection, he or she is better able to deal not only with the present but with the hereafter. Instead of restricting their thinking to the way they have been, age regression can help them see themselves as they could be.

While contemporary psychoanalysts and cognitive developmental psychologists maintain that returning to an earlier psychophysiological matrix is possible, perhaps even necessary, when treating certain types of pathology (Kohut, 1971; Stolorow and Lachmann, 1980; Gross, 1983), othes are more cautious. They might acknowledge that adult pathology can be understood in terms of developmental failure and repetition compulsion, but they argue that the psychic structure of the disturbed adult differs from that of the child and that developmentally previous modes of functioning are not retrievable in their pure form because they have been unalterably changed (Piaget and Inhelder, 1969; Nash, 1987; Denburg, 1990). Nevertheless, whether one views regression as vivid remembering or as actual reliving, practitioners from many theoretical camps have explored the use of hypnosis to produce age regressions of substantial depth quickly and efficiently (Gibson and Heap, 1991; Fuhriman, Zingaro, and Kokenes, 1990).

Theory and Research

Two core assumptions underlie the concept of age regression in clinical practice: early structures in human development are relatively imperishable, and regression, involving reinstatement of infantile psychological structures, has a healing effect. In classical psychoanalytic thought, psychopathology is viewed in terms of developmental arrest. These theorists maintain that returning to an earlier psychophysiological matrix is not only a possibility but a necessity if treatment is to be beneficial. Generally therapists from this orientation are concerned with the production of catharsis and insight from hypnotic age regression.

Later dynamic theorists maintained that although adult pathology could be understood in terms of arrested development, adult structures are essentially different from child structures and that previous modes of functioning are irretrievable. For these theorists, memory and therapy are viewed as reconstructed rather than actual. Typically, therapists from these orientations use hypnotic age regressions to induce cognitive reframing or to track down the source of a problem for later use in conscious therapy modes. It is important to note that the last two methods of healing do not require an actual reliving of the event (with primitive structures intact).

Nash (1988) provides theoretical support for the reconstructionist position by pointing to Freud's theory of topographical regression. Freud postulated that a regressive shift from thought to imagery carried with it a shift from secondary to primary process. This perspective on regression seems to fit better with the experiences of clinicians as reported in the literature.

Overall, the research in age regression seems to center on two questions:

1. Given that adults, when hypnotically regressed, do not become actual children, to what extent do their responses resemble those of children?
2. Do hypnotically regressed adults shift from sequential and secondary process modes of experience to imaginal and primary process modes?

Actual Regression to Primitive Structures

Clinicians and researchers have observed that highly suggestible subjects, when hypnotically regressed, exhibit dramatic changes in behavior, affect, and communicative style (Fuhriman, Zingaro, and Kokenes, 1991; Denburg, 1990). Does hypnotic age regression enable subjects to exhibit developmentally previous modes of mental functioning? Most of the research on hypnotic age regression has focused on cognitive, affective, and physiological sequelae to an actual relived regression. These researchers hoped to establish the existence or hoax of hypnotic age regression based on these objectifiable markers. The results are mixed.

Nash (1987), in a comprehensive review of sixty years of literature, grouped findings into four types of physiological markers that could conceivably be proof of a return to more primitive cognitive structures:

1. *Physiology.* While early studies indicated a return to infantlike electroencephalograms and childlike reflexes, they were poorly designed and

controlled. Nash noted that despite advances such as the computed tomography scan and nuclear magnetic resonance, no adequately designed experiment comparing child structures to adult structures has been published. In fact, most studies using advanced technologies fail to show a clear one-to-one relationship between the measured brain structures and specific functions (Horton, 1991). In the face of this evidence, it seems unlikely that support for actual physiological markers of age regression will be found.

2. *Cognitive and memory processes.* Two types of processes have been explored in the literature: recall of remote events and reinstatement of earlier cognitive processes. The best-controlled studies compare the results of the hypnotized subjects with "motivated" controls (control subjects who have essentially received the same suggestions as the hypnotized subjects but without a hypnotic induction) and then compare both groups with the results of actual children.

To test for recall of remote memory, researchers instruct hypnotically regressed subjects to relive a past event and then verify the subject's report with a third party. Nash (1987, 1988) noted that properly controlled studies failed to find a difference in accuracy of recall, even in the most hypnotizable of subjects.

To test for a return to earlier cognitive structures, researchers have typically administered either IQ tests or Piagetian-type tasks to discover whether regressed subjects perform at the cognitive-developmental level appropriate for the age to which they were regressed. In both types of studies, Nash found that the intellectual functioning of the regressed adults was no different from that of "motivated" controls and that both groups differed significantly from the performance of children. Researchers observed that although the adult performances may appear to be similar to the children's on the surface, the processing was essentially adult in nature.

3. *Perceptual processes.* Comparisons of hypnotically regressed adult performance with child performance have been explored with the Ponzo illusion, the Poggendorff illusion, and size constancy tasks. All well-designed studies showed that the hypnotized subjects performed like adults, not children. A study by Denburg (1990) on the autokinetic effect showed similar results.

4. *Personality processes.* Early studies using various projectives such as the Rorschach and the Thematic Apperception Test suggested that actual personality regression had occurred. However, these studies were poorly controlled and frequently single subject in design. Later studies, which were properly controlled, found that hypnotically regressed adult responses were easily distinguishable from child responses. Also, a study by Fuhriman, Zingaro, and Kokenes (1990) found a similar result using drawings.

Nash noted that the literature presents convincing evidence that hypnotically regressed adult subjects do not produce markers identical to those of children and that when these markers are similar to those of children, motivated controls can perform as well as the hypnotized subjects.

Shifts in Process Modes of Experience

Given that there is no support for actual retracing of early developmental structures, is there a difference in the experience and thought of a hypnotically regressed subject and a motivated control? Nash's review indicates that there is substantial evidence that, although primitive structures may not be revisited, a shift from sequential, secondary processing to imaginistic, primary process may be occurring during a hypnotic age regression. He pointed to four areas of research:

1. *Changes in thought processes.* Well-designed studies, using both nonhypnotized baseline responses of the hypnotized subjects and motivated controls, on projective tests revealed an increased incidence of primary process material, as well as a shift of thought processes in the direction of prelogical, symbolic, and primary process mentation. Additionally, Nash noted evidence that a relaxation of defenses occurs during hypnotic age regression. These results are obtainable only if the dependent measure is administered by a hypnotist. This seems to indicate that the relationship between the client and the hypnotist has an important impact on the quality of the age reduction.

2. *Increased availability of affect.* Nash (1988) cited his own research in reviewing the literature concerning this marker. In one study, Nash and his colleagues explored whether a transitional object reported by a hypnotically age-regressed subject was the same as the subject had had as a child. They compared the reports of hypnotized subjects and motivated controls with reports of their mothers. Hypnotized subjects showed an increase in spontaneous, specific, and intense expression of emotion; however, these subjects were significantly less accurate than the control subjects in identifying their specific childhood transitional objects. From this, Nash concluded that although hypnotic age regression may enhance access to important emotional material, it does not imply an accurate reliving of a specific event.

3. *Fluctuations in body experience.* Although there are many reports of both induced and spontaneous feelings of changes in the body (shrinking, swelling, loss of equilibrium), these experiences are not universal. Nonetheless, Nash suggests that there may be a link between this phenomenon and age regression, since it is theoretically similar to primary process mentation.

4. *Transference relationships with the hypnotist.* While Freudians have always considered hypnosis a regressed relationship, only recently has this concept been empirically investigated. The results have been mixed. Nash

cites several studies that did not show a difference in the quality of the subject-hypnotist relationship, as measured by semantic differentials and subliminal activation of symbiotic fantasies. However, in a departure from the heavily analytic orientation of most age regression research, he points to Sheehan's line of research, which has shown that hypnotized subjects more often spontaneously expressed feeling cared for, protected, and supported by the hypnotist.

It is possible that the difficulty in exploring this construct lies in the elusive nature of transference. Until a better methodology is invented, the importance of the transference in hypnotic age regression can only be guessed at.

Conclusions and Implications

Does hypnotic age regression exist? Nash (1987) concluded that just as hypnotically suggested amnesia, deafness, and other states are not functionally equivalent to their organic counterparts, hypnotic age regression is not a return to childhood. On the other hand, the research has demonstrated a shift from sequential, secondary cognitive processing to imaginistic, primary cognitive processing. Whether this shift facilitates the process of therapy is not empirically clear, though the testimony of therapists who use age regression techniques is consistently positive.

Psychodynamic theorists would argue that this shift in cognitive processing might enable a lowering of defenses necessary for "end-running" treatment-destructive resistances, such as memory blocking and repetition compulsion (Gross, 1983). Unfortunately, the therapeutic outcome literature is confined to case studies (discussed later in this chapter), which deliver little truly generalizable information.

For now, the broad-spectrum therapeutic utility of hypnotic age regression remains scientifically unestablished, and its selection as a modality of therapy is largely directed by theoretical orientation and clinical judgment.

Using Age Regression in Therapy

Choosing a Candidate

There are specific problem areas for which hypnotic age regression is not the treatment of choice. For some clients, exclusion is the result of unrealistic expectations. For others, the shift from secondary to primary cognitive process appears to create singular hazards that may require specialized training and technique to combat problems that may arise during and after the regression. Therapists who do not have this specialized training should not attempt to do age regression techniques with these clients without obtaining thorough training followed up by colleague counsel and supervision. The following are broad problem areas for which hypnotic age regression is contraindicated:

The person who has unrealistic expectations. This is a client who is often an appropriate subject for treatment but believes that hypnosis is a magic cure-all. Generally these clients have sought other types of therapy, with unsuccessful results. They are looking for something quick and easy ("I want to understand why I hate men in three sessions or less"), or they expect hypnosis to achieve the impossible ("I want to lose all memories of my father").

The borderline personality. Borderline clients sometimes cannot endure or experience the anxieties that will accompany the exploration of their problem, and age regressions can be especially threatening to them. They may have difficulty understanding that the hypnosis is part of a comprehensive treatment plan but may instead try to view the information obtained as compartmentalized, rather than integrated into several behavioral areas. Additionally, they may be receiving secondary gain from the perceived exotic nature of hypnosis, which may foil attempts to become healthy as they become comfortable with their discomfort.

The psychotic. Clients suffering from severe thought or mood disorder may react to a hypnotically induced age regression with a variety of intense, uncontrolled emotions. They may have tics, lack of physical coordination, or sensory disturbances. Some clients experience hallucinations, amnesia, and erotic impulses. Hypnotic age regression, especially if used as the primary treatment of such severe disorders, may intensify the existing condition, create negative side effects, or have no effect at all.

Initial Preparation

Before attempting age regression, the hypnotist should have some understanding of the client's personality and history. At the same time, it is also necessary to educate the client about hypnosis and what he or she can reasonably expect from the process.

An essential element to the regression's success is the trust the client places in the therapist. The client must be convinced that his or her well-being is an important consideration in the hypnotic situation. For this reason, the process of regression should be unhurried, communicating to the client that he or she is safe, protected, and in control.

Frequently therapists have the subject write his or her name or draw a simple picture (say, a house or a person) before beginning the regression. This can be done on a chalkboard or a large pad of paper mounted on an easel or lying on a table in front of the subject. It is important to provide a large drawing space and large, easily grasped markers or chalk because the subject may have some impairment of fine motor control while age regressed.

During the regression, the subject may be directed to write his or her name or draw the same person or object. If the subject initially appears confused, gentle direction ("here . . . use this chalk . . . yes, that's right, draw on this board right here") will orient the subject to the task.

If the subject is sufficiently regressed, the drawings will reflect the primitive nature of a child's illustration or shift from an adult's cursive signature to a child's awkward printing. The therapist may elect to have the subject draw at different "ages" during the regression. These tasks can be used as tests of the depth of the trance. Additionally, these drawings can be used after regression for comparison of age differences and to help the subject gain confidence in the hypnotic regression.

Building an Induction

It is generally agreed that age regression requires a deepened state of hypnotic trance. Accordingly, time and care should be taken to create a deep trance before beginning the regression induction. The first four steps of this induction use standard techniques found elsewhere in this book. A model regression induction is then provided, with variations on the model given in the next section.

Beginning the induction: "Take a nice deep breath, close your eyes, and begin to relax. Just think about relaxing every muscle in your body."

Systematic relaxation of the body: "Begin by letting all the muscles in your face relax, especially your jaw; let your teeth part just a little bit and relax this area."

Creating imagery of deeper relaxation: "Drift and float into a deeper and deeper level of total relaxation. You are feeling lighter and lighter."

The initiation of the age regression induction requires special attention in order to create a deeply relaxed state. This will include instructions to the client as to what will happen and what to expect, followed by deep breathing and systematic relaxation of the body. It is important to take time with this part of the induction for new clients, as it helps them shift their focus from the anticipatory anxiety of a new experience to their inner sensations and states.

Since clients can have dramatic expectations of their experience in age regression, some therapists prefer to limit the initial session to relaxation and deepening, without attempting a regression. This can help clients gain confidence in their own ability to relax and fully experience the trance without the pressure of an actual regression.

For clients experiencing difficulties opening themselves up to this level of trance, it can be useful to explore the feelings and thoughts they had during the induction. Since victims of abuse and trauma are frequent candidates for age regression hypnotherapy, there may be substantial issues of trust that must be addressed consciously before they can allow themselves to enter the deep relaxation of hypnosis. Allowing clients to articulate these feelings and reassuring them that they will be able to enter hypnotic trance "when they are ready" can often alleviate their anxieties. Asking them if there is anything that might make it easier for them can provide valuable clues as to what is inhibiting their ability to relax.

Deepening the trance: "Drift and float into a deeper and deeper level of total relaxation. You are feeling lighter and lighter . . . imagine a luxurious elevator . . . you float into this elevator and look up and see the numbers changing . . . you are going up, up one floor, then a second floor [continue to ten floors] . . . when the doors open you see a special and peaceful and beautiful place."

Deepening the trance requires patience and skill in the hypnotherapist. Care must be taken to not rush this stage, allowing clients the opportunity to explore their capacity for visual imagery. For more on deepening trances, see the previous chapter.

Getting Permission and Establishing Communication Signals

When it is clear that the client is in a state of deep relaxation, the therapist encourages the client to gain permission from the unconscious to review the targeting memories. This can be particularly helpful for victims of abuse or for clients whose trust level is very low and who need complete assurance that they are in control and will not be coerced in any way. It is also a way of deepening the trance.

Therapist: I want you to ask your unconscious self if it will be all right to go back to when you were younger . . . ask that part of your mind if it will agree to allow you to see, hear, and feel what happened, remembering that you are completely safe, that it is in the past, and that it is not happening to you right now . . . raise your finger if your unconscious self agrees with you that it is good and helpful for you to go back and review what happened.

Clients who do not acquire permission from the unconscious to proceed must be reassured that this is all right and that they will proceed only when they feel it is safe and that they are ready for the experience. Sometimes it is useful at this point to ask these clients, while still in trance, if their unconscious will tell them why they are not ready and let them remember that reason after they finish the trance. Then the therapist and the client can review what may be inhibiting the latter's ability to accomplish hypnotic regression. If the unconscious does not give permission to know (or remember) why they are not ready, give the following direct suggestion:

Therapist: It's okay that you won't remember why you weren't ready. You will feel confident in your decision to wait until you feel safe; however, your unconscious will begin to let you know, through dreams and images, why you aren't ready to go further.

At this point, the client is brought out of trance to talk about his or her feelings. The therapist continues to meet and induct deep trances, but stopping here, until the client is ready to move further into the regression.

For clients who do receive permission to proceed with the regression, this is the time to establish finger signals for communication with the hypnotherapist. (Talking can be difficult while in a deep trance.) Some therapists prefer to direct the client to raise a forefinger if they want to say yes, or designate one finger for yes and another for no. Other therapists allow the client to choose fingers for signaling. This can be done by either direct suggestion—"I want you to lift your right forefinger to signal yes"—or by a nondirective suggestion—"sometimes I will ask you questions and I need you to answer me. Choose a finger that, when lifted, means yes. Just let that finger naturally rise and that will be your 'yes' finger . . . that's it . . ."

Finding a Focus for the Regression

Since hypnotic age regression is generally used to address specific symptoms or problems, it is necessary to direct the client to search out memories that directly pertain to the therapeutic goal. Otherwise, client and therapist may go off on endless, fruitless fishing expeditions that accomplish very little and ultimately can become an unconscious defense against regression to the most pertinent points in time. It is important not to lead the client in any way; the client must choose the most important memories. The therapist's job is to provide a safe and supportive environment for that choosing. A good technique for this is similar to the child's game, "Is it bigger than a bread box?"

> *Therapist:* Remember how you told me that you are afraid of cats? [Wait for a signal after each question, repeating the question if necessary.] Remember that fear of cats? . . . did something happen to you that is related to this fear, that maybe started this fear? . . . it did? . . . let's think, how old were you then . . . were you ten years old? . . . younger than ten years old? . . . were you nine? . . . [Keep going until you get to the age.] . . . okay, good, you were five years old . . . and let's see where you were, were you at home? . . . at a friend's house? . . . were you by yourself? . . . [Keep adding details until a time, place, and setting are generally established.]

Another way of focusing on regression is to ask the client to visualize a television set and change channels until he or she sees a scene that has to do with the therapeutic target—for instance:

> *Therapist:* We know that you are afraid of water, and now we are looking to see if something happened that is related to this fear . . . are you ready to look? . . . I want you to see a television set . . . it is a friendly TV set and perfectly under your control . . . I want you to practice changing channels on this TV set . . . are you changing channels? . . . good . . . now, I want you to change channels and watch each screen as much as you want, but when you see a picture that has to do with your fear of the water, I want you to signal me . . . that's right, signal me when you see a picture that relates to your fear . . . [When the client finds a scene relating to the therapeutic focus, the therapist asks questions to establish age, time, setting and people present.]

Variations on this method can include flipping through a calendar, looking out a train or car window, or looking through pages of a picture book. The method should feel comfortable and familiar for both client and therapist. If a client gets stuck or cannot find an appropriate memory, the therapist can go back to the elevator (or cloud, or some other deepening technique) and then "get out" at one of the other methods mentioned in this section. If nothing works, the client is reassured that the experience has been worthwhile and that he or she will awake feeling quite refreshed and relaxed.

Reviewing the Focused Memory

At this point, the therapist must decide whether the client should experience this memory actively or passively. Therapists advocating an active experience generally view the client's symptoms as being the result of repressed emotion. Accordingly, they urge their client to "relive" the memory, strong affect and all, in hopes of catharting the repressed emotion that is crippling them. Therapists who support a more passive regression are helping a client to experience a heightened and vivid memory, which, when viewed from an adult perspective, will be reframed to a less threatening interpretation of that event.

Active regressions often take a form similar to this:

Therapist: You will now begin to enter the scene you see before you . . . you are floating toward the scene . . . floating and entering, and now you are there . . . you are six years old . . . take a minute to look around . . . that's right, look around and perhaps you'll be quiet and really listen to what's going on . . . that's right, you are there now, you are six years old . . .

A more passive approach encourages the client to be a spectator of the scene or invites the client to "wrap yourself in a magic shield that will keep you from any harm." At all times, the client is reminded that he or she is not actually experiencing the memory and can leave the scene at any time. A typical passive induction might be the following:

Therapist: Now I want you to turn on the TV set, and I want you to turn the channel until you get to the scene where you are eight . . . that's right, you're watching yourself be eight years old, and you know that it's just a TV program and that you have the channel selector and can change the channel anytime you want, but perhaps right now you find yourself very curious, very interested in seeing what happened, and so you pay very close attention . . .

Sometimes, especially for new clients, regression proves difficult. When resistance is met, it can be useful to remind the client "not to work so hard." Hadley and Staudacher (1985) suggest an instruction similar to the following:

Therapist: Your subconscious will be doing the work. I want to tell you a story that I think you will be able to enjoy. And while you are listening, your subconscious will still be working for you, looking further and further into the past, bringing things together for you, helping you to integrate it all. But you can relax, let go, and listen to the story. And when your subconscious has the scene ready that sets the stage for your problem, your "yes" finger will rise.

At this point, the conscious mind is distracted by describing a bicycle trip, a walk on the beach, or a trip to the mall. The story should include careful description of minute details:

Therapist: You know how it is to ride the bus. As it pulls up, its brakes hiss and squeal and the door folds open and the bus driver looks at you and smiles. You step up onto the bus and hear the door close behind you and feel the lurch as it pulls into traffic. You reach into your pocket and pull out your change. It's hard, isn't it, to put the money in the little slot. First one coin and then another. It beeps at you when you are through . . .

Alternatively, some variation of the Ericksonian techniques described in chapter 5 can be helpful in coping with subjects who manifest some resistance at this or other stages. The client should now describe the scene to the therapist, possibly in a thick, slow voice. The therapist can ask simple, direct questions. The client may not answer them. If the client does not initially answer the questions, the therapist waits. It is possible that the scene being viewed is complex or traumatic, and the client needs time to absorb it before speaking. After a minute or two, the therapist repeats the instructions, including the count to three. If the client is still silent, the therapist asks the unconscious if there is a specific reason for the silence and even asking again for permission to reveal the scene to the therapist. If all of this fails, the therapist suggests again that the unconscious may work on the problem without revealing it and brings the client out of trance.

As information surfaces, the therapist should seek to reassure the client by a reminder that he or she is an observer and can keep safe, comforted, in control, and so on.

Dealing with Catharsis Reactions

Sometimes clients experience intense feelings of fear, rage, or sadness. Some hypnotherapists believe that a catharsis of such emotion is healing and beneficial. Toward that end, they furnish and arrange their offices to minimize danger to a client who is rocking, pounding the floor, or pacing while experiencing the scene. They may have pillows on hand to give to clients, encouraging them to vent their emotions on the pillows or hug them for comfort. They may speak to the client, encouraging a venting or release of emotion:

> *Therapist:* Yes . . . yes . . . you are really angry now . . . let it go . . . who is it who hurt you? . . . what did they do? . . . that's right . . . you hate him, you deserve to hate him . . . let it all out . . . let go of it.

Other hypnotherapists believe that catharsis is of little value or perhaps even countertherapeutic and place an emphasis on maintaining an atmosphere of safety for clients, helping them modulate and reframe the intense emotion they may be feeling. Anderson-Evangelista (1980) proposes suggestions similar to the following.

> *For anger:* "Of course you felt very angry and upset after what happened to you. No one should ever treat a child that way. But now that you are grown up, you can look back with a different perspective, you can understand what they did, you can see them as the unhappy and disturbed people they were."
>
> *For grief:* "Naturally you were confused and upset and had tremendous feelings of loss, and you know, you really did survive it all, even when you thought for sure you wouldn't. You've gained so much strength through all that. When you are little, saying good-bye is hard, but now that you are so much older, so much wiser, you can say good-bye in peace. You can now let it go."
>
> *For guilt:* "You can certainly understand the confusion and the feelings of guilt, and, you know, you've suffered enough through the years to make up for that mistake. You can now forgive yourself, gradually even forget it, and let it go."

All camps agree that when the reaction becomes dangerous or abnormal (seizures, vomiting, unusual changes in skin color), immediate intervention is required to gain distance from the memory. This may be facilitated by suggesting something like the following:

> *Therapist:* You are in my office; you are *not* back then, but you are only remembering . . . that's right, you are safe and I am with you and this is only a memory . . . and you will leave

> this memory and come out of the trance when I count three
> . . . one, two, three . . .

If this does not appear to have a quick positive effect, medical intervention is mandated immediately.

Concluding the Induction

It is important for the therapist to ask if it is all right for the client to remember the traumatic scene. Otherwise, the therapist makes a suggestion that the scene will remain forgotten until the client is stronger and ready to know. The induction concludes with a standard conclusion script.

Variations on Age Regression Inductions

Many aspects of the model induction can be varied to accommodate the needs and personality of the client. Judicious selection of voice, script, and timing within the overall therapy can heighten the usefulness and reduce resistance for a specific client. Modifications to the basic regression induction can be made around several factors.

Authoritative versus Permissive Style. In authoritative inductions, the therapist assumes a directive role, instructing the client as to what he or she will do next, see next, and feel next—for example:

> *Therapist:* You will now begin to travel back in time, you will see the pages of a calendar flipping back in time, page after page, and you will feel excited by this . . . you will want to find out what happened that year, your fifth year . . . now you are there . . . you are five, and you are watching them riding in the boat and you feel detached and safe as you watch . . .

It is important to assess each client's needs and receptivity. Clients whose motivational investment lies principally in the therapist's expertise may need an authoritative figure. Clients who have been abused, terrorized, or abducted (or who tend toward passive-aggressive personality styles) may be quite resistant to such directive methods and may require a permissive style on the part of the hypnotherapist.

In permissive inductions, the therapist assumes a nondirective role, suggesting possible paths to explore or directions to go in. The therapist frequently reminds the client that he or she is in control and may not have the images or feelings the therapist is suggesting, but that he or she is free to go at any pace or use the most comfortable imagery. It is important, when using this style, to keep the wording as vague and open-ended as possible, allowing the client to choose the imagery or response most natural for him or her:

> *Therapist:* If you like, you may choose to go back in time now . . . back to an earlier time . . . perhaps even to the time you were five, if you like . . . perhaps to another time . . . but as you travel back in time in a sort of conveyance, whatever travel method feels safe to you, you may notice that you feel curious about what happened, curious about going back in time . . . if you are going back in time, signal with your "yes" finger . . . good . . . you may begin to see a picture soon, perhaps a picture of the boat, perhaps not . . .

Directed versus Nondirected Regressions. in directed regressions, the client is instructed to "go back to" the appropriate age or incident, when a time or event is known. For instance, a twenty-six-year-old man wished to find out if a memory of a childhood molestation was real or imaginary. He believed the act happened when he was around eight years of age. He was induced into a deep trance.

> *Therapist:* Your mind is like a storehouse. Everything you have ever experienced is stored accurately and completely in your mind and is available for review now or at any time you want. I'm going to count from twenty-five back to eight. As I do, you'll move back in time, back in time so that when I reach eight, you'll be eight years old. Your mind will provide all the details of that time, all the information you wish to know from that important event. Going backward in time, twenty-five . . . twenty-four . . . twenty-three . . . [counting back for each year, leaving enough time between numbers to get the image of that year firmly in place before moving on] . . . nine . . . eight. The number eight, the age of eight. Notice your surroundings [and other phrases to help the client establish his location and time]. What's happening? [present tense].

In trance, the man replied that he was in a locker room with his soccer coach, who was showing him some pictures of men engaged in sexual acts with children. He expressed a wish to leave, and the coach grabbed his waist with both hands. He was able to escape relatively unharmed but had never been able to tell anyone about the incident.

An alternative semidirective technique uses metaphor to help the client gain access to prior memory storage:

Therapist: Imagine a pad of white paper in front of you . . . on the top sheet your present age is written, and on each following page is written the age before . . . As I count backward, each page will fall off the pad until you reach the number [X] . . . You will think as you thought then, feel as you felt then, able to experience fully the events and feelings which occurred then . . . thirty-five [current age] . . . thirty-four . . . thirty-three . . . X.

It is helpful to begin inquiry with a birthday. Returning the client to the current age is accomplished by a counting-forward suggestion. It is advisable to suggest that the client will "bring back" only those memories she or he wishes to or feels to be important.

In the nondirective approach, the client is instructed to regress to a time just prior to the onset of a presenting problem. Theoretically, the client's unconscious will present the event most concerned with the production of the problem. For example, a woman presented complaining of a fear of flying that had persisted since her adolescence. After relaxation induction, the therapist suggested the following:

Therapist: Your inner mind has its own time line, its own understanding of each event in your life, what caused it and what the outcome was. As you rest comfortably, your unconscious mind can move back effortlessly through the years to something important happening just before you noticed you were afraid of flying. Something important, and your unconscious knows how to point out to me just when it has found that something.

When the therapist received an affirmative finger signal, she asked, "What's happening?" The client described riding to the airport with her grandmother, who was nervously patting the child and murmuring that she would never see her family again. When they arrived at the airport, the grandmother slowly kissed the client good-bye and boarded the plane. The client described looking up at her mother, who was crying, and thinking that her mother knew her grandmother would never return. When the client was brought out of hypnosis, she was able to review the episode from a new perspective, giving herself the necessary insight that planes bring people home as well as take them away.

Unconscious versus Conscious Work. Many hypnotherapists assert that a great deal of work can be accomplished by the unconscious without the direction or awareness of the conscious mind (Gibson and Heap, 1991; Bodden, 1991). They propose that hypnosis can be a catalyst for such unconscious work, especially in very resistant clients. In such work, the decision of modality for work is made by the client's unconscious.

Such an induction begins with relaxation and deepening; at the point at which permission is sought from the unconscious, if permission is denied, a second question is posed: "Can the unconscious work on the problem without exploring it in the trance?" If the answer is affirmative, the therapist instructs the unconscious to work on the problem and, when the problem is resolved to its satisfaction, to release the symptoms associated with the problem (since they are no longer needed). For example, a client suffering from bulimia was regressed to a time important to the symptoms of bulimia.

Therapist: Are you there . . . do you see a picture of a time important to your symptoms . . . if you do raise your "yes" finger [client does so] . . . now I want to ask if it's all right for you to share that scene with me [client raises "no" finger] . . . oh, it's not safe to tell me about this scene you are watching? [client raises "no" finger] . . . that's okay, you don't have to tell me . . . I need to ask another question now, I need to know if your unconscious can work on this problem without us exploring it together? [client raises "yes" finger]. That's fine, that's good. I want to suggest that your unconscious will work on this scene and work on how it is related to your symptoms of bulimia, and when it has worked it through and solved this problem, it will let go of your bulimic symptoms, because you will no longer need them. They were useful once, but they aren't useful anymore, once this problem is solved . . . and you can let them go and feel safe about letting them go . . .

Use of regression material can be maximized by giving a posthypnotic suggestion that encourages the client to retain as much as the unconscious mind will allow. It can be suggested that the unconscious will make memories available at the rate that feels most comfortable to the client, possibly through dreams.

In general, regression appears to be most effective when there is some conscious acceptance of past issues. Where there is no conscious memory of a hypnotically induced age regression, it typically indicates the material or incident covered was too traumatic for the conscious mind to deal with.

Age Regression with Self-Parenting Techniques

Price (1986) describes an approach that combines regression to an age related to the symptoms or pathology and the application of the self-parenting techniques found in transactional analysis (TA). Such self-parenting (or use of the adult ego state as a substitute parent for the child in the memory) can allow the client to access repressed memories while serving as a protective, nurturing adult figure to the childhood self. Price suggests that for those skilled in TA techniques, age regression (and its accompanying shift to primary process) can provide a powerful tool for overcoming resistances to treatment that are primarily manifested in blocked memories.

Age Regression to Birth

While many hypnotherapists maintain that there are limits to how far back remote memories may be retrieved by regression, Scott (1984), in a series of case studies, describes a technique for regression back to the natal or even uterine period. This technique involves the stimulation of specific areas of the body that "may have an early mechanical memory by which traumatic incidents make an impression on the soma cells . . . which record the trauma and, later, replay the original impression."

Scott proposes that such age regression is an important therapeutic procedure, recovering the early trauma that can mark preoedipal conflicts. However, such approaches are met with a great deal of skepticism in the scientific community, and there are no independently produced verifications of such a regression.

Problems Associated with Hypnotic Age Regression

Individuals quite naturally produce idiosyncratic responses to hypnotic age regression. All responses require judgment and discipline on the part of the therapist.

Role Playing

Resistant clients, in an attempt to please or frustrate their therapist, may role play instead of actually regressing. They will act out whatever they believe the therapist requires. This may be a way of avoiding traumatic memories. This type of resistance is best handled by slowing down the rate of regression and stopping at a time close to the incident. A nonauthoritarian approach, using vague wording, is also helpful in obscuring from the client the wishes of the therapist. Later, the therapist may gradually return to the desired age—for example:

> *Therapist:* You will want to rest now, you will leave this scene and begin to drift . . . drift . . . you are resting and drifting on something, something good and safe and comfortable . . . you

may be resting and drifting toward something, or perhaps you are not . . . it is up to you, it is always entirely up to you . . . you are breathing and drifting and when you are ready you will come to rest at a very special place . . . and when you arrive at that place, you may want to just be there for awhile, without talking, perhaps noticing what's going on around you, perhaps not, perhaps just resting comfortably . . . and when you are ready you will move on . . .

Leading by the Therapist

Therapists must avoid leading the client during an age regression. Leading is the asking of questions that advance the action of a regression by offering alternative memories. "Are you talking to your mother now?" is a leading question, and for some suggestible subjects it can act as an instruction: "Talk to your mother now." In these situations a client will either recall a different situation, one where he or she spoke to mother, or fantasize speaking to mother.

Lawrence (1986) found that highly hypnotizable subjects are particularly vulnerable to the creation of pseudomemories by the hypnotherapist (in his sample, 50 percent of his highly suggestible subjects retained such memories as veridical after hypnosis). Not only will such sloppy technique compromise the therapeutic effectiveness of regression, it can also invalidate criminal proceedings and age regression experiments (Coons, 1988). As always, the client's own memories are what is important, not the therapist's theories or hopes.

To reduce leading, the therapist must use noncommital phrases to advance the action in the regression, such as, "What happened next?" or "Something important happened next. What is it?"

Special Applications

The hypnotic age regression literature provides some examples of specific applications for differing therapeutic tasks. These articles tend to be grouped in two types of therapeutic utilities: finding a hidden cause of the presenting problem and meeting a treatment destructive resistance.

Finding a Hidden Precipitant to the Presenting Problem

Often clients seek hypnotherapy because other forms of therapy have not worked. Others may seek validation of vague feelings that "something happened to me" or that "something is wrong" through hypnotic age regression. In both cases, it may facilitate treatment to discover if there is an actual event or series of events that led to the presenting problem. In dynamic schemas, this may include the recovering of repressed memories or the discovery of an event that arrested development. In cognitive-behavioral schemas, such regressions involve a search for the original learned association or distorted cognition that is currently causing the problem (Bodden, 1991).

For dynamic therapists, the regression is used to provide insight and catharsis. Eisel (1988) reported the use of hypnotherapy with age regression in a program for state prison inmates. The hypnosis was incorporated into a cognitive therapy program for inmates with a documented history of explosive anger disorder. Eisel and his colleagues used regression to establish a "first significant event" that was presented to the inmate as a "cause" of his anger disorder. This was followed by a catharsis of the feelings for the original event. The perception/interpretation of the event was then reframed through hypnotic suggestion. Eisel reported a reduction of acting-out behaviors and a decrease in self-report of anger after the treatment.

For cognitive therapists, the regression is used to reframe the distortion or unhook the paired association through posthypnotic suggestion. Types of problems that can be addressed in this way include compulsive and/or self-destructive behaviors, eating disorders, phobias and other anxiety disorders, dissociative disorders, and sexual disorders.

In their review of the literature on the use of hypnosis in the treatment of eating disorders, Vanderlinden and Vandereycken (1988) noted that age regression appears to be especially useful in dismantling the dissociative state usually triggered by a binge, through regression to the first binge and hypnotic suggestion of a different (fully aware) response. Gross (1983) describes the use of hypnotically induced regression to uncover the past traumatic events that may have led to the illness, followed by the direct hypnotic suggestion to substitute other feelings and activities (such as sports) for the binging. Additionally, Gross extended the cognitive-behavioral model to include the posthypnotic suggestion of specific healthy eating habits.

Finding and Dismantling Resistance

Clients often seek hypnotherapy because more traditional forms of therapy do not seem to help. Indeed, many hypnotherapists will turn to hypnotic age regression when other forms of hypnotherapy are not working. In these cases, it is presumed that the symptoms fill some useful purpose or need, which must be identified and addressed before any therapy can be useful.

This approach is often used in phobias and other anxiety disorders that are proving resistant to standard cognitive therapies. It is also used for treatment of compulsions or self-destructive behaviors that appear to be immune to behavioral treatment.

In a series of case studies involving the treatment of trichotillomania, Hynes (1982) described the use of hypnotic age regression in patients for whom pharmacotherapy and behavior modification alone were not working. By using regression to target the traumatic events and reframing (with direct suggestion) the interpreted "needs" that arose from them, Hynes reported an increased efficacy of traditional treatment modes for three of five patients.

In the case of particularly resistant vaginismus (resulting in twenty-two years of unconsummated marriage), Oystragh (1988) reported that age regression and automatic writing enabled the woman to give up her need to resist sex and, with additional hypnotherapy for relaxation and desensitization, resulted in a positive outcome.

Additional Uses

The case study literature provides ample examples of the inventiveness of hypnotherapists in the use of age regression to solve thorny problems.

Spiegel and Rosenfeld (1984) described the treatment of a sixteen-year-old girl who spontaneously regressed in age, particularly when under stress. Although they were careful to distinguish her problem from that of individuals with multiple personality disorder (MPD), they borrowed techniques from hypnotherapy of MPD in order to access and control the age regressions.

Jue (1988) described the treatment of a twenty-eight-year-old patient with Stein-Levanthal syndrome (hermaphroditism) who was raised as a female but wished to assume a male identity. Regression therapy was used to explore his developmental patterning and the parental introjects that prevented the successful acquisition of the male identity.

Goldberg (1990) suggests that "guiding therapy patients into past lives and future lifetimes through hypnosis can aid in the resolution of self-defeating sequences." While few hypnotherapists are ready to embrace this construct of human anxiety and depression, Anita Anderson-Evangelista (1980) suggests that all therapists be prepared for such a client request. She describes a spontaneous "past life" regression of a client during a regular hypnotherapy, which was later put to good use as the fantasy material was mined for symbolism of what was causing the neurosis.

One observation I have made about alleged regressions to past lives is that most who claim such an experience assert they were interesting characters like nobility, Druid priests, or warriors. Few claim to have been a lowly serf, a scruffy peasant, or a sharecropper. But statistically, there should be about a hundred of the latter experiences for every one of the former.

Ethical Considerations and Professional Concerns

Just as each therapeutic approach has its own technique, it also has its own foibles for unsuspecting or careless therapists. Expertise in one area of therapy never automatically confers skill in another. Accordingly, the following suggestions are offered for the most effective hypnotherapeutic experience.

Therapist Attitudes

A therapist who believes that anything and everything is possible through age regression may become overly ambitious. This ambition may fuel a desire to exert boundless influence. If this becomes the case, the goal of the age regression shifts to one of client compliance, with the therapist's motives distorted by a thirst for power.

On the other hand, overly skeptical feelings harbored by the therapist attempting age regression may result in a negative attitude being unconsciously conveyed to the client, defeating the goals of motivation and trust.

Maintaining a Frame

Characteristics that appear to be conducive to positive regression experiences include the following:

- Approaching each client as a unique individual whose problems cannot be quickly categorized.
- Having the ability to identify therapeutic problem areas and determine the type and scope of the induction to be used.
- Maintaining an objective view of the hypnotic age regression experience.
- Preventing personal aspirations or values from distorting treatment goals.
- Accepting and dealing with emotional displays that arise during and after the regression.

Fraudulent or Abusive Use of Hypnotic Age Regression

As with other therapeutic modalities, clinicians must guard against even an inadvertent misuse of hypnotherapy that could create loss or injury to the client. This loss or injury can range from the relatively benign use of a technique that is clearly not helping to fraudulent claims of assistance or healing that cannot be realistically obtained.

Hypnotic age regression is particularly vulnerable to abuse in forensic cases, custody and injury cases, and treatment of minors. In these cases, participation by the client may be less than voluntary, and a third party (often the one who is paying the therapy bills) may have a vested interest in a specific outcome.

Coons (1988) described a case in which a female police officer, whose children had been shot during the night, was hypnotically regressed to the night of the shooting by a police hypnotist before being charged. The resulting taped induction revealed a flagrant attempt on the part of the hypnoist to lead the subject in a series of confabulations and suggested distortions that ultimately resulted in her admission of guilt.

With the tape as the only evidence, the woman was charged with attempted murder, lost her job, and lost custody of her children, who denied that their mother had shot them. No evidence was collected to support her original story (she reported being hit on the head yet was not examined for bruises), nor was her father (who lived next door and had a documented history of domestic violence) seriously questioned.

Presumed guilty and suicidal, the woman was hospitalized until examined by Coons for multiple personality disorder. His examination of the taped induction and the woman's current status led him to conclude that the woman was not mentally ill and that the "confession" was hypnotically induced. Subsequently, the police dropped charges against her. Nonetheless, she never regained her job or custody of her children.

While an apparently powerful tool for healing, hypnotic age regression can also be an instrument of harm, deception, or narcissism. Clinicians must guard against abusing the public trust and client naiveté when using this mode of intrapersonal exploration.

8
Self-Hypnosis

"Where's the rest of me?"
—Ronald Reagan, referring to his missing limbs in *Kings Row*

S elf-hypnosis, like hypnosis and various forms of concentrative meditation, could be characterized by focused attention within a constricted
stimulus range. Indeed, most of the techniques that are demonstrated
throughout the rest of this book can usually rather easily be adapted to
self-hypnosis. However, self-hypnosis differs from heterohypnosis in that
the induction does not rely on another person separate from the client.
Self-hypnosis differs from other forms of concentrative meditation mainly in
the way that it is used. Many forms of meditation are used for religious
purposes or for clearing one's mind. For example, in transcendental meditation, an individual must go through a ritual induction and be given a
special mantra, to repeat over and over to achieve a trancelike state. The
goal of such meditation is usually to achieve some higher level of cosmic
consciousness. Similarly, "self-hypnosis is an altered state of consciousness
that is self-induced" (Sanders, 1987, p. 29). Self-hypnosis as a therapeutic
technique is less mystic and ceremonial, and the goals are more diverse.

Brief History

Self-hypnosis was introduced by one of two Frenchmen: A. A. Liebeault, in
1888, or Emilie Cour, in 1922, depending upon how one interprets their
techniques. Self-hypnosis was not widely addressed in scientific research
until the early 1970s, but it has been used extensively in therapy for a
variety of problems since the 1950s (Levitan, 1991).

Shirley Sanders (1987), a renowned expert in self-hypnosis, presented
the following case, which represents a typical problem for which self-
hypnosis is useful:

> Ed, a 34-year-old white male with a diagnosis of adult asthma, was re-
> ferred for hypnotherapy to reduce his anxiety about his response to asthma
> and to learn ways of reducing his attacks through relaxation. This patient
> experienced great fear and impatience during stress—fear that he would
> not be able to breathe and impatient at having to wait his turn in line, when
> driving and in many other life situations.

138

After discussion of relaxation and hand warming as a way of monitoring, the patient was instructed to close his eyes and to describe a warm, comfortable scene. After he described the scene, he was asked how he felt. He described himself as relaxing, more quiet, and breathing easily. In addition, his temperature rose.

The therapist reinforced the comfortable images and suggested that the patient practice at home, thinking of the comfortable scene and monitoring the temperature before and after the practice. (p. 38)

Sanders reported that this patient had fewer asthma attacks and experienced less need for medication after six sessions and the continued practice of self-hypnosis. This case is representative of the long-recognized clinical utility of self-hypnosis, especially as an adjunct treatment.

Self-Hypnosis versus Heterohypnosis

Dimensions of Sociality

Self-hypnosis is obviously distinguished from heterohypnosis by the presence or absence of a hypnotist. London (1967) suggested viewing hypnosis on a dimension of sociality. "Sociality" refers to the "extent to which hypnosis is induced in one person as a direct consequence of acts involving the observable participation of another person" (p. 48). Self-hypnosis and heterohypnosis are polar opposites when viewing the hypnotic induction on this dimension, and the distinction between the two is easily made. The distinction becomes clouded, however, when self-hypnosis is aided by the use of audiocassettes or other devices designed to induce hypnosis, as is common in clinical practice. Such techniques occupy an area in the intermediate range on the sociality dimension.

Theorists have even debated the existence of self-hypnosis and heterohypnosis as separate entities. A widely held belief is that all hypnosis is self-hypnosis and that the external hypnotist is merely a guide. It is commonly argued that the client is responsible for the result in carrying out the concepts presented, regardless of where these ideas come from. Some theorists hold to the extreme position: hypnosis always requires an identifiable external hypnotist (London, 1967). Others, at the opposite extreme, assert that heterohypnosis is simply aided self-hypnosis with an external hypnotist present (Hilgard, 1979).

McConkey (1986), in a study that examined opinions of 173 college students regarding hypnosis, and self-hypnosis found that the majority of students saw self-hypnosis as "a variation of hypnosis with a hypnotist, and for both hypnosis and self-hypnosis they considered that the experience depended on the ability of the individual rather than on the ability of the hypnotist" (p. 315). Thus, general opinion seems to lean toward the importance of the client and his or her abilities and away from the role of the separate hypnotist.

Phenomenological Differences

Certain phenomenologial differences beween self-hypnosis and heterohypnosis are hypothesized by the Chicago paradigm (Fromm and Kahn, 1990):

1. Surrender versus control and mastery.
2. Spontaneously arising visual imagery and idiosyncratic fantasy.
3. Depth of hypnotic state.
4. Ease in achieving depth.
5. Cognitive activity.
6. General reality orientation.

Clients using self-hypnosis should be prepared to experience these differences:

> They should be given training in the ability to "let go," and to become more ego-receptive to imagery. They must also come to understand that whereas attention is concentrative in heterohypnosis, they must allow for the use of a different type of attention in self-hypnosis—namely, free-floating, expansive attention. That is, we need to explain to our patients that they should allow themselves to "experience effortlessly" and not try so hard. (Fromm and Kahn, 1990, p. 215)

Result of Posthypnotic Suggestion

It is often supposed that self-hypnosis is merely a response to a posthypnotic suggestion. Although the easiest way for a client to learn to self-hypnotize is for the trance to be induced by someone else and for the client to be given posthypnotic suggestions for induction, research has shown that a person can easily engage in self-hypnosis with a minimal amount of instruction (Hilgard, 1979). There are no statistics available, however, that indicate what percentage of people can learn self-hypnosis without having previously been hypnotized by someone else or who have directly witnessed an hypnotic induction.

Central Executive Functioning

Hilgard (1979) presented the idea that central executive functions involved in the process of hypnosis are divided between the hypnotist and the hypnotized client. He presented self-hypnosis as a strong illustration of such a division of the executive functions. The client must divide attention between the internalized role of the hypnotist and the process of being hypnotized.

Technique for Self-Hypnosis

Introduction

When instructing a client in the use of self-hypnosis, the therapist defines a straightforward, detailed formula for the client to follow. For some clients who report feeling awkward with the idea of self-hypnosis, the more structured technique of autogenic training (see chapter 4) is often a useful precursor. Alternatively, helping clients to design and record their own home practice tape while they are in the office is a good lead-in procedure to having them later practice true individual self-hypnosis further along in the course of treatment.

The formula must be designed with the client in mind, so that the particular method chosen will be quick and easy for the client to implement—for example, identifying specific imagery that the client finds relaxing or, conversely, that the client finds troubling (for example, suggesting to a hydrophobic client that she sees herself floating on a raft in a swimming pool will be counterproductive).

It is often helpful for the prescribed formula to contain a key word or phrase that the subject can repeatedly say during the induction phase. When such a suggestion is made while the client is hypnotized, the therapist must be sure to add that the key word or phrase will have no hypnotic effect on the client unless he or she intentionally uses it for the purpose of self-induction. The self-induction formula may be presented to the client (and is usually most effective) while he or she is hypnotized. Once the formula is presented, the client is awakened immediately and allowed to self-hypnotize using the new formula.

Induction

Several different types of induction techniques are mentioned in the literature on self-hypnosis. Rothman, Carroll, and Rothman (1976) advocate the use of an arm gravitation technique or an eye rollback technique, which are commonly used in heterohypnosis. They suggest combining these techniques with simple muscle relaxation and/or visualization exercises.

Hyperventilation is another helpful technique. A client can be instructed to take several short breaths at a very rapid rate and continue this breathing pattern until a slight amount of dizziness is felt. The feeling of dizziness should be followed by as much relaxation as possible. Next, a formula, such as the repetition of a key word or phrase, should be implemented.

Following is a technique suggested by Kroger and Fezler (1976). They recommend that the client practice this induction technique for at least ten minutes, three times a day, because rapidity and ease of induction will increase with practice. Other authors suggest different schedules. It is best to negotiate and contract with the client a schedule that includes at least one daily practice and on a schedule the client feels he or she can keep. Kroger and Fezler suggest that the client sit in a comfortable chair with hands in lap and feet on the floor. The client should fix his or her eyes on a spot on the ceiling above eye level and then

> begin counting to yourself slowly from 1 to 10. Direct your attention to your eyelids and, between numbers, tell yourself repeatedly that your eyelids are getting very, very heavy. Again and again say: "My eyelids are getting heavier and heavier. I feel my lids getting so heavy, and the heavier they get, the deeper relaxed I will become . . . My lids are getting very heavy. It will feel so good to close my eyes."
> By the time you count to 2, think of enough suggestions like the ones just mentioned so that you actually feel the heaviness of your eyelids. When you are sure that your lids are indeed heavy, count to 3 and let your eyes roll up into the back of your head for a few seconds. Then say "My lids are now locked so tight that I doubt very much that I can open them . . . I begin to feel a nice, calm, soothing relaxed feeling beginning in my toes, moving into my legs, and into my thighs as I keep counting." . . . Then double back for repetition . . . and continue in this way.
> . . . When you finally reach the point where, by the count of 7, your limbs are sufficiently relaxed, you repeat again all the suggestions you have given yourself. (p. 36)

Depth of Trance

Similar to heterohypnosis, a deep stage of trance is not necessary for most purposes. A trance of medium depth is probably ideal for self-hypnosis, and the lethargy associated with deep levels of hypnosis may actually be counterproductive in some situations.

Depth of trance is important in some rare circumstances, including hypnosis for dentistry work, childbirth, or anesthesia for some other purpose. Depth also becomes a factor when clients will be opening their eyes during the hypnotic trance or if the self-hypnosis is being studied for research purposes.

Deepening Techniques

Most of the deepening techniques utilized by hypnotists in heterohypnosis may be used effectively in self-hypnosis also (Sanders, 1991; Walker, 1991). Cheek and LeCron (1968) suggest that some type of movement, such as the lifting of one hand to the face, may be useful as a deepening technique. Such a technique should first be presented to the client as a posthypnotic suggestion. The imaginary escalator technique, which is commonly used in heterohypnosis, may also be quite useful as a deepening technique in self-hypnosis.

The use of imagery has been found to be an effective deepening technique; however, the effectiveness appears to be confounded with level of hypnotizability and personality characteristics and gender (Lombard, Kahn, and Fromm, 1990). Thus, imagery may not be effective for all clients, and it is difficult to predict who will be able to use imagery to deepen the hypnotic trance.

Many theorists believe that the technique of fractionation is the most effective deepening technique used for hypnotic involvement, both heterohypnosis and self-hypnosis. The observation, as well as the theory, is that each hypnotization makes the subject a little more suggestible and favors the induction of a deeper hypnosis on the next "trial" (Hammond, Carroll, and Hammond, 1987, p. 119). The following case exemplifies this technique:

> A twenty-four-year-old female presented for therapy complaining of debilitating asthma attacks. When under stress, she reported feeling as if her chest constricted, and it became difficult to breathe normally. Her breathing difficulties quickly escalated to a full-blown asthmatic attack.
>
> Deep relaxation has been shown to increase parasympathetic activity and stabilize the activation of the autonomic nervous system in response to stimuli. Thus, the goal of hypnotherapy was to help the client enter deep levels of trance to enhance deep relaxation.
>
> The client was hypnotized in the first session. She appeared to have difficulty achieving depth. While in a light trance, she was awakened and then quickly rehypnotized. This process was continued a few times in the first session, and the client was given the suggestion to practice the technique at home between sessions.
>
> During the second session, the client reported that she had practiced the technique successfully several times a day and that the number of full-blown asthmatic attacks had decreased near the end of the week. She was hypnotized during this session and appeared to achieve a deep level of trance easily and quickly.

Hammond et al. (1987) examined the effectiveness of fractionation as a deepening technique in self-hypnosis and contrasted it with the effectiveness of the commonly used technique of imagining descending a ten-step staircase. These authors found essentially no differences reported in the depth level of the self-hypnotic trance between subjects who utilized fractionation and subjects who utilized the imaginal staircase technique. In fact, some subjects clearly preferred the fractionation technique, and others clearly preferred the imaginal staircase technique. Based on the finding of virtually no differences, the authors concluded that there is a definite need to individualize the specific techniques utilized to the unique needs of the client.

Practice

Once a client is familiarized with an induction formula, he or she should practice this technique for ten to fifteen minutes at least once a day. Some clients may need to practice more often, so instructions should be phrased so that clients will feel comfortable doing that. When self-hypnosis is a newly acquired skill, regular practice is a necessary part of the normal learning process. As with autogenic training, which has a self-hypnotic component, regular practice is the key to success.

The goal of the practice in the early stages of treatment is for the client to be able to reach a state of light hypnosis fairly quickly and with a minimum amount of effort. The ease with which this goal can be achieved will vary with the individual client. Little practice is needed for some clients; others require much more time and effort. Even clients who are excellent hypnotic subjects sometimes have great difficulty learning self-hypnosis (Rothman, Carroll, and Rothman, 1976). It is best for clients not to perform any tests or try to produce any phenomena, such as anesthesia, until they have practiced the induction effectively several times and have continuing access to a hypnotherapist.

Client Problems

When a client seems to be having a great deal of trouble learning to do self-hypnosis effectively, an audiotape can be a helpful tool (Hammond et al., 1988; Sanders, 1991). The therapist can record a hypnotic induction performed during the therapy session with the client and allow him or her to use the tape to practice self-hypnosis outside the therapy session.

Hammond et al. (1988) examined responses to behavioral suggestions and subjective experiential ratings of clients and compared heterohypnosis, tape-assisted self-hypnosis, and self-directed self-hypnosis. Results indicated no differences among them in response to behavioral suggestions. However, tape-assisted self-hypnosis was consistently rated as superior experientially to self-directed self-hypnosis by newly trained subjects. These findings suggest that an audiotape may be especially useful in the beginning stages of self-hypnosis training.

While practicing self-hypnosis, some clients exhibit a strong tendency to fall asleep. This can usually be prevented with the posthypnotic suggestion that a client will remain in a hypnotic state for a specified period of time or until ready to awaken.

Another difficulty in the practice of self-hypnosis is that time seems to pass very quickly for most clients. In order to deal with conflicts or problems that this may present, it is suggested posthypnotically that the client will awaken spontaneously at the end of a specific time period or at a certain time (Cheek and LeCron, 1968).

Clinical Usefulness

"Many psychotherapists feel that there is insufficient time in one therapeutic session per week to produce and establish lasting attitudinal, emotional, and behavioral changes desired and needed by patients. Patients, too can be discouraged and their resistance enhanced by their feelings of regression into unhealthy behavior patterns over the time between appointments" (Rothman, Carroll, and Rothman, 1976, p. 244). Self-hypnosis provides a viable and useful adjunct to treatment. It enables the client to work and progress between sessions. Most therapists find that self-hypnosis is quite useful in combination with homework assignments of a behavioral nature, especially because it helps to reinforce newly acquired behavior.

Another useful property of self-hypnosis is that it somewhat empowers the client. This property makes self-hypnosis a useful technique for clients who are having difficulties terminating therapy. Through self-hypnosis, the client learns to generate help himself or herself and becomes less dependent on the therapist.

Following is a list of five ways that Fromm and Kahn (1990) have outlined to use self-hypnosis effectively:

1. The therapist can teach patients to practice true hypnotist-absent self-hypnosis at home and, if possible, in the workplace.
2. In self-hypnosis, in the hypnotherapeutic hour, the therapist can intertwine heterohypnosis and hypnotist-present self-hypnosis for a patient's benefit.
3. The therapist can encourage a patient to do self-hypnosis at home, alone, and then to bring in material that came up in self-hypnosis during the therapy hour.
4. The therapist can let a patient make tapes in the patient's own voice in the hypnotherapy hour. The patient can then, at home, listen to those tapes and use them for self-hypnosis.
5. The therapist can make a tape, in the therapist's voice, for a patient to take home and to use for self-hypnosis.

Indications and Contraindications for Use

Certain characteristics of both therapists and clients seem to increase the success rate of self-hypnosis. Therapists who ask clients whether they have been practicing at home seem to be more successful than those who merely teach the client the skill, instruct the client to practice at home, and then do not monitor and stress the importance of practice after the initial session (Fromm and Kahn, 1990). Self-hypnosis requires certain characteristics in the client in order to be successful (Sanders, 1991; Fromm and Kahn, 1990; Rothman, Carroll, and Rothman, 1976):

- Willingness to participate in self-hypnosis.
- Motivation and a certain amount of self-discipline.
- Self-confidence and persistence.
- An ability to work effectively independently.
- Little need for external support or validation.
- Willingness to take risks.
- A tolerance for ambiguity.

In addition to a relief of symptoms, clients receive certain benefits when they are able to employ self-hypnotic techniques successfully that they may not gain from standard therapy:

- Clients often will experience a feeling of pride and an increase in self-esteem because they remove the symptom through their own efforts.
- Clients will not be as dependent on the clinician to remove troubling symptoms.
- If the original symptoms return, clients can quickly employ the same formula that first removed the symptom.
- The same formula can be employed should any substitute symptoms appear, giving the clients even more independence and self-reliance.
- The level of relaxation attained from the use of self-hypnosis may help clients stay more relaxed and free of tension while going about daily routines.
- Regularly practicing self-hypnosis often improves concentration in general.

There are certain contraindications or disadvantages in the use of self-hypnosis:

- When the technique may result in further dissociation or withdrawal on the part of a particular client or the client shows borderline characteristics.
- When a client presents with passive-aggressive tendencies.

- If the client is receiving some strong secondary gain for the identified symptoms.
- When the client exhibits resistance to change.

Self-Hypnosis and Therapist Orientation

Based on a survey of therapists in the American Society of Clinical Hypnosis, Sanders (1987) identified four categories of clinical self-hypnosis orientations, and in each, the therapist's role, the goals of therapy, and the types of problems addressed were found to be different:

1. *Eclectic.* The majority of the therapists surveyed identified themselves as eclectic. Eclectic therapists utilize a variety of theories and techniques. Therapeutic goals vary from behavior change to insight to support of adaptive functioning. It is difficult to characterize the use of self-hypnosis by eclectic therapists because such therapists tend to use their creativity to generate techniques that work with individual clients.
2. *Behavioral.* Behaviorism was the second most commonly endorsed orientation in this survey. The typical goals identified by behaviorists were eliminating deviant behavior and building up new adaptive behavior in small, progressive steps. Cognitive behavior therapists especially reported that they often find that self-hypnosis is well suited for these goals because it facilitates the strengthening of contingencies and behavior rehearsal through the use of imagery. Behaviorists tended to view themselves as either teachers or prescribers in the utilization of self-hypnosis and commonly employ it to treat long-standing habit problems, such as smoking, performance anxiety, and pain.
3. *Physiological.* The third most commonly endorsed orientation to self-hypnosis was the physiological orientation. Therapists identifying themselves as physiologically oriented tended to view themselves as either healers or prescribers. This orientation assumes that the mind and the body interact and that self-hypnosis is useful in accessing that interaction. The goals in physiological self-hypnosis are usually to access the physiological level of functioning, such as reducing physical tension or lowering blood pressure. The basic techniques used in physiological self-hypnosis require the client to imagine certain organs or metaphorical ideas that represent organs. It is hypothesized that such imagery triggers physiological reactions. Another emphasis is on deepening the hypnotic state; it is hypothesized that a deep trance will affect physiological functioning.
4. *Psychoanalytic.* The fourth most commonly endorsed orientation by practitioners of self-hypnosis was the psychoanalytic orientation. The goals in psychoanalytic therapy are usually to uncover cognitions, feel-

ings, and memories. Self-hypnosis is useful with such goals because the altered state of consciousness that is produced tends to decrease censoring and fosters free association. Psychoanalytic therapists tend to see their role in self-hypnosis as nondirective and benign guides, who are mainly interested in personality reconstruction and self-growth experiences. They tend to monitor but not direct the client in self-hypnosis.

Treatment of Specific Disorders or Problems

Self-hypnosis is widely used in a variety of settings and to treat a wide variety of symptomatology. It can be easily adapted and individualized and is useful with both children and adults. For example, Cheek and LeCron (1968) asert that self-hypnosis is the best means of treating insomnia, unless the insomnia is a "deep-seated neurotic symptom." Habit disorders, such as smoking and also overeating, are responsive to self-hypnosis, as are alcoholism and drug addiction (Kroger and Fezler, 1976), a broad range of psychosomatic and psychophysiological disorders, frigidity, impotence, pain anxiety (Kline, 1976), and many other medical and psychological disorders (Sanders, 1990). Self-hypnosis is commonly used to aid relaxation and improve concentration, and it can be useful in producing self-anesthesia and in treating a variety of physical symptoms (Cheek and LeCron, 1968). In most cases self-hypnosis is used as an adjunct to ongoing psychotherapy or hypnotherapy.

Following is a brief sampling of how self-hypnosis is employed in treatment. Specific examples are related to illustrate the utilization of self-hypnosis procedures within the given treatment protocols.

Habit Control

Self-hypnosis is commonly employed to treat habit control disorders. Such disorders are one area where self-hypnosis is often virtually the only, rather than an adjunct, technique. Typically, one to three sessions are held during which time a client is hypnotized and may be given a self-hypnosis formula and posthypnotic suggestions to aid the self-hypnosis. These sessions may be done individually or in a group setting. The client is often given a series of audiocassettes to listen to in order to aid self-hypnosis and gain control over the specific symptoms (Kline, 1976).

The American Lung Association periodically publishes a manual that provides the basis for a one-session group hypnosis program designed for smoking cessation. In this program, clients are hypnotized in a group. During the hypnosis, the group leader emphasizes the importance of self-generated imaginal experiences, relaxation, urge management, coping strategies, positive self-suggestions, and practice. Clients are encouraged to visualize themselves as "transformed" by the decision to quit smoking. Further suggestions include visualizing:

- A favorite spot associated with feelings of protection, security, and relaxation.
- The self as a nonsmoker in a variety of situations.
- The health benefits of being a nonsmoker.
- Successfully coping with urges to smoke, along with the development of self-rewards that can be administered daily.
- High-risk situations along with instructions to utilize coping mechanisms other than smoking.

At the conclusion of the session, each client is given a cassette tape with a self-hypnosis induction recorded on it and a set of suggestions that recapitulate the treatment highlights. The importance of daily practice is strongly emphasized.

Neufield and Lynn (1988) followed twenty-seven subjects who had gone through this group session treatment. They found that the treatment yielded an abstinence rate of only 20 to 25 percent. However, the public often views such an intervention as a panacea. In reality, the effectiveness of such an intervention is questionable. Abstinence rates for different types of smoking cessation interventions that utilize self-hypnosis range from 0 percent all the way up to about 95 percent. Certainly such an intervention can be helpful in treating habit control disorders if the client is highly motivated.

Psychological Symptoms

Self-hypnosis can easily be integrated into treatment for a variety of psychological symptoms. For such symptoms, self-hypnotic techniques are probably most useful if used as an adjunct to ongoing psychotherapy or hypnotherapy. Following are a few of the more specific circumstances in which instruction in self-hypnosis may be helpful for a client and/or situations in which self-hypnosis is often the only treatment employed.

Self-Injurious Behavior. Self-injurious behavior is a symptom that accompanies many disorders and takes on many forms. Behavior therapy is usually the treatment of choice; however, self-hypnosis has proved to be a somewhat useful adjunct to behavioral therapy in dealing with self-injurious behavior (Orian, 1989). Behaviors such as hair pulling, self-mutilation, nail biting, and head banging have been effectively treated using behavioral techniques and/or hypnotherapy. The following case study, reported by Carmia Orian (1989), illustrates the useful combination of behavioral techniques and self-hypnosis to treat self-injurious behavior.

The client was a 22-year-old female who repeatedly injured the skin on her face and legs with tweezers and the sharp edge of a pendant. She scratched her legs to the point that they developed sores. Then, she concluded that the hairs on her legs were the cause of her sores and she would penetrate the skin deeply in an attempt to remove the hairs. She reported feeling no pain during this activity and stated that it gave her some satisfaction. She inflicted similar wounds on her face. Her legs and face were covered with scabs and scars.

The principal goal of the hypnobehavioral treatment was the removal of symptoms by interrupting the habit and raising the level of the patient's self-control. The treatment was conducted in 13 weekly sessions with the therapist. The client was hypnotized and it was suggested that she was in control of her body and her behavior patterns. For example, while her fist was clenched, she was given the following suggestions: "Your will-power is as strong as your clenched fist. You are in control of all your body and its processes. You are responsible for your own behavior patterns. You can initiate them and terminate them. You want your legs and face to get better and be smooth and beautiful; therefore you will stop injuring them . . . You want to conquer this bad habit you have of injuring yourself and you will succeed in this. Every day you will find yourself more and more in control of your behavior." (p. 87)

During the hypnosis, she was also instructed to relate positive messages concerning her future behavior to herself—for example, stating that she could regain control over her body and its processes and that she would have beautiful legs. After the hypnotic trance was terminated, the client was told to keep a daily diary and record the number of times she injured herself daily, when she did this, and how she felt when doing it.

The next session, the client reported that she felt she was fighting an "internal war of conflicting needs." The therapist instructed her in self-hypnosis and asked her to practice it once a day while she continued to keep her diary. As the treatment continued, the practice of self-hypnosis at least once a day was emphasized and directive imagery was introduced. The client was instructed to imagine herself in three months with a healthy face and legs and to imagine herself feeling proud of her appearance and satisfaction at the end of treatment.

At the end of the thirteen treatment sessions, the client was reminded to practice self-hypnosis daily. A year after the end of the treatment, the client reported that the symptoms had disappeared. Such a treatment protocol could be easily adapted to treat other forms of self-injurious behavior.

Multiple Personality Disorder. Hypnosis has been used increasingly to treat multiple personality disorder (MPD) (Shapiro, 1991). (See chapter 11 for a more detailed presentation of the application of hypnotic techniques to MPD cases.) Actually, more attention "has been focused on the conceptualization of MPD as a condition in which autohypnotic capacities are mis-used and form the substrate of the psychopathology" (Kluft, 1988, p. 91). However, Kluft at the same time suggests that the dissociative capacities of MPD patients could be transformed into skills.

Kluft (1988) advocates teaching MPD clients the skill of self-hypnosis. He reported that several of his clients had been taught self-hypnosis for symptom relief and "to allow the continuation of internal dialogues among the personalities between sessions" (p. 91). Braun (1984) advocates the use of instruction in self-hypnotic techniques for only certain MPD clients, primarily those who have been integrated. Such clients may find self-hypnosis helpful for purposes of relaxation, assertiveness training, rehearsal in fanstasy, and protection from overstimulation. Also, many MPD clients appear to use self-hypnosis spontaneously for relaxation and anxiety relief.

A case reported by Kluft (1988) exemplifies the use of self-hypnosis with MPD clients who have been integrated. One client spontaneously be-gan to use self-hypnosis for anxiety reduction. She had been in therapy for many years and was quite psychologically minded. Kluft taught her to use self-hypnosis between scheduled sessions and whenever she thought she might be experiencing a return of dissociative symptoms: "She was in-structed to place herself in a relaxed state with a brief eyeroll induction and by silently saying a cue word, and then to allow whatever concerned her and needed her attention to form as an image on a visualized screen. Thereafter she was to inquire as to whether any other alter was present, inviting any such to respond by saying a 'yes' that she would hear within her head, or by raising a finger" (Kluft, 1988, p. 93). On one occasion, the client asked if an alter was present, and her finger lifted. She was able to ask the alter about itself and found that the personality was a nameless eight-year-old girl who had witnesses a traumatic event when the client was young. The client was able to talk to the alter and tell her that the core personality would not avoid the pain of these events and that she would ask the new alter to rejoin her. "Shortly thereafter, the patient was flooded with intense affect and had a spontaneous abreaction. . . . When she recovered her composure, she could not reach the alter. She repeated the autohypnotic inquiry about the pres-ence of others and got no response" (p. 94). Kluft reported that the client was able to practice this technique reliably for several years and had no positive signs of separateness.

This case illustrates the potential for use of self-hypnosis in the treat-ment of MPD. Kluft (1988) reported, however, that many of the clients with whom he had tried to implement self-hypnosis were too afraid to use the technique properly, fearing to monitor for the presence of an alter person-ality because they were afraid of what they might find.

The use of self-hypnotic techniques in the area of treatment for MPD remains largely unexplored and certainly controversial. The individual client's and also the therapist's feelings of comfort with using the techniques should receive utmost consideration before the treatment is utilized.

Stress Management. Self-hypnosis is commonly used in an effort to manage tension or anxiety due to stress. Many promote self-hypnosis as an effective and relatively risk-free technique for coping with stress. Self-hypnosis is often taught to clients by teachers outside the professional mental health fields in an effort to deal with the effects of stress, an unfortunate but increasing trend (Sanders, 1990).

Although many support the use of self-hypnosis as a panacea for the effects of stress, the empirical data present a more realistic view of the effectiveness of self-hypnotic techniques. Most studies find that self-hypnosis, similar to meditation, yields only a moderate degree of success in the treatment of stress-related symptoms (Soskis et al., 1989). In fact, it is likely that only about 40 percent of clients show improvement in the management of stress symptoms (Raskin, Bali, and Peeke, 1980). Clients who are well motivated to relieve the stress are more likely to be successful.

Soskis et al. (1989) examined how clients seem to employ self-hypnotic techniques and the results they achieve. They first found that nearly half of the subjects in their study experienced a significant problem in scheduling even a brief uninterrupted time to practice the self-hypnosis. "Part of the problems appeared to be internal, related to difficulty allocating resources explicitly for self-care. Other problems were more prosaic. Ringing telephones were the chief culprits in providing serious interruptions, even if an answering machine was used" (Soskis et al., 1989, p. 288). Nevertheless, the importance of practice should be stressed. Self-hypnosis is actually the acquisition of a new skill and, like any other new skill, requires regular practice in order to become effective. Perhaps the therapist and the client could work together to find a time when the client would not be interrupted. For example, the client may be able to identify a short period of time during which he or she does not usually receive important telephone calls and could unplug the telephone during this time. Helping the client identify priorities is also useful. Perhaps the client's own personal well-being and relaxation are not as important to him or her as fulfilling the expectations of others. This may be a sensitive area to explore, but it is important to do so. Social desirability becomes a factor because many clients will not willingly admit or even recognize that their own personal well-being is not a top priority for them.

Soskis et al. (1988) found that a significant proportion of the subjects in the study experienced discomfort with the technique itself. They suggest that a clinician work with the client to design a strategy that may effectively avoid this problem. In this case, other alternatives may be meditation, biofeedback, or autogenic training, methods with a similar success rate as self-hypnosis (Raskin, Bali, and Peeke, 1980).

Physical Symptoms

Chronic Pain. Hypnosis is often used in the treatment of chronic pain. (See chapter 12.) Self-hypnosis can be a useful adjunct here. Self-suggestions may be quite helpful in shifting a client's self-concept away from identification with a physical illness, thus decreasing awareness of accompanying symptoms. Large and James (1988) found that with clients who practiced individualized formulas for self-hypnosis daily, a bigger shift in self-concept away from physical illness was associated with the most pain relief.

It is important, however, that the self-hypnotic formula be individualized. For example, if a client has severe pain in his knee for which there is no medical reason, training the client to use glove anesthesia can be helpful. Once the client becomes able to produce anesthesia in his hand, it can be transferred to his knee. Regular practice is also important (Large and James, 1988).

Tourette Syndrome. Gilles de la Tourette syndrome is a complex tic disorder. Symptoms of the disorder are often treated quite effectively with hypnotherapy, and self-hypnosis may be a useful adjunct treatment. Kohen and Botts (1987) utilized a combination of self-hypnosis, progressive relaxation, and imagery in treating this disorder. They typically induced hypnosis and then allowed the client to imagine a "favorite place." The trance was usually deepened with progressive relaxation. Then the client was given specific suggestions regarding awareness of and control over the various tics. These suggestions were tied to the imagined favorite place in some manner. For example, one child reported that his favorite place was playing football. During hypnosis, the child was given suggestions such as to "imagine that he was the quarterback and directed his own movements, those of the other players [his muscles metaphorically], and also gave the right signals at the right time in order to win" (Kohen and Botts, 1988, p. 232).

Based on an analysis of four case studies, Kohen and Botts (1987) concluded that self-hypnosis may successfully allow children to ameliorate and/or completely control the motor tic components of this condition. Also, vocal tics appear to diminish substantially with the continued practice of self-hypnosis. The importance of individualizing hypnotic suggestions and involving the parents in treatment in an effort to maintain practice of self-hypnosis is stressed.

Medical Emergencies. Self-hypnosis may be helpful for the rapid reduction of anxiety in emergency situations. Following is a case history, presented by Daniel Kohen (1986), that illustrates the use of self-hypnosis in a pediatric emergency situation. The client was an eight-year-old boy who had sustained a laceration to his forehead that required suturing. The child liked to play football and reported that he had a lot of daydreams. The therapist explained that [the boy] could close his eyes and daydream so well that he could forget about being here until it was time to go home, and that nothing would have to bother him. He closed his eyes and entered trance. . . . As suggestions for imagining playing football were given, he was assured that all procedures would be explained as they were performed. As I guided [him] in the imagery of playing football, I suggested that he make sure he concentrated on getting the signals correct.

I told him that I was going to wash the cut. I gave a direct suggestion for absence of discomfort saying, "As I wash it, all of the hurt can be washed away . . . your muscles can get loose, soft, and comfortable. . . . I then told [him] that he might be able to notice a "small touch" as the local anesthetic . . . was injected but it did not have to bother him, and that as he paid attention to his football game, he might see that he might not even notice it at all. . . . No subjective complaint of discomfort or withdrawal was evident throughout the repair of the laceration. (Kohen, 1986, pp. 284–285)

Individualizing the self-hypnotic formula and imagery is of great importance.

Conclusion

Self-hypnosis is distinguished from heterohypnosis by the presence or absence of an external hypnotist; however, the debate over the importance of an external hypnotist is ongoing.

Self-hypnosis may be effectively used for a variety of different symptoms, only a few of which have been discussed in this chapter. Self-hypnosis is commonly used as an adjunct to heterohypnosis and can easily be adapted for virtually any symptom that can be treated with heterohypnosis. Self-hypnosis is the learning of a new skill and requires much practice. Certain clients will respond better to these techniques than others. Self-hypnotic induction and self-suggestions should be individualized to be most effective. Self-hypnosis is not a panacea for any symptom and is most effectively used in the context of ongoing treatment.

Part II
Applications

This part examines hypnosis in specific applications: habit disorders; psychological, dental, and medical problems, including chronic pain; hypnosis with children; hypnosis as an aid to performance enhancement; and forensic hypnosis. Although applications were discussed in part I, it was primarily in the context of technique. In this part, many additional techniques are elaborated, now within the context of specific applications.

Each chapter in part II explores a wide variety of potential applications. The exception is chapter 9, which presents a number of issues and suggestions that apply generally throughout the rest of this part, although these suggestions are mainly couched in the context of smoking cessation, one of the most chronic habit disorders.

9
Hypnosis and the Habit Disorders

No doubt Jack the Ripper excused himself on the grounds that it
was human nature.
—A. A. Milne

The habit disorders most frequently encountered are habitual abuse of
tobacco, alcohol, illicit drugs, and foods. Since problems such as
alcohol dependence and overeating show marked similarities, some
common approaches for the varied problems are effective. Many common
principles and techniques for eliminating substance abuse can also be
adapted to address compulsive syndromes such as pathological gambling,
kleptomania, pyromania, and sexual addiction (Citrenbaum, King, and Cohen, 1985).

This chapter differs considerably from the following ones in this part.
Rather than elaborating on a wide range of specific applications, as is the
case in the other chapters, the focus here is on a set of general strategies and
techniques that are directly applicable to smoking cessation, to a slightly
lesser degree to substance abuse problems, and to a lesser though still significant degree to the habit-control issues often embedded in and/or accompanying the disorders discussed throughout the other chapters in this part.

The Facts on Hypnosis and Habit Control

Clinical research and clinical reports establish hypnotic interventions to be
effective aspects of habit control even when certain aspects of the results are
debated. The following brief synopsis suggests that when hypnotherapists
practice with skill, conviction, and common sense, clients can find relief
from habits and addictions. However, people beset with such habit disorders can change only when they are ready to admit that their own choices
and behaviors are the root of their problems. This chapter explores the
professional's use of hypnosis in the motivated client's process of change.

Tobacco

Tobacco use has the distinction of exhibiting the highest lifetime prevalence
rate of any mental disorder, with approximately 35 percent of the population having been directly affected at some time since birth (Maxmen, 1986).

157

Cigarettes are the most abused form of tobacco, and cigarette smokers frequently approach hypnotherapists with requests for aid in quitting. Reports on the use of hypnosis over the years show that as few as 20 percent of the clients ever achieve abstinence from tobacco use, and other reports estimate almost 90 percent of clients meet the goal (Edmonston, 1981). A recent report claims a 70 percent abstinence rate of former smokers after a brief therapy intervention involving hypnosis (Carlson, 1989).

These figures, and the studies that produce them, are impossible to compare due to wide differences in measures and methods employed. For example, one review of the literature abstracts at least sixteen different treatment procedures, divided into single-session, multiple-session, and group-session formats, and crossed with variables such as hypnotic susceptibility, client motivation, therapist characteristics, degree of telephone contact, and degree of individualization of the program (Agee, 1983).

Many people are able to quit smoking without the use of hypnosis. Studies using random assignment to varied treatments, such as those by Hyman et al. (1986) and Lambe, Osier, and Franke (1986), show virtually no difference between hypnosis and other active treatments, placebo, or no-treatment control groups, especially at a six-month follow-up. Those results could fuel doubts as to the efficacy of hypnosis. An alternative interpretation simply highlights the fact that a clinician should never randomly accept a person as a hypnotherapy client. Selection effects—the bane of controlled studies—are the key to successful clinical practice. Random assignment of subjects to varied treatments may be a clean way of detecting absolute effects, but the very process dilutes the two major components of hypnotic intervention: belief and expectancy.

Alcohol

Attempts to treat alcohol dependence with hypnosis run into theoretical arguments from the outset. Many therapists with experience in hypnosis claim that alcoholics constitute one of the most intractable groups for trance induction. Controlled studies comparing hypnosis treatment efficacy among alcohol abusers and alcohol dependent populations are lacking. Indeed, few clinical case reports appear in the literature, especially when compared with reviews of tobacco use cessation and obesity reduction treatments.

One fact is obvious: for any success to occur, an alcoholic who states that he or she wants to stop drinking must make that presentation to the hypnotherapist when fully sober. Detoxification, whether in a residential unit or in an ambulatory detoxification program, must precede any recovery intervention. Hypnotic intervention requires a client who can focus attention, selectively dissociate, and encode deep memories. Intoxication interferes with each of those processes.

Another fact is equally clear: no treatment for alcoholism, especially when follow-up measures are made after several years, works any better than Alcoholics Anonymous. A hypnotherapist can provide valuable aid to an alcoholic intent on recovery, but the professional should always insist that she or he will work only with a client who also works within an AA program.

Drug Addiction

Little literature exists on the application of hypnosis to the control of habitual abuse of illicit drugs. One report of treatment proposes that an age regression use of hypnosis can facilitate recovery by healing an allegedly causal birth trauma (Hull, 1986). A suggestion more consonant with mainstream theory notes that the relaxation effects of hypnosis might effectively mimic the relaxation effects of cocaine use such that hypnosis might have value in substance abuse treatment (Resnick and Resnick, 1986). A case study of a heroin addict's recovery program that includes hypnotic intervention appears in Vandamme (1986). An eighteen-month follow-up showed no apparent relapse for that client.

Obesity

The literature on hypnotic treatment of obesity indicates results similar to the studies on tobacco use cessation. Many of the earlier reports were primarily anecdotal, with little critical rigor. The earlier studies that attempted to meet canons of empirical method showed mixed results and such varied design and component content that meaningful comparison was impossible (Mott and Roberts, 1979). More recent reports of the anecdotal or clinical case style continue to report positive results in the treatment of obesity with a hypnotic component (Cochrane, 1987). A study with a rather limited number of subjects showed remarkable results in favor of both hypnosis and high hypnotizability (Anderson, 1985). Those results are confirmed by more recent studies replete with control groups and varied levels of treatment. Results indicate that hypnosis is a significant component in such treatment and that a subject's measured hypnotizability correlates positively with degree of weight loss (Barabasz and Spiegel, 1989; Holroyd, 1990).

Other Habits and Compulsive Syndromes

As the hypnotherapist encounters habits with less public awareness or behaviors with a very low base rate of occurrence, the research and report literature provides even less insight and guidance. A search in the journals will reveal a few happy, odd accounts of successful use of hypnosis treatment of such quirks as tongue thrust (Golan, 1991). Undoubtedly, the less successful efforts are less likely to reach print. Application of hypnosis to the amelioration of more disturbing habits deserves both clinical and experimental attention. For example, hypnotherapists are likely to see a sharp increase in presentations for relief from compulsive sexual behavior as public awareness of the problem increases (cf. Carnes, 1989).

Facts Summary

Four points from the literature on the hypnotic treatment of all habit disorders are important (and in fact, are so in a more general fashion to most of the disorders discussed throughout this book):

1. Highly hypnotizable clients respond with better abstinence rates than do less hypnotizable clients.
2. Several sessions of heterohypnosis treatments (commonly set at four sessions) produce better abstinence rates than single-session treatments.
3. Suggestions tailored to the individual, whether delivered in vivo or by recordings, produce a better outcome than generic suggestions.
4. Treatment packages that combine hypnosis with some other intervention produce better outcome measures than hypnosis-alone treatments.

Therapist Characteristics

Clients show better abstinence rates at long-term follow-up when the therapists performing the hypnosis have extensive experience with hypnosis and extended contact with the client (Barabasz et al., 1986). It is impossible, however, to attribute this effect strictly to the experience level or the contact length per se since the reports do not guarantee that clients' awareness of the therapists' experience levels and expectations of contact lengths might not have influenced the outcomes. As often appears in any other aspect of hypnosis, existence of belief may be just as important as (or perhaps much more important than) existence of an actual foundation for the belief. The salient point, however, is that good portions of confidence should be present on both sides of the coin for the hypnotherapy to have its maximum effect (Orman, 1991). This fact is as true for the hypnotherapist as it is for the client.

Client Characteristics

Clients should have (or have the potential to develop) adequate faith in the hypnotic procedure for maximum efficacy. A thorough assessment prior to any treatment will enable the therapist to provide the client with a clearer picture of cessation success probability. A measure of hypnotizability can aid in prediction of results: clients who score higher on scales of hypnotizability also show better abstinence rates at long-term follow-up after hypnotic treatment (Frishholz and Spiegel, 1986; Citrenbaum et al., 1985). As in all other screenings related to the use of hypnosis, the therapist should remain alert to the possibility of uncovering or excerbating psychotic features in clients. Such clients should not be accepted. Some savants of the field note that clients who use a substance, food, or compulsive behavior to compensate for a neurotic need will be particularly resistant to change even if they are highly susceptible to hypnosis (Crasilneck, 1990). This opinion, however, may be considered a patent truism since only a neurotic organism would maintain a behavior known to be perniciously maladaptive. The issue is not so much the neurotic need per se, but the depth of the person's desire to stop the neurotic behavior.

Paradox: The Core of Hypnosis and the Source of Recovery

Some approaches try to alter or strengthen the client's "willpower" to cease the targeted behavior. Other approaches manipulate the contingency relationships in the client's environment so that the reinforcers for the targeted behavior are removed (Jordan, 1989). Regardless of the theoretical position held, hypnosis can serve as a useful adjunct in treatment. Both heterohypnosis, under the direction of a professional, and self-hypnosis, as learned from the professional, can aid clients in changing behavior through new choices (Davidson, 1985).

The Paradox of Recovery

The hypnotherapist does not have to resolve the theoretical debates about "willpower" and "disease models" when contributing to clients' recovery. No matter what theoretical orientation the therapist might hold on the issue of will and determinism, the exhausting academic squabble can be transformed into a functional therapeutic paradox for clients who seek relief from the problems of habit and compulsion.

This recourse to paradox dovetails neatly with a major explanation as to why hypnosis is effective at all: that hypnosis is an exercise in paradox, as demonstrated by the influence of the remarkable work of Milton Erickson (Citrenbaum et al., 1985). Paradox also characterizes the essence of many self-help programs for recovery from addictive and compulsive behaviors, such as Alcoholics Anonymous (AA). In the first step of AA's Twelve Steps, members admit to being "powerless" over alcohol and admit that their life has become unmanageable. In the recognition of that foundational powerlessness and chaos, the person first finds the strength to refuse the next available alcoholic drink and to restore order to living in that very moment.

Veterans of Twelve Step programs of recovery readily announce to inquirers and new members that most people find the demands of the program to be too rigorous. The programs implicitly recognize that members have resistance to change. Rather than attacking the resisting defenses, the programs simply declare that such fears are common to all and that they will not automatically sabotage recovery since recovery depends on progress rather than perfection. The programs rather neatly sidestep the resistances, acknowledge members' right to own their individual resistances, doubts, and fears, and assure members of their progressing ability to change according to their own pace.

Hypnotherapists can learn from such proved wisdom. They must be able to use clients' resistance to change as the very opportunity for change (Orman, 1991). They must eschew attempts to strip resistances from clients. Most direct assaults on the defenses fail, and the few that succeed may leave clients in pain or distrust.

Rather than forcing the client into some posture of doctrinal purity on recovery or denuding the client's psyche of long-entrenched defenses, the hypnotherapist begins using the paradox as soon as the client presents for treatment with both a behavior targeted for change or extinction and certain indicators that the client is indeed amenable to change. The inherent paradox is two-pronged: (1) the habit is so strong and compelling that it appears to the client that he or she will never be able to alter the habit, but (2) the client's solicitation of help from an expert suggests that he or she believes that the habit can be altered. These two facts are in distinct contradiction. The therapist must take the force of the contradiction and turn it into momentum for change rather than opportunity for shame and ridicule.

Both aspects of the paradox, however, must be clearly present before any recovery can begin. If the first condition is absent, then either the inquirer does not have a problem or still denies that the designated habit is a problem. People who present while still indulging significant denial are often on the telephone or in the office because they are placating loved ones, employers, or legal systems. They are not convinced they have a habit control problem. A person in this category might say something like, "Actually, I can cut down on smoking [drinking, eating, gambling] at any time, but I hear that hypnosis is an easy way to help me bring it under control" (that is, "I'll be able to cut down somewhat—that will make me [or them] feel better, but I won't really have to give it up"). When the hypnotherapist hears such ideas, she or he must immediately explain to the person that the total treatment package, including hypnosis, is demanding and rigorous and that the person does not appear to be a suitable client for that clinic or office.

Such clients also readily resort to the statement that they "will try to" make the overall change, carry out some required therapeutic task, or something else. They should be confronted with the admonishment that "trying is lying." When decisions are needed, "I'll try . . ." is an inevitable predictor of eventual failure.

If the second condition of the paradox (the belief that change can occur) is absent, the inquirer either is not actually soliciting help (even if other people or systems are pushing the person to change) or has become so demoralized as to lack hope for any change. If the screening process reveals that the motivation appears to flow first and foremost from other people rather than from the individual, the inquirer should be told politely, but directly, that no one has ever recovered from endangering habits because of another person's motivation.

If the inquirer lacks any real hope for change, the therapist is probably faced with a significantly depressed person who should be referred for an appropriate treatment—perhaps a time-limited cognitive-behavioral package focused on elevating the triad of thoughts, behavior, and feelings. The combination of depression and substance abuse (especially alcohol abuse, cannabis abuse, or sedative abuse) is particularly tricky because of the strong interaction of the substance and the depression. A key characteristic for success with hypnosis is the client's ability to focus and to dissociate selectively (Barabasz and Spiegel, 1989), and an active episode of a mood disorder is likely to impair these essential abilities.

When both elements of the paradox are clearly present, the hypnotherapist can highlight this paradox to the client in the following manner (in this case for smoking cessation, but the model is appropriate for virtually all habit disorders):

Therapist: Yes, Bill, you are right. Smoking is certainly driving, persistent, and annoying. It seems deceitful: one moment you find extreme pleasure in a cigarette; soon, however, you feel bad because of it. The habit seems so strong that some people might despair of any release from its grip. Bill, you want to quit smoking, but that change seems distant. It is an odd quirk, that even while you acknowledge that the smoking habit is so strong, you have come to this place at this time to see me so that you can quit smoking, Bill. Obviously, Bill, part of you feels that you can become a nonsmoker, and we will work together to amplify that clear voice from that part of your person. I also think that part of you has some doubts but that those doubts are not strong enough to keep you away from our session. Bill, you are a remarkably complex person, as revealed by these facts.

In such a manner, the therapist reflects both the client's feelings of hopelessness and the client's feelings of hope implicit in the act of presentation.

Screening Clients

The inquirer's history of attempts at cessation or modulation of the presented behavior must always be reviewed. In particular, a clear picture of any prior hypnotic treatments must be obtained. A history of relapse after hypnotic intervention does not automatically disquality an inquirer, but the hypnotherapist must discern the manner in which the client presents at this moment. Does the client have the attitude of, "Hypnosis did not work before, but I will give it another try" or is the attitude one of, "Hypnosis worked to help me change before, and maybe I can use it again along with some other tools to extend my success"? The former admission is a certain prelude to failure; the latter is a fairly good predictor of success. In general, a long history of failed attempts at quitting, whether such attempts did or did not include hypnosis, and an expressed dependence on powerful others to control health, indicates poor prognosis for a client (Horowitz, Hindi-Alexander, and Wagner, 1985).

A review of previous attempts at hypnotic management should determine the following variables:

1. Mode (one-on-one versus lecture hall group).
2. Use of an explicitly orchestrated induction versus subtle use of relaxation and focus.
3. Use of aversive imagery and pairing versus pleasant experience amplification.
4. Number of session of heterohypnosis.
5. Frequency of use of self-hypnosis.
6. Other components (for example, self-monitoring, environment changes).
7. The defined target (for example, cessation versus reduction).

If the survey shows that the inquirer actually experienced a hypnotic program similar to the only one the screening hypnotherapist is prepared to offer, the inquirer should be referred to some other mode of treatment or to a hypnotherapist who offers a significantly different package. It is unlikely that a change in therapist alone will render effective a program with a failed track record. If the hypnotherapist can offer a package with some significant differences, the match of therapist and client is more auspicious.

The screening should determine if the inquirer presents with a problem of such magnitude or repercussion that other professional referrals must be pursued. The occasional need to send a person who uses drugs or alcohol for detoxification will arise. People beset with compulsive gambling habits may need the aid of a competent financial adviser. Although people with obesity should not have excuses of endocrine imbalance reinforced, the possibility needs to be ruled out. People with a sexual addiction or compulsion that has involved intercourse with multiple partners may need testing for sexually transmitted diseases.

Inquirers should be told very clearly, and at the outset of an interview, that most state governments limit confidentiality. This fact is particularly pertinent to inquirers who seek to change certain patterns of compulsive sexual behavior but can apply to most of the habit disorders.

Transition from Screening to Treatment

Whether the screening is carried out on the telephone or in the office, that contact should be clearly demarcated from actual entry into treatment. The screening should be the hypnotherapist's opportunity to decide whether to accept the inquirer as a client.

That decision may depend on the inquirer's willingness to comply with the therapist's initiation requests. For example, an inquirer who reports smoking three packs of cigarettes a day may be told that the hypnotherapist will begin treatment when the inquirer reports back to the office that usage has been reduced to one pack a day for a period of three days. An inquirer concerned about alcohol use may be told that the treatment will begin when the person is able to report twenty-four hours of sobriety and attendance at three separate AA meetings. An overweight inquirer may be asked to schedule treatment after losing five pounds prior to treatment. For all of the habit disorders, some detailed monitoring of the disorder should be a precursor to any treatment—to get clearer data and to start to confront the client's self-protective delusions about the extent of the disorder. Also, anyone in any predicament should be asked to pay for at least one-half of a standard treatment up-front.

These methods present several paradoxical messages. The inquirer has to do something in order to become a client. That is, the initiation of a healing relationship with the professional depends on a behavior change in the inquirer. When the inquirer changes a behavior, he or she finds a positive consequence: positive attention from the professional. When the inquirer makes the step to become the client and to experience attention from the professional, the client knows that the professional's attention is valuable because it costs hard cash. Finally, the inquirer who previously thought that he or she had no control over a habit has already learned as a new client that he or she does have some control.

Perhaps as important, this type of initiation protects the hypnotherapist from delusions of power and/or a tendency to "fix" other people. Both traps are avoided when the clinician realizes from the outset that the client is the one who will change the client's behavior. Clearly maintained rules about payment improve the therapist's security so that her or his issues are not as likely to emerge in a passive-aggressive manner and to hamper work with the client.

Building the Hypnotic Component of a Treament Package

Definitions and Targets

The first step requires a clear definition of the problem behavior and a clear target for the proposed change. When the issue is use of a substance not required to maintain normal human life (tobacco, alcohol, illicit drugs) or a behavior not an integral part of social or intimate relationships (such as gambling), the most effective target is absolute abstinence. Definitions related to overeating are a little more complicated. Abstinence obviously cannot be defined as "not eating." For some people, the eating of a particular class of food might be targeted for total cessation. For others, the target is controlled eating of all classes of food. Measurement might be strict, in terms of numbers of calories per day, or more relaxed, as in numbers of eating episodes a day (traditionally designated as "three normal meals").

Good results, however, have been demonstrated by using hypnotically enhanced states to teach the client to trust the body's own healthy, accurate, and discernible signals for when a good portion of the right foods have been ingested (Ronan, 1988). This approach treats fat as an organ of the body that can be regulated by relaxed, conscious attention, just as biofeedback training allows a person to learn control over autonomic processes.

For behaviors related to compulsive sexual intercourse, the parameters must be set according to the individual client's most heartfelt values. Absolute abstinence is absurd in the case of food and usually contraindicated in the case of sex. The client can use the concept of abstinence in terms of "no sexual activity except in the context of a significant relationship" or "no sexual activity that incurs risk of injury or arrest to self or to others."

The period of time for a target should be manageable and conceivable. "Never again" is simply too threatening, because any slip or relapse will be considered a permanent stain on the remainder of the client's life. There is much wisdom in the AA adage, "One Day at a Time." With such an approach, each day of nonuse is a success, and any day with a slip is always followed by another day of potential success.

Clients are never told to stop craving; they are simply told that they will eventually notice fewer instances of craving and with decreasing intensity as they successfully meet each day's task of "not using" or "not doing." This distinction between the client presenting with a "desire to stop [drinking, smoking, gambling, overeating]" and a client requesting a hypnotherapist to instill a "desire to stop desiring [alcohol, tobacco, a big win]" is crucial. The first condition is a necessary but nonsufficient state for ensuing success. The second wish is not only unnecessary and insufficient; it is in fact detrimental. It is not surprising that one of the most successful scripts for smoking cessation, as presented by Spiegel and Spiegel (1978) and adapted to address overeating by Barabasz and Spiegel (1989), explicitly dissociates the client's desire for the object from the client's willingness to act toward the object. Those scientist-practitioners applied well in hypnosis a key fact of Twelve Step recovery: recovery comes in "not doing," not in "not wanting to do."

A quick review of basic learning processes clarifies the pitfall of placing primacy on desiring not to desire. The long-established pattern of addictive or compulsive abuse means that a "desire to desire" a substance or activity has been heavily, consistently, and frequently reinforced by delivery of the substance or the experience. That "desire to desire" will never begin to dissipate until it is no longer reinforced, and reinforcement will be cut off when the behavior that supplies the substance or sensation ceases. The "desire to desire" will eventually die of natural causes (though, admittedly, the death throes will not be pleasant) if the reinforcer is withheld.

On the other hand, the hypnotherapist will always want to use both hypnotic suggestion and clinical conversation to reinforce the client's discovery that his or her anxiety level is markedly low during the deep relaxation that attends both heterohypnotic and self-hypnotic treatment sessions. Such suggestions can be phrased as:

Therapist: And, so, Sherry, as you walk serenely in that pleasant place, finding plenty of comfort space for your truest self and your body, you come across a clear, clean pool in the meadow. You look into the shining water and see yourself. Sherry, you like the way you look in the reflection. You realize that you are very pleased with your ability to enjoy the clean odor of fresh air and to see the clear, blue sky. For the first time in a long, long time, you do not want a cigarette at this moment, Sherry. You also know that in the future, after you have left this quiet place of comfort and joy, and when you are engaged in the daily demands of work, life, and love, Sherry, you will know that if a desire to smoke a cigarette appears in your mind, you can simply find this place of reflection; this place where you see yourself calm and pleased, in a meadow of peacefulness and freshness. You will find that you can have the same experience of relaxation and the same pleasure of experiencing yourself without having a cigarette. And, Sherry, you will always be able to return to this pleasant meadow whenever you want to, because you will always walk with this pleasant place inside of you.

Session Length and Numbers

The number of hypnotic sessions in the office should be set as soon as the therapist accepts the client for treatment. Programs vary from single-session smoking cessation to multiple-session packages. Packages with at least four heterohypnosis sessions seem optimal. The decision is based on the hypnotherapist's personal style, client history, and the nature of the problem. If success is not reached in the first "package," another may then be negotiated, with reasons for failure being critical to the negotiated contingencies.

Explaining Hypnosis

The hypnotic component of the treatment must be carefully and accurately portrayed to the client. The client's concerns and beliefs about hypnosis are the issues to be considered. If the client expresses fear and suspicion that hypnosis can be used against the client's best interests, the therapist reflects those feelings while offering statements that generally allay the fears. If the client expresses convictions that hypnosis will work like a magic spell, the therapist reflects the client's feelings of strong hope and belief while subtly introducing the facts about the natural functions (including the natural limits) of hypnosis. Once again, paradox should be explored and used, not resisted or dismissed. The therapist should explain that all hypnosis is in part self-hypnosis and that the therapist's role is to teach the client the technique that opens the resource. If the client attributes the power of habit control to the therapist, the therapist should accept the attributed power on a surface level and yet return it to the client in gentle statements that highlight the client's abilities to choose and to change. Most important, the therapist must avoid any hint of arguing with the client over "who is really in control." Relational congruence in preparation for the hypnotic treatment is much more important than doctrinal purity, even if such a consensus about the nature of hypnosis actually existed in the literature.

Choosing Inductions

The therapist should choose the mode of induction with which he or she is most comfortable and effective and considers to be most effective. When the studies report information on induction, they do not suggest that the in duction mode contributes to the outcome efficacy. The use of eye fixation with eye closure, accompanied by the suggestion that the client is entering a sleeplike trance, is reported in Baer, Cary, and Meminger (1986). Arm levitation induction techniques are also reported (Edmonston, 1981). When a therapist intends to instruct the client in the use of self-hypnosis as a supplement to the treatment provided in the therapist-led sessions, the therapist should use an induction modality an individual can operationalize on his or her own. For example, inductions that require a person other than the client to manipulate a pendulum or some other device are not advised. Continuity in method between the therapist-assisted sessions and the client practice session away from the office will always strengthen treatment efficacy. Such treatment packages are reported in many clinical studies (Agee, 1983).

A classic induction may not actually be a necessary preparation for hypnotic suggestions. One former smoker attributed her smoking cessation to an auditorium-sized, single-session hypnotic intervention. The session was advertised explicitly as a venture into hypnosis, and she attended it with friends. She enjoyed a two-year abstinence from cigarette smoking after a thirteen-year history of heavy smoking. Her report puts this in context:

> We were told to sit upright in our chairs with both feet on the ground and both arms on the rests of the chair. We were told to imagine ourselves walking through a very pleasant place; a sweet, gentle place; like a meadow of soft grass and bright flowers. As we walked we felt the breeze blowing gentle across our faces; and I was able to imagine the sweet smells of the meadow brushing my nose. We were directed to the billowy, puffy clouds in the sky; and to imagine ourselves sharing in the lightness. We were to find ourselves noting that the more we considered the clouds, and their wondrous buoyancy, the more we ourselves would find ourselves to be cloudlike and light, ready to float and bounce above the meadow's surface.
>
> Our leader then told us to remember the distance we were walking, and to note that even as we were enjoying this pleasant meadow, we were now back on the ground, and our legs were becoming heavy as we walked, and our arms were becoming heavy as we walked. Then we would stop walking, and we would count numbers for awhile; and then we would continue to walk even more through the meadow, with heaviness in our arms and legs increasing with each step. And then we would stop our steps again to count; and then move on with our arms and legs now almost numb like deadweights. Finally, we were told to give in to gravity, and rest ourselves in the soft meadow grass; to lie down and relax, letting our heavy, leaden arms and legs sink deep into the softness of the turf as we stretched ourselves prone. To relax more completely than even sleep itself ever would allow.

Obviously such a presentation could have been delivered in one-on-one therapy, with the many added potentials that mode offers, but this approach was sufficient for this former smoker.

Using Challenges

The literature pays little attention to the role of challenges as a measure of trance depth in the outcome efficacy of hypnotic treatment, although it often suggests that trance depth per se is not as crucial to outcome as client belief that the procedure is effective. If a therapist feels that some type of challenge is needed in a particular case, challenge selection should probably reflect the modality of habit performance. For example—

> *Therapist:* Bill, you find that the index finger and the middle finger of your right hand are parallel and touching. You are aware that they are together as your arm lies on your chair's rest. With your eyes closed, Bill, you can visualize the fingers together, and you begin to realize that the two fingers are becoming increasingly cool despite their closeness. The cooling of those two fingers increases, and you are increasingly aware that the two fingers are icy cold, Bill; you feel no pain, but you feel the fingers now frozen together. You find that you cannot separate the fingers due to the frozen feelings. You lift your arm and bring the icy, frosty finger pair to your lips. You touch your lips with the flat, frozen fingers, and as they touch your lips, Bill, you find that the fingers stick as tightly to your lips as they stick to each other. And now you cannot move them from your lips, Bill; when you pull, they will not come free. And when I tell you, Bill, but not yet, your fingers will release from your lips, and the frozen feeling will melt away, with all warmth and feeling returning just as before. And when I tell you, but not yet, Bill, and when the fingers release and the warmth returns, your arm will drop back gently to your chair, and you will find yourself even more deeply relaxed and in trance.

This challenge is offered because it leads the client into a counterintuitive experience of the same body parts and range of motion so often associated with smoking (or any of the other hand-to-mouth habit problems). The induced loss of control in hypnosis is the paradoxical avenue for a new exercise of control.

Using Suggestions

Suggestions are most effective when fitted with dual prongs: one pointing to the aversive aspects of the habit and one to the benefits that will derive from ending the habit. Some of the suggestions offered the client who was induced through the meadow scene are as follows:

Therapist: Your eyes are closed, but your ears are open, and you can hear me clearly. You hear clearly that cigarettes are poison to your body. The nicotine hurts you; burns you; turns you into a person you do not want to be. Your eyes are closed, but you can see clearly, Irma. There is a saucer of tar; it is thick, sticky, and icky. It globs in the dish; it seeps over the edge of the bright white porcelain, soiling it and ruining the cloth on the table beneath. You are seeing a laboratory; a table with a bowl of tar squeezed from cigarettes and a vial of concentrated nicotine leached from a pack of cigarettes. The nicotine is more poisonous than cyanide, Irma; you see a rubber-gloved hand reach into a cage and remove a frightened white rat; the hand shaves the hair from the rat's back; the hand pours three drops of the nicotine on the pink skin. Irma, you see smoke rise, and the rat flinch. You smell the stench of the chemical burn on the animal's flesh; you see the blisters bubble up on the skin. The gloved hand now smears cigarette tar on the raw wound; the blisters now expand and spread, changing into blotches traveling far beneath the skin, under the fur; the blisters become tumors.

Now, Irma, you see that you are a nonsmoker. You are able to taste subtle flavors of favorite foods; Irma, you can smell delightful aromas of culinary delights; you can catch a whiff of a favorite cologne. You see yourself as a nonsmoker three weeks away. Irma, you see your teeth in a mirror: they are bright white, for the dentist has just cleaned them. And they will stay white with the normal brushing that suffices for you, a nonsmoker. You are a nonsmoker four weeks away. An elevator in a tall building is not working, and your friends complain of the walk up the stairs. But you are a nonsmoker, and you easily climb to the fourth floor; you scale eight flights of steps, and you breathe with ease; you feel your blood pumping and surging with strength; the effect is your own reward for being a nonsmoker.

Alternative Scripts

Apparently logical reasons for dissolving a habit may not always be the most meaningful ones for a particular client, so alternative scripts should always be considered. Even when the obvious ones are effective, an alternative script can often be helpful as a booster. For example, in one case I saw, a smoking cessation client had shown little response to scripts similar to those above. The script that finally moved her, leading to an eventual, total success, was an amplified version of the following:

Therapist: Now, Monika, you have an image of yourself looking in a mirror. You notice some wrinkles at the base of your neck and near your mouth and eyes. You are aware that smoking increases the wrinkling of your face. [Indeed, there is solid evidence that smoking more than triples the average person's likelihood of premature facial wrinkling.] As you look at yourself in the mirror, you notice some cigarette smoke wafting about in the air. As this smoke floats about, notice your skin begin to wrinkle even more. You can see what it will be like as the wrinkles become more obvious, as they make you look older, much older than your actual age.

After developing that theme, one can reverse the procedure, having the person visualize moving away from smoking in various ways, perhaps by destroying any smoking paraphernalia or refusing the offer of a cigarette from a co-worker. As the client does this, have him or her visualize the smoke gradually disappear, and the wrinkling disappear, as a more youthful look returns to the face.

Such alternative-motivation scripts—for example, with an older alcoholic, an increased loss of memory and the consequent confusion and embarrassment—often are effective where standard scripts have little or no impact.

Supportive Scripts

It is also worthwhile to develop scripts that indirectly support the main target behavior, especially when there is any good reason to believe one of these secondary factors will come into play. For example, there is clear evidence that cessation of smoking causes a lowering of metabolism, with an average eventual weight gain of six to eight pounds even when there is no rise in caloric intake. This is a negative reinforcer for most people trying to stop smoking. Hence, it is worthwhile to develop an adjunct script similar to the following:

Therapist: As you know, Monika, when you stop smoking, as you will be able to do, your body's metabolism will slow down, which will have a number of positive effects on your general health. But it also means it will be easier for you to gain some weight.

The good part is knowing, both consciously and down

deep in your unconscious mind, that your body is going to feel more alive and energetic as you slough off the effects of smoking. You are going to feel an increasing need to get exercise. [Amplify on images of various exercise patterns that have been discussed earlier.] You feel your energy go up, you really enjoy getting more exercise, and because of the exercise, you know from past experience that you will feel less need for food. The more you exercise, the less need you will have to eat, especially to eat junk food or fattening foods and sweets, as you know this is a signal to you that you are bored or frustrated rather than hungry.

Habit disorders are usually supported by a number of inadvertent and/or secondary reinforcers. Developing strategies to counteract such effects is often crucial to success.

Building the Rest of the Package

Although the client may be keenly convinced that the hypnosis sessions as conducted by the therapist will alone turn the trick in a habit change, the treatment package should include several other important features that increase the probability of abstinence after extended times. Quitting a behavior is not difficult. Remaining abstinent is.

Walking the Twelve Steps

Adaptations of AA's Twelve Steps to address other addictions, compulsions, and habits appear to be limited only by the number of descriptors people can prefix to the word *anonymous*. Although such programs operate with policies of attraction rather than promotion, the benefits they provide can certainly be touted as consistent with a complete recovery package that includes hypnosis. Most urban centers offer a full menu of "alphabet recovery," and although the problems addressed and the social subgroups served can sometimes seem humorous, the success members enjoy is nothing to be laughed at. If there is a program that corresponds to a client's situation and enough available meetings so that it is likely that the client can find at least one amenable to his or her schedule and personality, the client should attend the program.

Self-Hypnosis

An efficient means of aiding the client's ability to achieve a self-induced hypnotic state is to provide him or her with an audiotape of one of the office sessions (see chapter 8). The client and therapist should contract for a daily self-hypnosis practice schedule, and a record of such practice should be brought to the sessions. Also, the client should be able to access some degree of heightened relaxation at any time in a day when a strong craving to indulge the habit arises.

Changing the Environment

The client should remove all paraphernalia and supplies of the targeted materials from living and working spaces. If the client has even the slightest idea that a particular item could be a stimulus to return to the habit, the item must go, at least in the early stages of recovery. The rule of thumb is, "If you suspect it's a problem, it is a problem, so get rid of the problem before it becomes a problem that you cannot get rid of." Contracting with significant others to help in this process is critical.

Replacing the Behavior

A contract for instituting adaptive alternatives to the old habit should be drawn up. Physical activity is often an effective way to reduce the anxiety many people feel as they abandon an entrenched, destructive habit. The contract should call for regular practice of some such activity, recourse during times of particular stress and relapse risk, and a careful monitoring of activities that might become harmful if amplified as a replacement response. For example, a client who has just quit smoking cigarettes should reduce intake of caffeine and alcohol (and calories) at the very time when he or she would probably like to increase both. In fact, no matter what habit is targeted for extinction, it is wise to require the client to contract to drink no alcoholic beverage and to use no recreational drug for thirty days, beginning twenty-four hours before the first session. If he or she cannot agree to such a contract or cannot maintain it after one is set, another seriously detrimental habit has been revealed.

Follow-up

The client should have the opportunity to contact the hypnotherapist to check in daily on recovery status during the first week. Telephone contact, limited to a few minutes, is excellent, but sending the client away with a set of postcards is another way to encourage the contact. The client should feel encouraged to talk with other people who are recovering from the same habit. Therapists who have any reservations about Twelve Step programs might give them more attention on this component alone—that is, the ease of contact that these informal systems allow among members and program sponsors' willingness to talk on the telephone at any time far exceeds what is practical or even appropriate for professionals.

Acknowledging the Client's Central Identity

Note the frequent use of the client's name in the sample scenarios of individual treatment. The use of a preferred name is a powerful and free reinforcer always ready in the mind and on the tip of the tongue. A visit to any meeting of a Twelve Step program of recovery reveals the importance of naming. The practice may seem at first to approach absurd limits. Yet each time a person offers to speak, that person will usually say, "Hello everybody, I'm Bill, and I'm a(n) [alcoholic, nicotine addict, sex addict, etc.]." In turn, like a Greek chorus, the other members acknowledge that person by saying in unison, "Hi, Bill." That same interchange might occur as many times in an hour as that person speaks up.

Learning Theory and Name Calling

What purpose could such overworked verbalizations serve? In the daily life of a person with an active addiction or habit disorder, the substance or the behavior becomes the center of all existence. In effect, the person revolves around the addiction or habit disorder. The person's core of being is shunted aside, and the person's self-esteem and identity is replaced by compulsion. In the course of an hour-long meeting, the greeting-response repetitions in the meeting restore the person's central identity and shunt the addiction or compulsion to the side so that it now revolves around the person. The syntax demands that the person is prior to the problem. Also, the member offers the group two pieces of information: (1) "My name is Bill," and (2) "I'm alcoholic." The group reinforces only one of the information packets—the packet that carries the name: "Hi, Bill." The problem ("alcoholism") is not denied; it is simply put in its proper place as one key aspect of the person's life rather than the single center of the person's existence. As in the physical world of levers and fulcrums, where a person stands in relation to a task makes a big difference in the ability to do the job, and frequent naming in positive context lets the person stand at the best vantage point.

The hypnotherapist functions much like the group of members. What the therapist lacks in number, she or he adds in prestige, skill, and situational power. In the scenario presented, the client's name is carefully invoked only in the syntax that carries a positive message to the client. For example, the name is used in direct connection with the words "you are right" and "you want to quit smoking." When the negative aspects of the habit are mentioned, they are separated as much as is possible from the named identity of the client.

Most likely, no one in our busy world ever in the course of a day hears his or her name enough times spoken by others in positive contexts. Other people usually invoke our name when they have either a request for our services or a complaint about our behavior. Even when compliments are offered, they are rarely prefaced with our name. (You can collect your own data on these points. Note how often you hear statements like, "Brook, could you bring that book here?" and "Robin, I think you need to work on this proposal some more" but only, "I like the way your hair looks" and "You did a great job on that project.") The therapist is able to restore some of those gifts of "naming without shaming" to the client in the course of the therapy.

Practicing the Technique

This insight means that therapists must actively choose to interact with a client in a way different from street conversation. In short, the therapist must "unlearn" the socially conditioned pattern of invoking names primarily in situations of demand, correction, and shame. Therapists do not have to be perfect at providing invocations in positive contexts; they just need to be better than the environment in which the client functions on a day-to-day basis. Therapist self-reflection may reveal that she or he has a particularly tough time being positive toward a particular client or a particular class of habit-disordered people. An indicator of such resistance would be withholding clients' names in general or speaking the names primarily in the context of negative and/or demanding situations. Such discovery is aided by a good collegial supervision relationship or listening to tapes of one's therapy sessions.

The therapist must follow up this insight with practice. As with clients, insight provides the will to do good work, and practice provides the skill to do good work. The patter of language as used in hypnotic discourse differs from speech enjoined in most social situations. The ability to include the frequent invocation of the client's name as an artful, integral part of the discourse can be strengthened when the hypnotherapist actually practices a set speech.

The topic for the therapist's practice may not have anything to do with a habit control problem; it may, in fact, be the opportunity to affirm his or her own abilities as a professional and as a hypnotherapist. For example, an abbreviated scenario follows, which can be practiced:

"[Your name], you are a well-trained professional who wants to learn even more. Sometimes hypnosis seems odd and its techniques foreign; but, [your name], you can master the techniques that provide the best presentation of your skills to your clients. [Your name], you know that you are important to yourself and to other people. But it is hard for you to accept the sound of your own name so many times. Yet, [your name], you also know that it starts to feel good, natural, and normal to hear your name."

Expand the speech to the point where anxiety peaks and calm ensues. You will find that you at first feel awkward and embarrassed at hearing your name so frequently; then you may even feel rather warm and tingly, and, finally, you feel simply matter-of-fact and comfortable with who you are, what you are hearing, and what you are doing. As the hypnotherapist garners clinical experience and confidence, the interaction with actual clients will supplant the need for separate practice.

The therapist who only rarely engages in hypnotherapy should be particularly willing to maintain a rehearsal schedule (for all components of hypnosis), since skills become rusty through lack of application. Athletes and musicians never confuse training and practice with playing and performance. They know that they cannot do the latter without the former and that several weeks away from the court or the keyboard means that a few drills or trills are in order.

Summary

The scenarios provided here are samples. Knowledge of a few standard scripts, such as the four provided by Walker, Collins, and Krass (1982), will help therapists build their own repertoire of intervention patter. The best scripts grow from the therapist's knowledge of the potential client as garnered from the screening procedure. The attentive hypnotherapist is able to pick out the main themes and topics of the inquirer's concerns. Those might fall in the negative field of the targeted habit's ruinous end. Other clients may present with more positive goals and aspirations. Such form and content provides the frame and stuffing for the hypnotic inductions and suggestions. In providing a battery of change-oriented options (including hypnosis), the client caught in a pattern of destructive habit can have access to the experience, strength, and hope needed to escape the cycle.

10
Hypnotherapy and Psychological Disorders, I

> It's all in your head, Buster, but don't get the idea it's any of that
> psychological crap.
> —Major Frank Burns,
> from the television show, "M.A.S.H."

The use of hypnosis as an aid in healing psychological disorder has a history stretching as far back as three thousand years. Scientific and clinical interest in hypnosis waxed and waned throughout the nineteenth century but first clearly focused on psychological disorders near the middle of that century. In 1851, a Dutch physician, Andries Hoek, was the first to use hypnosis as an uncovering technique in his treatment of a young woman suffering from what today would probably be diagnosed as post-traumatic stress disorder. The patient, Rita van B, had suffered several traumatic experiences, including repeated abuse, rape, and the witnessing of the accidental death of one of her uncle's servants (van der Hart and van der Velden, 1987).

The use of hypnosis as an uncovering device for psychological disorder was popularized by Freud and his colleagues as a means to reach the unconscious. When the psychoanalytic school abandoned hypnosis in favor of free association, the use of hypnosis again became unpopular. The discovery that hypnosis was valuable in treating combat fatigue in World War I led to a renewed interest in the technique, and this has continued to grow to the present day (Morgan, Darby and Heath, 1992; Sarbin, 1991). The focus of this chapter is on ways in which hypnosis can be used to treat specific psychological disorders.

Rationale for Using Hypnotherapy

Hypnosis has been used in the treatment of many psychological conditions, with varying degrees of success. A large body of clinical literature exists documenting the successes—and failures—of hypnotherapy, but there are not many well-designed, carefully controlled research studies. Hence, it is not always easy to judge the validity of hypnotherapy for a given client.

Research

One of the better studies (Gould and Krynicki, 1989) examined the comparative effectiveness of hypnotherapy on different psychological symptoms, including depression, phobic anxiety, somatization, and psychoticism. The subjects, who received three hypnotherapy sessions one week apart with intervening self-hypnotic training, showed significant improvement on all nine variables measured. The greatest improvement occurred with anxiety symptoms, less with affective symptoms, and the least with symptoms involving ideation. The researchers attributed the improvement to a decrease in the fight-or-flight reactions common to periods of arousal, pointing to the relaxation component of hypnosis as the key to the obtained effects.

Mechanisms of Change

Given the clinical and research documentation that hypnosis can be an effective means by which to bring about positive change with psychological symptoms, it is still unclear by what mechanism this change is brought about. Holroyd (1987) reported a list of nine characteristics of the hypnotic trance state that she believed acted to potentiate psychotherapy with psychological disorders:

1. Attentional changes, both in narrowing the focus of attention to concentrate on a specific topic, and in allowing more free-floating attention to improve free association.
2. Use of imagery to increase awareness of affective reactions and to help with creative problem solving.
3. Dissociation, used to help access the unconscious and to allow clients to reexperience traumatic events in their lives.
4. A decrease in reality orientation, allowing improved cognitive reframing and more work with primary process material.
5. Increased suggestibility, improving the efficacy of direct interventions.
6. Strengthening of the mind-body interaction, leading to successful hypnotic treatment of such physical problems as pain and skin diseases.
7. A heightening of clients' willingness to follow the directions of the clinician and surrender a degree of their own initiative.
8. Increased affective intensity, allowing more access to repressed or defended emotions.
9. A stronger rapport between clinician and client, resulting in a closer working relationship.

Although she admits that these nine are not necessarily inclusive, she states they may serve some clinical usefulness.

Hypnosis and Other Psychological Treatments

Modern hypnotherapy originally flourished in the psychoanalytic school. As new theories of dysfunction and psychotherapy emerged, however, hypnosis was blended with these therapeutic approaches more and more frequently. With today's movement toward a more flexible and eclectic therapy style, hypnosis has been combined with a number of distinct models of therapy, including rational emotive therapy (RET) and cognitive-behavioral therapy.

Hypnosis and RET

Albert Ellis's Rational Emotive Therapy (RET) has been used with hypnotherapy in several ways. Stanton (1989) described using a hypnotic induction and suggestions based on RET in his work with high school teachers who wished to reduce their levels of stress. The subjects showed a marked decrease in stress measures at the end of the study and at a twelve-month follow-up. In this case, RET was the main focus of the treatment, with hypnosis used as the medium by which the intervention was carried out.

Another combination of hypnosis and RET was described by DeRoos and Johnson (1983). This paper, which discussed several obstacles encountered by some individuals using RET, used hypnosis as a means to enhance the effects of RET. The authors stated that hypnosis helps clients with problems such as resistance to treatment, easy distractibility, and excessive anxiety.

Hypnosis and Cognitive-Behavioral Therapy

Hypnosis has commonly been used in conjunction with behavioral and cognitive-behavioral therapy (Golden, Dowd, and Friedberg, 1987). Hypnosis is seen to potentiate behavioral therapy chiefly through strengthening such variables as credibility of treatment and the client's expectation of success.

Risks in Hypnotherapy

As with any other form of psychotherapy, hypnotherapy carries the risk of negative effects if used incorrectly or without proper planning and insight. An extreme example described by Haberman (1987) involved a psychotic male patient who was treated with hypnosis for relief from erectile dysfunction. A lay hypnotist (who provides a strong testimonial for requiring more training, not to mention common sense, to do hypnotherapy) gave him a posthypnotic suggestion that the thought of performing oral sex on females would lead to arousal. Although this treatment did result in improvement of his physical condition, intrusive, repetitive thoughts of performing oral sex on women led to increased anxiety and obsessional rumination—not surprising, since due to severe facial mutilation from a prior suicide attempt, the man had no tongue.

Anxiety

Uses of Hypnotherapy with Anxiety

The anxiety disorders are a popular target for hypnotic intervention (Meyer, 1992). From an overall perspective, there are three major ways in which hypnosis has typically been used to treat the various anxiety disorders. The first is the use, under hypnosis, of relaxation and systematic desensitization. The relaxation and focusing of concentation inherent in hypnotic trance are diametric opposites to the tension and out-of-control feelings common to those suffering from anxiety. For example, a client suffering from a simple phobia who finds it difficult to face even the mildest form of an anxiety-provoking stimulus can often use hypnosis to relax to the point of enduring the feared stimulus so desensitization can successfully proceed.

The second common method is the use of hypnosis with cognitive restructuring, following the theory of cognitive therapy. In this case, the clinician conducts the basic work of cognitive therapy with the patient in a hypnotic state. This is done by suggesting replacement cognitions for irrational thoughts while the client is in trance, thereby intensifying the impression of the new thoughts on the client's mind.

Finally, hypnosis may be used to uncover the sources of anxiety and stress and allow direct interventions to be directed at these targets. For example, a client whose anxiety has resulted from a traumatic experience she has repressed from conscious memory can use hypnosis to break through the defenses protecting the memory. In this case, the clinician can direct the client through an age regression to reexperience the original trauma and thereby make it accessible to working through in a nontrance state (Golden, Dowd, and Friedberg, 1987).

Phobias

Phobias are patterns in which chronic avoidance behavior is combined with an irrational fear of a particular object or situation. A classic phobia is disproportionate, disturbing, disabling, and marked by a response to a discrete stimulus (Meyer, 1992). Treatment is focused on learning to experience the stimulus with reduced anxiety and being able to function normally in its presence. Kelly (1984) demonstrated that phobic subjects scored highly on three measures of hypnotizability, providing evidence that they may be particularly good candidates for hypnotherapy. Given this evidence, it is not surprising that the literature includes a large number of reports of successful hypnotic treatment of individuals suffering from phobias (Bodden, 1991; Sarbin, 1991; McGuiness, 1984; Seif, 1982; Van Dyke and Harris, 1982).

Ego-State Reframing. Several theories of the etiology of phobias underlie distinctly different treatment methods using hypnosis. Stanton (1986) describes a technique called ego-state reframing in which the clinician uses hypnosis to communicate with the part of the client's mind that is responsible for the target behavior. This technique is based on a theory that posits the existence of a number of different ego states within a client, each with its own desires and motivations and each pulling the client to behave in a different way. Treating a phobic process from this perspective involves contacting the ego state responsible for the behavior, discerning the motivation for the behavior, and finding alternative, adaptive behaviors to replace the problematic patterns. An example of this treatment follows.

> Jack was a thirty-eight-year-old single male with a moderately severe case of acrophobia, the fear of heights, which stemmed from a childhood experience of falling from a treehouse, which resulted in multiple fractures and a fear that he was dying. For a number of years, he had been aware of the condition, but as it caused him no difficulty to avoid high places, he had ignored it. Three months before he came for treatment, he had met a young woman, and they had become romantically involved. This woman had a hobby that caused some conflict in the relationship: she enjoyed hang gliding and wished Jack to share this activity with her. Jack wanted to participate.
>
> Treatment started with a standard induction and proceeded on to establishing communication with the ego state responsible for the phobic behavior. This was accomplished following Stanton's (1986) procedure: by Jack's asking if the "part of me that controls my avoiding heights will communicate with me now." Usually some physical or affective sign is forthcoming; Jack felt a tingling sensation in his hands. This was confirmed by asking the ego state to repeat the sign if it indeed meant "yes." Once this was accomplished, a sign for "no" (a tingling in the feet) was established in the same manner.
>
> At this point, Jack asked the ego state directly to reveal the purpose of the phobic behavior to his conscious mind, saying, "Will you tell me why you are keeping me afraid of heights, what you're trying to do for me with this?" Because he already knew what the causal event was, it was no surprise that the purpose that "came to him" was linked to his terrifying experience as a child: the control-

ling ego state told him that it was keeping him safe from such dangers. If the ego state does not provide an answer, it may be necessary to repeat this process at a later time or to approach the process more gradually.

Once the reason for the phobia was confirmed, the next step was to generate alternate behaviors. Again, the ego state was asked to go to work—in this case, to help generate ideas for behaviors that would accomplish the purpose of keeping Jack safe while still allowing him to experience the pleasures of hang gliding. Several alternatives were generated, including educating himself about the safety procedures involved in the sport and learning what weather conditions were the safest for gliding.

When the alternatives were defined, the ego state was asked if it would be responsible for activating them when appropriate, just as it had activated the acrophobia in the past. A "yes" signal was received and repeated for confirmation. If this agreement is not received, it is necessary to bargain for a trial period of several weeks, which usually produces a "yes" response. As a final check, Jack then asked if there was any other ego state that objected to the new behaviors. There were none; if there had been, it would have been necessary to repeat the process with the new ego state (Stanton, 1986).

If a second ego state had responded with a "yes" signal at this point, the clinician would have had Jack ask this state what purpose it was serving in maintaining the symptoms. If the reason revealed was the same as that initially discovered, the clinician could give this second ego state the same responsibilities as the first in an attempt to improve functioning. If a second purpose emerged, the process of having the ego state brainstorm alternate behaviors would be repeated, and it would be charged with implementing them at the appropriate times, just as the first ego state was assigned to find and utilize ways to keep Jack safe from the "dangers" of heights.

Stanton admits that this process may stretch the belief of many clinicians. He defends his intervention by noting that his experience has shown most clients to be quite open to this explanation of their behavior and also noting that whether the theoretical constructs here truly exist or not, they serve their purpose by acting as a useful framework for an effective intervention.

Systematic Desensitization. A more direct and less counterintuitive approach to the hypnotic treatment of phobias is based on the relaxation aspects of hypnosis, using trance to enhance a systematic desensitization type of treatment (Wolpe, 1958). The client is taught systematic relaxation and gradually is exposed to the fear-evoking stimulus, using the relaxation skills to decrease the discomfort associated with the stimulus until the fear is extinguished. Hypnosis is used to potentiate the relaxation, to add imagery to the relaxation process, or to view how pleasant the future will be without the phobia to limit activities (a case of progression rather than regression).

This intervention can be used more easily with a resistant or skeptical client than the ego-state reframing technique (Seif, 1982). Seif describes how the induction and suggestions can be reframed as "simple relaxation" or imagining a peaceful scene. For example, a client who balks at the idea of hypnosis will often be more agreeable to using visual imagery to relax. By imagining a favorite location and picturing himself or herself relaxing in this setting, the client may pass into a trance state and find the desensitization more effective without going through a formal induction. This is valuable for use with clients with issues of control or who have negative stereotypes about hypnosis.

One young woman who steadfastly refused to have anything to do with the "mumbo-jumbo, voodoo stuff" she saw as the basis of hypnosis readily agreed to work with guided imagery. The clinician asked her about memories of favorite places and discovered that she had spent many enjoyable vacations at a resort on the gulf coast of Florida. Visualizing herself on the beach at this resort and concentrating on the peaceful, secure feelings she had felt there, the client achieved a deep state of relaxation and was able to work rapidly through a hierarchy of her feared situation—in this case, thunderstorms. Neither she nor the clinician mentioned the word *hypnosis* again, but they were both pleased with her progress in what appeared to the clinician to be a moderately deep trance state.

Psychodynamic Therapy. A third approach to the treatment of phobias with hypnosis follows traditional psychodynamic theory. In this method, hypnosis is used to accomplish age regression and uncover the cause of the phobia, which is assumed to be based in a traumatic event in the past. This approach, with some variation, has been used to treat fears of insects (Domangue, 1985), the dark (Lamb, 1985), hypodermic needles (Nugent, Carden, and Montgomery, 1984), and even mayonnaise (Van Dyke and Harris, 1982).

With this method, a standard induction and regression to the age of trauma is used. When the age of interest has been reached, the client is encouraged to relate the experience to the clinician, both while in trance and afterward.

A classic example of this method is in the case of adult survivors of child abuse. Although the actual incidents of abuse may be repressed and not accessible to the client's conscious mind, the effects of the trauma may still be profound. Using age regression, possibly coupled with relaxation to make the remembering itself less traumatic, the clinician can help the client to relive the abusive experience. From this point, exploration and interpretation of the experience are conducted, using further hypnotic sessions to allow exploration of the unconscious for hidden associations between the initial event and the phobic behavior, if necessary. After this point, treatment continues within the standard framework of psychodynamic theory.

Obsessions

Obsessions, whether as a symptom of obsessive-compulsive disorder (OCD) or some other psychological disturbance, are usually difficult to treat. Hypnosis has been used as an adjunctive treatment for obsessional thinking in several ways.

Systematic Desensitization. A variation of systematic desensitization treatment using hypnosis was reported by Taylor (1985). His client, an eighteen-year-old woman, described recurring intrusive thoughts of knives and cutting her father's face. Taylor used a television screen image in trance and had the client visualize a beautiful field of flowers, which was employed to teach relaxation and decreased psychomotor arousal. He then had the woman visualize a split screen; on one half, the flowers appeared, while the image of a knife appeared simultaneously on the other half. By concentrating on the flowers, the woman learned to relax in the presence of the knife image. As the image of the knife became less and less threatening, her obsessional thoughts gradually decreased.

Taylor's intervention used the pairing of the anxiety-provoking stimulus (the knife) with relaxation to lead to a decrease in negative thoughts. Hence, the structure of the treatment followed the paradigm of systematic desensitization (Wolpe, 1958), with the addition of the hypnotic imagery to strengthen and expedite the relaxation training.

Self-Esteem Enhancement. Another approach to treating obsessions involves the use of hypnosis to strengthen a weakness a client perceives in himself or herself that leads to the obsession. Johnson and Hallenbeck (1985) describe such a case involving a female client with obsessive fears of being in danger. The fears were not rational in their degree or focus and had led to years of rituals in an attempt to stave off the imagined threats.

The authors framed the client's problem as a lack of self-confidence and a feeling of weakness or lack of efficacy. Hence, their treatment involved instilling a sense of power in her that would counteract the fears. This was accomplished by using guided imagery in which she experienced several power fantasies, including flying, skillfully riding a large, white horse, and finding and wielding a magic power source. For example, the last fantasy might involve the client's undertaking a perilous journey, overcoming many dangers and difficulties along the way, and entering at last into a castle where she finds and claims a magic amulet or stone that is both protective and gives her powers and confidence far beyond that she believes she now has. Simultaneously, the direct suggestion was made that she would gradually and imperceptibly become more powerful as an adult woman. The images were also blended with relaxation exercises. In this way, the clinician succeeded in helping reduce the obsessions without fostering feelings of incompetence and dependency in the client (Johnson and Hallenbeck, 1985).

In a paradoxical approach, one can provide a type of antidotal mantra, such as "letting go" or "change calms me" and ask the client to repeat it (a task obsessives take to with relish):

> *Therapist:* Let the word(s) repeat themselves in your mind. Feel the word(s) stroke you as with a feather. As the word(s) strokes you softly, you slip deeper and deeper into this focused, relaxed state. The word(s) becomes part of yourself—you accept it—let it become a part of your being, and start to live it . . .

Panic Attacks

Panic attacks apparently respond to treatments involving hypnosis much in the same way as other anxiety disorders. Hypnosis is used as an adjunct treatment to increase the effects of the main therapeutic modality, such as RET (Der and Lewington, 1990) or chemotherapy. In this study, the trance state was used to teach relaxation, imagery, and the A-B-C-D-E theory of Albert Ellis (1962). The client used the television screen technique to examine unpleasant experiences from a safe emotional distance, allowing the relatively rapid use of RET to challenge and alter the irrational cognitions leading to her panic attacks.

After induction into a hypnotic state, the client was asked to visualize a peaceful, secure place where she could be safe and was led through progressive relaxation. She then visualized a television screen on which she viewed an incident she had experienced that had resulted in negative feelings. She was to see herself in the situation on the screen rather than to reexperience it directly, thereby allowing her to remain at a safe distance and avoid the intense negative affect associated with the experience.

At this point RET was used to show her the irrational components of her thoughts and her self-defeating behaviors. The A-B-C-D-E paradigm (A = situation, B = cognition, C = emotional response, D = physiological response, and E = behavioral response) was implemented by identifying the components in her thoughts and tendencies that were irrational and allowing her to see and understand the dysfunctional elements therein. This was followed by a second "visit" to her scene of relaxation.

When she had regained her condition of calm and relaxation, she was instructed to revisualize the stressful scene, this time inserting more rational thoughts about it and eliminating the self-defeating factors present earlier. For example, she could be guided into more realistically evaluating the possibility of dying or "going crazy" in the stressful situations. This allowed her to confront the threatening situation with less anxiety and to challenge her own irrational and self-defeating tendencies, leading ultimately to a reduction in her symptoms of panic.

Stress

A common complaint today is that of excess stress in a client's life. Whether this complaint refers to something as formal as the symptoms of a generalized anxiety disorder or to an overall feeling of being overwhelmed by the pressures of life, the client is likely to request help in the form of regaining control and a feeling of security in life.

Hypnosis is a valuable tool in the treatment of stress (Golden, Dowd, and Friedberg, 1987). The relaxation and focusing of attention in hypnotic induction act to counter the discomfort of stress. Further, hypnotic treatment has been shown to be an effective intervention for stress in experimental studies.

One study compared the effectiveness of hypnotic suggestions, waking suggestions, and passive relaxation in treating stress experienced by medical students (Palan and Chandwani, 1989). Suggestions designed to strengthen the students' self-images and improve their study habits were made, including such suggestions as that their interest in and motivation to study would increase, their concentration would improve, their memory for the relevant material would improve, and they would have less anxiety when facing examinations. The researchers found that the students in all conditions showed a significant increase in motivation to study but that only the students in the hypnosis group reported a signifiant improvement in such well-being variables as general health, sleep, pleasant mood, and self-confidence.

A case example may serve to clarify the procedures useful for treating stress.

Julie was a twenty-one-year-old college student who requested treatment for complaints of decreased concentration, increased subjective anxiety, and difficulty sleeping. She reported that she was working thirty hours each week at a telephone sales job while carrying a full load of classes, some of which required extensive library research and other out-of-class time commitments. A recent illness had put her behind in her classwork and raised doubts in her own mind about her ability to succeed in school. This self-induced pressure served to frustrate even further her attempts to catch up with her work.

Julie's case was conceptualized as a need to regain her self-confidence and learn more effective ways to manage her heavy work load. Organization and study skills were the first focus of treatment, using a cognitive-behavioral approach to overcome her newly emerged doubts about her ability to perform as she had in the past. Simultaneously, her therapist used hypnosis to teach her relaxation skills to use when she felt "stressed out" and unable to concentrate.

Hypnosis was introduced using a systematic relaxation induction that allowed Julie to feel and recognize the experience of a nonstressful state. Because she named test situations and long stretches at work as peak stress times, Julie was also taught to relax without using a formal induction, so she could apply this technique to these more public situations.

While Julie was in the trance state, her therapist asked her to visualize a situation wherein she felt powerful and in control of everything around her. Julie described being in the role of an air traffic controller, guiding huge jets safely in and out of a busy airport, coordinating a potentially chaotic flow of planes in an organized, efficient manner. Rush hours, conflicting demands, difficult decisions about priorities, and other stressors were all seen as manageable and nonthreatening.

Using this self-designed image, the therapist had Julie identify each of the stressors in her life as a plane in her imaginary airport. Instead of the names of airlines, Julie soon described a scene of jumbo jets labeled "Homework," "Research," "Quality Control Supervisor," and other stressful constructs in her life. Each "airplane" was focused on in turn. With the clinician's help, Julie would imagine situations wherein the stressor demanded immediate and full attention. For example, her plane labeled "Supervisor" demanded that all the other planes be cleared from the airfield, mirroring the demands for all of her time and energy that Julie felt from her supervisor at work. In this scenario, Julie was able to maneuver this plane skillfully around and through the other planes and bring it safely to its hangar.

This treatment continued for several weeks. Each time Julie reported a new or particularly difficult stressor in her life, her therapist had her practice shuttling the corresponding plane through takeoffs and landings, taxiways and hangars, until she felt confident in her ability to control it. He invented scenarios that required her to develop and describe solutions: "Your main runway has three planes jockeying for takeoff position at once. What are you going to do?" In this case, Julie assessed the size of each plane (the magnitude of each problem), the passengers aboard (the other people in her life involved in the situation), and the value of the cargo (the importance of each task) and reported her solution: "Term Paper is given clearance for immediate takeoff. Work Schedule will taxi up behind it and wait for further instructions. Daily Reading will remain behind for the next available opening in outgoing traffic."

After eight weekly sessions, Julie and her therapist agreed to terminate treatment. Julie reported being caught up with her work and no longer intimidated by her responsibilities. She had found ways to schedule her responsibilities that not only let her complete them successfully but gave her time to pursue a more active social life, which she had previously thought "I just can't fit in."

Julie's case was relatively smooth and uncomplicated. She had the imagination to create a helpful image that could be directly applied to her problems and the motivation to carry through with her work in therapy. More difficult cases, however, can still be approached using the basic form described here. As with all other hypnotic treatment, constructing the intervention to the client's specific situation is of paramount importance.

Posttraumatic Stress Disorder

The clinical picture of posttraumatic stress disorder (PTSD) is a complex one, including such symptoms as reexperiencing the traumatic event through memories, dreams, or flashbacks; avoiding potentially threatening stimuli by social withdrawal or decreased memory and/or affect; and symptoms of increased physiological arousal common to all anxiety disorders (Meyer, 1992; Kingsbury, 1988).

Given this complicated pattern of complaints, the focus of treatment for PTSD depends on which symptoms are the most distressing for an individual client. The hypnosis literature describes the treatment of recurring dreams (Eichelman, 1985), hypersensitivity to olfactory stimuli (Monaghan, 1985), exaggeration of the startle response (Mutter, 1987), as well as the common focus on generalized anxiety among other symptom clusters.

Specific treatment techniques for PTSD vary depending on the symptom(s) of major focus. Kingsbury (1988) divides the common symptoms of PTSD into two groups. He labels the first group denial symptoms and describes these as featuring defensive characteristics such as amnesia and social withdrawal. The second group is labeled intrusive and includes images such as flashbacks and dreams.

Treatment of denial symptoms generally involves cathartic techniques such as age regression to reexperience the trauma. Examples of this technique are described by MacHovec (1985). In his cases, clients remember abusive or otherwise threatening situations that occurred anywhere from one week to twenty years prior to the treatment. In one example, a twenty-seven-year-old man with severe anxiety underwent age regression to seek the source of his disorder. Upon returning to the age of seven, he reexperienced an episode in which his mother punished him by putting him in a yard with a flock of chickens. The birds aggressively pecked the boy's feet and legs, bloodying them and sending him into a state of terror. When his mother returned, she showed no sympathy and ignored his feelings. After recalling this incident, he was able to vent the emotions connected with it and experienced a rapid reduction in his anxiety and improvement in his social functioning. Several treatment modalities were used concurrently and subsequently with the hypnotherapy, but it appeared that the hypnosis was the key to his uncovering the block to previous treatment.

Intrusive symptoms, on the other hand, are best treated with interventions of transformation, by which the frightening experiences are reframed in a way that allows the client to achieve mastery of the memories. A case example will be used to illustrate this technique.

Pat was a thirty-nine-year-old, unemployed veteran of the Vietnam War. Formerly a sergeant in the Marine Corps, he received several commendations for bravery in combat, including the Bronze Star. During his tour of duty, he spent most of his time with a unit that conducted frequent reconnaissance missions into enemy-controlled territory. Much praised by his commanding officer, Pat prided himself on being a resourceful and reliable field leader.

During one mission, Pat's squad was ambushed by a group of North Vietnamese guerrillas. Pinned down by enemy fire, he was unable to escape the area himself and was helpless to assist his fellow soldiers. He witnessed the slaughter of his friends without being able to do anything to stop it.

After his discharge, Pat was unable to cope with any situation involving decisions that affected other workers. He lost several jobs requiring supervisory work because he could not trust himself to make decisions, regardless of how innocuous they might be, about his co-workers. At the same time, he was plagued with nightmares in which he relived his experience in the ambush, along with a number of other dreams in which he found himself helpless to avert a certain disaster. A Veterans' Admininstration social worker referred him to a hypnotherapist for therapy.

The therapist quickly identified Pat's feelings of loss of competence as a key issue. Pat seemed obsessed with his failure to find a way to save his comrades and viewed this as a sign that he would never again be competent in any situation. Challenging this belief was a formidable task, as he firmly and repeatedly stated that the squad had been his responsibility and their deaths rested on his shoulders alone. This belief was so strongly embedded in Pat's mind that he was unable to hear any of the alternative views of the incident that the therapist suggested.

Consequently, the therapist decided to use hypnosis to get Pat past the overwhelming guilt and self-blame he felt so he could consider more reasonable assessments of the cause of the traumatic experience. A sample of this process is as follows:

Therapist (T): Pat, you've told me you're sure that your friends died because of you. I don't think it's that simple. What I'd like to do is help you to look back at that time in a way that will help us both understand just what happened and why.

Pat (P): I think you're wasting your time. I appreciate you trying to make me feel better, but that doesn't change what I did. But if you want to try, let's try.

After inducing trance, the therapist first worked to get Pat to recall the general experience of his time in combat: describing different tasks each man had, how the missions normally turned out, and the feelings that went with a successful mission. As Pat described the day-to-day routine, it became apparent that his feelings of complete responsibility were not reflections of the actual working of the group. He was one member of a well-constructed team in which each member had to rely on the others for safety in the field.

The therapist pointed this out to Pat, who was initially resistant to such a conclusion. Using hypnotic suggestions, the therapist worked on restructuring Pat's cognitions to reflect the reality of the situation more accurately.

T: You said you had to keep rechecking your squad's scouting reports yourself. Why was that?

P: I kept finding mistakes. They weren't big ones . . . but if they were screwing up on anything, how could I trust what they said?

T: So it sounds like you had far more pressure on you than you were supposed to. You were carrying more responsibility than a squad leader was supposed to have. I don't think anyone could keep up that kind of vigilance day after day.

P: But I had to! It was my job!

T: Pat, I think you were trying to do your job and everyone else's as well. I think *they* let *you* down.

As Pat described more and more memories that supported this accurate view, his self-criticism and despair changed to a deep sadness for the loss of his friends. He reported extremely painful feelings of emptiness and abandonment following the tragedy and eventually came in touch with feelings of anger with his squad members for not being as conscientious as he was and being caught in the enemy's trap as a result.

Pat was shocked by his anger and felt guilty when it initially emerged. With further help from the therapist, he discovered that it had been easier to blame himself than to feel the anger he had toward his dead comrades. With the emergence of this anger and subsequent working through it, Pat was able to reevaluate his own competency in a more objective light and began to regain his self-esteem and confidence.

Conversion Disorders

The conversion disorders, formerly referred to as hysterical neuroses, represent a type of disorder that has fit well with the traditional psychoanalytic theory of hypnotherapy since the time of Freud. Characterized by a loss or alteration of physical functioning with no apparent cause, conversion disorders are thought to be the result of a psychological stressor that leads to the physical symptom in an unconscious effort to relieve the psychic pressure without directly acknowledging the cause of the stress.

Treatment

The use of hypnosis in treating conversion disorders generally takes one of two approaches. The first is exploration, in which age regression is used to uncover the cause of the disturbance. This approach is used by analytic hypnotists. A second, and much simpler, approach is that of symptom reduction. In this approach, posthypnotic suggestions are made that the person will no longer suffer the relevant symptoms. Although it is disarmingly simple and obvious, success has been reported with its use (Van Dyck and Hoogduin, 1989).

Diagnosis

Another use of hypnosis with conversion disorders is in assisting with diagnosis. When a question exists as to the organic or functional nature of a disorder, hypnosis may be used to help with the diagnostic decision (McCue and McCue, 1988).

The approach used is to induce trance in the client and compare his or her ability to function under hypnosis to the ability to function in the waking state. A client with a one-sided paralysis thought to be of psychogenic origin can be hypnotized and given suggestions that there is actually more function on the affected side than he or she realizes. For example, the clinician can suggest to the client in trance, "You feel stronger than you have since your illness began [accident occurred]. Your mind has the power to move your left foot. I want you to show me now how you can move it just slightly."

This cannot rule out a conversion disorder, of course, but it can rule out such conditions as paralysis due to neurological damage to the motor cortex. McCue and McCue (1988) also note that this technique can be useful in testing for malingering; if the client is convinced that hypnosis can overcome organic deficits, he or she may show abilities under trance that are not apparent in the waking state.

Specific techniques for working with a classic conversion disorder are illustrated in this case.

Thomas was a married man in his late thirties with several children. He presented with complaints of weakness in his hands that interfered with his work as a plumbing contractor. Thorough physical and neurological examinations turned up no organic cause for the weakness and no history of trauma evident.

Upon taking a personal history, the clinician involved in Thomas's case discovered that Thomas had a history of psychiatric treatment for obsessional thinking, dating back to the birth of his first child, that focused on fears of not being able to fulfulll what he saw as his responsibilities to his family. Particularly disturbing to him was the inconsistent flow of work he received as a result of the normal fluctuations in the building industry. As this area was explored in therapy, Thomas revealed a persistent fear that he would not be able to support his family financially, despite the fact that he had done so for approximately fifteen years.

Concurrently with this therapy, the clinician used hypnosis in an attempt to remove the symptom of manual weakness. He made direct suggestions that Thomas would slowly begin to regain strength in his hands and had him visualize working at his job with skill and confidence. Although Thomas showed some increase in hand strength during periods of hypnosis, this effect did not generalize outside treatment. Feeling that further efforts in this direction would be futile, the clinician suggested that hypnosis be used to regress Thomas to the period when his obsessive fear began.

Subsequently the therapist induced trance and began a standard age regression technique. He directed Thomas to "go back in time and space to a time when you feel confident about your abilities. You're going back, back through time, getting younger and stronger." This took a surprisingly (to the clinician) long time; for the first three sessions in which this technique was used, Thomas never reported finding such a time. On the fourth attempt, he finally identified a time of security when he was three years old. After allowing Thomas to fix this point in time thoroughly in his mind, the therapist directed him to "come forward in time and space to a time when you first learned that responsibilities were scary things." Thomas identified a scene when he was four or five years old in which he overheard his father tell his mother that he had been fired and did not know if he would be able to find work again. His mother reacted with panic, and Thomas relived the fear of seeing his mother in a vulnerable, weak condition that frightened him very much.

After returning Thomas to the present and bringing him out of the hypnotic state, the therapist questioned him about the incident and found that he had had no memory of it before the hypnotic episode. Further exploration of the incident in waking sessions convinced Thomas and his therapist that this was the cause of his obsessions.

Several months of additional therapy followed in which Thomas explored his thoughts and feelings about his responsibilities and his fears of what could happen to his family if he "failed" them. Since it became apparent that a large part of his fear involved being rejected by his wife and children, the therapist, with Thomas's agreement, conducted several sessions of family therapy. In these sessions, Thomas was able to voice his fears to his family and was greatly relieved when they reassured him that they would love and respect him regardless of his success in the business world. With his anxiety lessened, Thomas gradually improved his self-confidence and trust in his own abilities, and to his delight he found the strength returning to his hands.

The therapist concluded that Thomas's disorder was a defense against what was to him a very real threat that he would be found a less than acceptable husband and father. By experiencing his fear as a physical weakness, Thomas could deny responsibility for his failure to support his family. After all, he wanted to work hard; he simply was not physically able. When Thomas had reexperienced and worked through the initial fear-causing situation, the threat of a similar problem happening to him no longer felt inevitable, and he was able to return to work.

This case illustrates the flexibility needed in the use of hypnotic treatment. When one approach failed, the therapist shifted the focus of treatment to uncover and resolve the block and thence work effectively to return Thomas to a functional state.

Sexual Dysfunction

> Drink, sir, is a provoker of three things: Marry, sleep, urine, and
> nose-painting. Lechery it provokes and unprovokes; it provokes the
> desire but takes away the performance.
> —William Shakespeare, *Macbeth*

Masters and Johnson (1970) set the standard for treatment of these conditions with their approach that combines cognitive, relationship, and behavioral components. Hypnosis can serve as a valuable adjunct to these interventions (Morgan, et al, 1992).

Golden, Dowd, and Friedberg (1987) identify four situations when the use of hypnosis is appropriate in treating sexual dysfunctions: (1) if the client spontaneously requests hypnotic treatment, (2) if the client is receptive to the idea of hypnotherapy when offered by the therapist, (3) when a high level of anxiety appears to be a factor in the problem, (4) when the client appears to have a problem with negative or insufficient positive sexual imagery. On a more practical note, hypnosis is also indicated when an individual comes to therapy alone and couples work is not possible.

Of these criteria, the first two are true of any case that potentially involves hypnosis. The last two represent areas that hypnosis is particularly well suited to address; the uses of hypnosis with anxiety have already been described, as has the ability of hypnosis to potentiate the effects of imagery.

Diagnosis

Hypnosis can be used in several ways to treat sexual dysfunctions. First, it can be a valuable diagnostic tool, useful in uncovering factors that cause or maintain sexual problems. In this role, age regression can be used as described in the section on conversion disorders to identify, and eventually to work through, the initial stressful event that led to the dysfunction.

Treatment

Hypnosis can be used with suggestions that increase the client's overall confidence and self-esteem or that work toward direct symptom removal. Direct suggestions are appropriate in this situation to restructure the client's cognitive self-appraisal and improve self-image. For example, if a man suffers erectile dysfunction as a result of an image of himself as weak and ineffectual, hypnosis as an adjunct to cognitive therapy can assist in building a more positive picture of his strengths and positive attributes. Hypnosis can also work to reduce anxiety and other emotional conflicts that block successful sexual relationships.

Hypnosis can be used to increase sexual desire in the case of disorders of inhibited desire or to decrease desire in cases of premature ejaculation.

For example, with a client presenting reduced sexual desire, the therapist can use imagery to help the client fantasize what a truly enjoyable, successful sexual encounter would be like, suggesting, "You find yourself thinking about your lover's body and how it will look and feel, knowing you will soon be lost in completely satisfying sensations." By building the client's ability to fantasize, sexual desire can be increased (Golden, Dowd, and Friedberg, 1987).

Techniques used in the hypnotic treatment of sexual dysfunction include enriching cognitive-behavioral treatments by the use of cognitive restructuring of negative sexual thoughts and beliefs (Araoz, 1983) and the use of Eriksonian metaphors in directed imagery (Gilmore, 1987). This latter technique involves an indirect approach to treating the dysfunction since Erikson believed that unconscious resistance would thwart any direct efforts. This method therefore uses metaphors or stories whose dynamics parallel those of the client, thereby allowing the conscious mind to hear them as nonthreatening while the unconscious mind works with them.

An example of this technique would be to hypnotize a female client suffering from orgasmic dysfunction and relate a story of a woman who knows a song capable of bringing great pleasure to those who hear it. The song has not been sung, yet it is well known to those closest to the woman that she has it in her possession, and these people grieve that it cannot be released and shared with them. The delight of the people when the woman finally sings the song and their adoration and gratitude toward her for sharing her gift is described in lavish detail. Erikson's theory would predict that the client's unconscious would hear and interpret the story and consequently work to release the "song" from its bondage.

Crasilneck (1982) described great (indeed, almost unbelievable) success with males suffering erectile dysfunction using direct suggestion that they could control the erection of their penises. He hypnotized them and demonstrated hypnotic catalepsy of one arm, having them feel the rigidity arm with the unaffected limb. He then emphasized that this powerful control could be equally effective with the penis. He explained the psychology and physiology of erection and repeatedly suggested that they had the power to control this reaction. This could be done by suggesting, "Feel how strong and powerful your arm is, and realize that all of your body is under your control, just like this rigid and powerful arm. Your mind has the ability to make your penis erect and strong and unbending, just like this arm." Using this technique, Crasilneck reported a success rate of 87 percent.

Two studies of women suffering from orgasmic dysfunction conclude that hypnosis is most successful with this population when age regression techniques to uncover causal dynamics are used rather than using direct suggestions (Obler, 1982; Steward, 1986). This differs from the findings of Masters and Johnson (1970), suggesting once again that careful assessment of the dynamics of each client is vital to planning and implementing an effective hypnotherapy. The following case study demonstrates a number of these prior techniques and issues.

James was a twenty-eight-year-old male who came to treatment complaining of an inability to maintain an erection during hetero-sexual contact. His history showed a late-blooming interest in girls during his school years and a general shyness and insecurity in dating and opposite-sex relationships.

The first several sessions of therapy were devoted to assessing James's views of men's and women's roles in sexual relationships and how he viewed himself as a sexual person. He revealed that he had been raised in a strict and strongly religious family where sex-ual matters were never mentioned, much less discussed. The only instruction he received from his parents was that "dirty feelings and thoughts" were sinful and should be avoided. Although James de-clared that he had long since rejected his family's religious beliefs and strict values, he admitted he was troubled by guilt over his sexual desires.

This became evident as therapy began, and James became so uncomfortable discussing his wishes and desires that he literally could not concentrate on the process of therapy. Having ascertained that he did indeed want to change this automatic negative response to sexual topics, the therapist began using hypnosis to teach James to relax during discussions of sexual matters.

Concurrently with the relaxation training, the therapist used the hypnotic state to explore James's deep feelings of anxiety and guilt around his sexual feelings. In trance, James reasserted that he had rejected the beliefs of his family about the sinful nature of sexual desires. However, when the therapist asked him, "What do you think of when you feel guilty?" he revealed that he believed his family would know that he disagreed with them and would reject him.

"A part of me that's still real, real little is scared," he told the therapist while under trance. "I don't know what's going to happen to me if my parents find out how I feel." When this fear was discussed in the waking state, James was surprised that "I still feel that way. I didn't realize how much control those old beliefs still have on me."

This revelation led to a change in the therapy. For several ses-sions, James and his therapist discussed his feelings toward his parents and how his need to have their approval as a child had never completely gone away. As he began to understand this and how it affected his life as an adult, James made several attempts to talk to his parents about more innocuous topics on which he knew he and they disagreed. He found that they accepted his views, although they still did not agree with him. At this point, he reported to his therapist that he felt more secure about working on his sexual problems.

When James had reached this point of being able to discuss sex without serious discomfort, the therapist introduced sexual imagery as a nonthreatening way to approach the experience of sexual pleasure. Using a hypnotic desensitization format, James progressed from imagining looking at fully clothed, attractive women to touching them, letting himself be touched, and eventually engaging in oral sex and intercourse. Whenever his guilt would reappear in this process, the relaxation techniques would be reapplied until he felt comfortable enough to continue.

As James became more comfortable with this therapy, homework assignments were added to generalize the effects outside the sessions. He found to his delight that he was able to ask out a woman he had admired for many months and eventually engage in a rewarding relationship with her, including successful sexual activity.

This case illustrates the care that must be taken when using hypnosis in the area of sexual dysfunction. Therapists must be sensitive to their client's values and feelings regarding sexual behavior, even if their purpose is to change these feelings. By letting the therapy move at James's pace, his therapist assured him that he was not "abnormal" or "weird" and allowed him to build self-respect and a sense of pride in his accomplishments.

Another important point in this case is the flexibility of the treatment modalities and even the focus of therapy as new information became available. The therapist realized that to continue working on sexual functioning without addressing the underlying issues of unresolved parent-child roles would be very difficult at best, and he shifted the therapy to address that issue. This once again highlights the use of hypnosis as a tool and a technique rather than a free-standing therapy approach.

11
Hypnotherapy and Psychological Disorders, II

> And indeed there will be time
> To wonder, "Do I dare?' and "Do I dare?"
> —T. S. Eliot, "The Love Song of J. Alfred Prufrock"

Hypnotherapy has considerable therapeutic utility with various psychological problems and disorders. Popular uses of it with major forms of psychopathology discussed in this chapter include applications toward mood disorders, dissociative disorders, especially multiple personality disorder (MPD), psychotic disorders, sexual trauma, and sleep disorders.

Depression

Hypnotherapy has a number of applications with respect to the treatment of mood disorders and depression. It can address what C. Rick Snyder (De Angelis, 1991) refers to as both the "agency" and "pathways" of depression. According to Snyder, hope is the critical antidote to psychological depression, and "agency" refers to the will or energy to set and achieve goals; "pathways" are the means to see and develop the several ways of attaining these goals. More specifically, hypnosis can be used to motivate and energize such clients, reduce phobic anxiety, and facilitate cognitive restructuring. It may also be used as an adjunct for clients with suicidal ideation and those suffering from bereavement.

Motivating clients with psychomotor depression can be facilitated by providing energizing suggestions and imagery. One might energize a client (that is, respond to the "agency" issue) by giving a detailed suggestion of taking a pleasant walk on a spring day:

> *Therapist:* As you relax, picture yourself walking down a path on a pleasant spring day. With each step you take, let yourself feel more energy, more invigorated, draining negative feelings from your body. Feel the warmth of the sun on your skin and the breeze blowing by you. Smell the trees and flowers in bloom as you walk past. Listen to the sound of the breeze

through the trees and the birds chirping as you walk, with each step giving you renewed vigor, energy, and motivation to handle any stressful task before you.

With each step, feel your energy and motivation increase. Let yourself continue walking down the path until you have sufficient renewed energy to return, with the ability to sustain yourself with this energy. When you feel yourself at this state, raise your right index finger. Keep walking down the path, with each step more energy returning. Feel the breeze and smell the flowers, with each step bringing more vigor.

This can be repeated until the client raises a finger, indicating that the goal has been met. Any scenario can be employed, with the scenario ideally chosen based on the individual client's perception of a scene that is found energizing.

Time projection techniques instruct the client to envision himself or herself in the future as more active and feeling better as time progresses, all which are antithetical to depression. The suggestions might include mention of previously enjoyed activities, perhaps before the onset of the depression). These techniques may be taught as an autohypnotic procedure. As an example, the therapist might suggest the following to a depressed client who is a sports fan:

Therapist: Picture yourself six months from now at a ball game with a few friends. Picture the team on the field, and listen to the sounds of the stadium. Feel the excitement and the thrill as your team makes a good play and scores. Notice how good you are allowing yourself to feel as you enjoy the game with your friends. When you begin to come out of the trance, allow yourself to continue to enjoy these feelings of excitement and energy. Let yourself continue to feel the energy as if you were at an enjoyable ball game.

Affect substitution may be used to elevate depressed mood. It is recommended that the suggestions and imagery utilized be maximally pleasant for the client. If this cannot be obtained, it is perhaps best to utilize general or ambiguous suggestions or images. For example, a middle-aged male who is depressed following unemployment, might, following induction, be given the suggestion:

Therapist: Picture yourself doing something you enjoy, something that brings you pleasure and satisfaction. Allow yourself to feel the enjoyment as you watch yourself engaged in this pleasant activity. With each image, let yourself feel the elation and pleasure that comes to you with this activity. As you open your eyes, allow yourself to maintain this feeling of pleasure and satisfaction that is evoked in you.

Cognitive-Behavioral Approaches

Hypnosis may be incorporated into a cognitive-behavioral treatment approach for depression. Hypnosis can be used to identify self-defeating thoughts and foster cognitive restructuring of these maladaptive cognitions. This is typically done in conjunction with other more typical cognitive-behavioral techniques. As an example, to identify self-defeating thoughts generated by criticism from an employer, the following suggestion might be given following induction:

> *Therapist:* Picture yourself with your boss, who is criticizing your work. Listen to the tone of his voice, notice the expression on his face as he criticizes you. Raise one finger if you have this in your mind. [Client raises finger.] Now concentrate on the thoughts that are running through your mind, the thoughts that automatically come into mind as your boss criticizes you and your work. When you have these thoughts in mind, again raise your finger. [Client raises finger.] As these thoughts come into mind, tell me your thoughts. Tell me what you're thinking as you watch and hear your boss criticize you.

Hypnotherapy may be used as a facilitator to restructure nihilistic cognitions, as well as an antianxiety technique in susceptible clients. To continue the example, the client may be given the suggestion to "notice and accept the positive messagees given by your boss. Accept the feelings of pride and accomplishment as you hear the positive messages from other people."

Retructuring nihilistic cognitions might be accomplished by hypnotically inducing the client to focus on positive rather than negative thoughts and messages from others and to increase attention to examination of the evidence upon which negative and self-defeating thoughts are based. The goal is to develop more accurate and less self-defeating cognitions.

For a client who persistently misperceives others as being critical, a posthypnotic suggestion might proceed as follows:

> *Therapist:* As you receive feedback, let yourself automatically examine the meaning of the feedback. Focus on the positive implications of the messages you receive, the good things that it

communicates to you. You may continue to relax, feeling positive about yourself as you hear the positive messages. Continue to let yourself feel more secure, confident, and able to continue to feel secure as the situation passes.

Specific Techniques

Another useful technique is the affect bridge—suggesting that the client recall a previous experience either similar or etiologically related to the current situation. For example, Amy, who shows characterological dysphoria and feelings of abandonment, might be led to recall an earlier or first experience of these feelings. Following induction, the therapist might suggest:

> *Therapist:* Amy, allow these feelings to carry you back to an earlier time when you also felt these emotions, when you felt the feelings of sadness and abandonment. Allow yourself to be carried back, as if on a bridge, and recall these earlier experiences. As these memories return to you, tell them to me. Tell me about these earlier experiences. [Amy begins to describe her first sexual relationship, following which she also felt depressed and abandoned.]

A related technique for uncovering previous experiences is the crystal ball technique, in which the client is told to watch a previous and important event be evoked out of the mists in the ball. Continuing the example:

> *Therapist:* Picture a crystal ball on a pedestal. Watch the mists swirl inside the ball, as if you are watching a thick fog. As you watch the fog, allow it to clear, allowing you to see a vision of the first time you felt abandoned. It may take some time to clear the fog, but as it does, tell me the picture evoked of your first experience of these feelings. [Amy relates watching her father leave, preceding the parents' divorce, during which Amy felt abandoned by the father.]

Therapeutic techniques include abreaction, in which the client is led, following induction, to express and cathart intense emotions. This technique should be utilized with a posthypnotic suggestion to remember only what the client can safely handle and can accept consciously. Other techniques include reframing and relabeling, which involves changing the meanings and labels attached to events. Television screen imaging can be used for depression. The suggestion is made for the client to control the thoughts by changing the channels and adjusting the volume and screen size.

It is important with depressive clients to emphasize internal strengths, give the client choice over the speed of recovery, phrase suggestions in the affirmative, and utilize self-hypnotic techniques to avoid dependency.

Suicidal Ideation

Hypnotherapy can be a useful adjunct in the treatment of suicidal ideation, which often accompanies depression. For Jack, who has been suicidal following a divorce, the therapist might provide a posthypnotic suggestion.

> *Therapist:* As you begin to feel suicidal, let your mind bring forth the image of a strong, safe place. Picture yourself in this safe place, harbored from your suicidal thoughts. Begin to focus on reasons why you don't want to die. (pause) Think of the things you enjoy, which the suicide would prevent you from doing and all the reasons you have to continue living. (pause) Begin to picture yourself doing something you enjoy, and let yourself experience the pleasure you have enjoyed.
>
> Focus on this pleasure and these positive feelings. Let these feelings fill you up, forcing out negative thoughts, forcing out depressed feelings and the desire to kill yourself. Each time you try to evoke this, let it come more quickly and easier as you learn to focus on this in place of your thoughts about killing yourself. Whenver you begin to feel suicidal, relax and think of these positive thoughts and feelings. How do you feel in this safe place, in this harbor from your depression?

The last question is used to gauge how well the client is able to distance himself from the suicidal ideation and the potential success of the posthypnotic suggestion. The posthypnotic suggestion should also be given to contact the therapist immediately should the suggestion be unsuccessful in warding off the desire for suicide.

Bereavement

Hypnotherapy may be used as an adjunct to treat traumatic grief (van der Hart, Brown, and Turco, 1990) by uncovering traumatic memories, neutralizing excessive affect, and substituting positive emotional reactions and imagery in the place of traumatic grief. For example, a client could be given the posthypnotic suggestion that instead of feeling grief, a memory of the beloved might instead induce a peaceful feeling of the belated at rest and at peace, with this peace flowing in the client as well.

van der Hart (1988) discusses an imaginary leave-taking ritual to assist the client to overcome the grief reaction and move on with her life. This includes having the client imagine under hypnosis peacefully confronting symbols of her relationship with the deceased, thereby abreacting the grief and allowing it to be put to rest. These confrontations might include memories of or objects symbolic of the relationship, such as a wedding band or a favorite gift from the deceased. For example:

> *Therapist:* As you relax in a safe, calm place, feeling tranquil and serene, calm and peaceful, begin to think about your deceased husband. Hear your husband give you permission to continue your life, moving forward with the pleasant memories of the times the two of you have shared. (pause) Now picture yourself in the future, performing activities you have previously enjoyed. Let yourself feel the pleasure as you engage in these behaviors, appreciating your husband's permission to continue enjoying your life.

Dissociative Disorders

Another major use of hypnosis is in the diagnosis and treatment of dissociative disorders, particularly MPD (Kluft, 1992; Shapiro, 1991). When working with clients who show dissociative tendencies, the use of a validated assessment scale (Frischolz et al., 1990) is recommended, not only for its diagnostic value but also to specify areas of progress (or lack thereof).

It is widely reported that clients with MPD are highly hypnotizable (Shapiro, 1991; Ross, 1984; Kluft, 1992, 1983), and some suggest that self-hypnosis is the central mechanism of MPD. Although most of the research articles involve case studies, there is some research support for the facilitative effect of psychodynamic psychotherapy and hypnosis on these disorders (Coons, 1986). There is some debate over the ability of hypnosis to foster development of alters, which are personality fragments with unique characteristics, distinct from the primary personality. However, it is important to distinguish between the personality fragments induced by hypnosis and the preexisting alters, the latter of which are relatively stable with fairly complete life histories.

Hypnosis may be used as a relatively rapid method of contacting dissociated aspects of the personality. One may use hypnosis to attempt to contact alters while the client is under hypnosis or use age regression techniques to access situations where alters were used to defend against severely traumatic events. Painful emotions may thus be abreacted, or hypnosis can be used to foster the primary personality's knowledge of the alters and the role they play in the overall personality. Kluft (1992) describes an inpatient program wherein nurses are trained and supervised in using specific techniques, such as ideomotor signalling and "safe place" imagery to work with inpatients with dissociative disorders. (Chapter 8 presents an example of the application of self-hypnotic techniques to an MPD case.)

Examples and Techniques

Examples provided in the literature include Ross (1984), who discusses a case where hypnosis was quickly used to contact an alter personality in a woman with MPD who presented complaining of frequent memory lapses. However, specific techniques used in the case were not discussed. An illustration of the use of hypnosis for an MPD is provided in the case of Diane, a twenty-five-year-old woman in treatment for about three years. Within the course of therapy, a major alter, Renee, is discovered. Whereas Diane is typically mild and shy, Renee emerges in situations requiring confrontational interpersonal interactions. Upon discovery of the alter, the therapist decided to use hypnosis for the purpose of exploration.

Following induction of the primary personality, Diane, the therapist used the following: "Diane, as you relax into a deeper and deeper state, allow that which controls you during your blackouts to temporarily come forward, taking control of your mouth. As this happens, watch and listen comfortably, staying in the deep, calm, and tranquil state you are now in. When you have given up control, raise your finger. Feel the tranquility as you allow that other force to come forward, temporarily taking control of your mouth. Who is coming forward? Who is in control of the mouth now?"

Once contact is made with an alter, the therapist can talk directly to the alter while in trance, allowing exploration of the personality structure and function of the alter. Future attempts may then call directly upon the alter personality to come forth, following induction of the primary personality.

As the therapist aids the primary personality in gaining knowledge of the alters and their role in the personality structure, the therapist aids in fostering reintegration of the alters with the primary personality. For Diane, this might initially involve getting permission from Renee to relinquish control to Diane in confrontational situations. As Diane learns to exert control in these interactions, Renee is enlisted to relinquish control. When addressing these issues with alters, interventions should be framed as being for the benefit of the primary personality. This process should be attempted gradually and may take months or years to come to fruition.

Hypnotic inquiry is also a potential tool to monitor treatment progress benignly. Kluft (1986) discusses this technique to gauge the restructuring of experiences and memories following integration. He asserts that memories and experiences of the alter are restructured into the memory of the primary personality following reintegration. This suggests that hypnotic access to the primary personality's memory may provide an index of the amount of reintegration.

To continue the illustration, Diane is asked, while in trance, the extent to which she is aware of Renee's existence. Inquiry across sessions can aid determination of the extent to which integration is proceeding. Increased awareness of memories experienced while under control of an alter is also an indication of treatment progress. For example, following reports of a blackout, the therapist asks, with the client in trance, "Diane, what do you remember about the blackout? Tell me what you remember happening." The extent of the primary personality's knowledge of events during blackouts is of diagnostic value, particularly as it changes over time.

A number of techniques are available for facilitating reintegration. Several are described in a case study presented by Confer (1984). He discusses using the alters to construct a hierarchy of traumatic situations, which is then used to reduce the intensity of the emotion on the primary personality. Hypnosis was also used to bring the alter and primary personality closer, directly talking to each other. Several seats were provided, with the suggestion given that each alter, when talking, should occupy a different chair. The component personalities were guided, along the lines of couples or group therapy, to express dissatisfactions, negotiate compromises, and express appreciation for each other. This ultimately facilitated reintegration of the alters.

An example, continuing the case illustration, utilizing a number of such techniques (following the induction of a hypnotic trance) is as follows.

Therapist: Diane, this is your seat, this is where you will sit when you talk. Do you understand? And Renee, this is your seat, this is where you will sit when you talk. Do you understand? [At this point, it might be beneficial to verify that each alter follows the directive as stated.]

Now, Diane, tell Renee about what it's like for you when Renee takes control, tell her how it makes you feel. [Diane expresses confusion, feeling scared, and out of control.] Now, Renee, what is your response to Diane? Why do you want to take control? [Renee expresses the desire to protect Diane by more effectively handling uncomfortable situations and protecting her from potentially painful interactions.] Now, Diane, are you willing to practice taking responsibility for the situations Renee has taken responsibility for? [Diane indicates agreement.] Renee, are you willing to let Diane practice taking responsibility for those situations, so Diane can feel relief from her comfort and fright? [Renee hesitantly agrees.] [Since the alter has functioned to protect the primary personality, suggestions are framed as being beneficial for the primary personality.]

Now, Diane, I want you to imagine yourself in a confrontational situation. Picture yourself with the other person, the surrounding environment, and hear the conversation. If you begin to feel uncomfortable, push your panic button, releasing all the stress, tension, and anxiety that builds up. Now, tell me about the situation, tell me about the conversation. [Diane describes an interaction with her landlord, telling him to fix a leaky faucet.]

This process is continued, having Diane role play the interaction, utilizing previously learned coping strategies.

Affect Titration

Due to the intensity of the affect evoked when treating MPDs (and it is a technique that can also be useful with depressives, borderlines, and others), the therapist must be careful in regulating the expression of emotions, both in the session and between sessions. A number of techniques can be used to titrate the client's affect and discomfort. This may be needed depending on the intensity of the affect being expressed and the available resources for modulating these emotions. These techniques are geared to increase the client's perceived mastery over the environment. They include alter substitution, which arranges in advance (through hypnotherapeutic interventions) for another alter to take over during stressful life events. The alter can be "put to sleep" or sent on a fantasy, for example, with the replacement being done with the permission of the replaced alter.

Another method is suggesting that clients push a panic button (developed in imagination) when emotions become too intense. For example, the therapist might suggest that Diane push a panic button that will allow her to relax and thereby inhibit the response that in the past served to mobilize Renee. Diane might be led to practice this by imagining a confrontational situation while in trance and using the panic button to induce relaxation.

The provision of a sanctuary ("safe room" or "secret place" techniques) may be employed and should be hypnotically suggested in such a way as to allow all alters to access the sanctuary in each alter's own way. For example, when all alters are hypnotized, one might place the suggestion of "each of you finding the safe place as you see it, just as it needs to be for you to feel safe. As you approach it, you will each start to relax, feeling comfortable and serene in each of the respective safe places."

Suggestions can also be used to bypass time (perhaps by hypnotically suggesting that emotionally excited alters fall asleep in their safe place until the next therapy session) and bypass affect (for example, keeping painful affect in a locked vault, set to open a few minutes into the next session). Autohypnotic use of these techniques may foster a sense of mastery and control by the patient. The hypnotherapist may want to attenuate affect (to increase recognition and coping of painful affect) or to regulate the flow of affect (by hypnotically suggesting that the affect be experienced as a "slow leak").

Hypnotherapeutic crisis intervention can be an important treatment component with MPDs (Kluft, 1992, 1983). These clients may require crisis intervention during times when high stress exceeds the defenses and coping mechanisms of the primary personality or alters. Factors that predispose MPD clients to an increased need for crisis intervention include masochistic and depressive personality features, lack of social support systems, and limited coping mechanisms. Interventions addressing suicide risks include helping the alter work through the feelings or yield control to an alter more capable of handling the crisis. Depression may be addressed by facilitating controlled abreactions and encouraging inner dialogue. Rejection from social supports may be addressed by facilitating the alters' giving support to one another by initiating a form of internal family therapy.

Amnestic States

Amnestic states, which are diagnostically similar to dissociative states, are also amenable to hypnotherapy. There are numerous case studies of hypnotherapy used with assorted dissociative disorders in the literature, including Eisen (1989) and Kaszniak and associates (1988). The latter case involved autobiographical retrograde amnesia following male rape. Hypnosis initially involved progressive relaxation and mental imagery (an elevator descending floor by floor). Age regression was used to facilitate early memories, such as the subject's first school and the house he lived in. Initial suggestions were provided ambiguously, to allow the client to fill in the memories based on his childhood experiences. Five sessions, which yielded progressively more information, were used to help the client remember the rape that preceded the amnesia. Although the initial recognition was reported to elicit strong emotions, the depression and anger reportedly lessened within ten days.

Eisen (1989) describes a number of interesting techniques. In one case, hypnotically induced imagery was used to establish a solid inner core in an effort to help rebuild the sense of self. This is not unlike the Japanese practice of developing *hara,* a focused point of stability and strength, pictured as a point in one's lower abdomen. While under hypnosis, the client is led to picture a special room in which a strong column represents the core of her own self. She is slowly led to approach the column (over a number of sessions) and gain increasing access to memories contained within. In this particular case, the emergence of a childlike figure in the room is approached by having the primary personality engage in "reparenting" techniques, by providing nurturance, and corrective emotional experiences to the "child-self." A strength in the approach used in this case study is the less active role of the therapist, which allows the client to progress at her own rate. This may also foster a sense of mastery over the recall of forgotten material.

Limitations

There are a number of limitations for the use of hypnosis in the treatment of dissociative disorders, especially MPD, with a partial list following. The importance of diagnostically differentiating MPDs from borderline disorders is stressed by Kluft (1983). For example, using hypnotically retrieved memories with borderlines with hysterical tendencies must be accompanied by an attempt to separate histrionic fantasy from fact. This differential diagnosis might be accomplished by assessing the blackouts, much more common in MPD, or the splitting more commonly observed in borderline clients.

Stress associated with emotionally intense hypnotically facilitated treatments may not be appropriate for older patients (Kluft, 1988). Kluft recommends consideration of the client's mental status and ego functioning and ability to manage severe stress to determine the appropriateness of hypnotherapy for these clients.

Psychotic Disorders

Although typically contraindicated for psychotic disorders, under some circumstances hypnotherapy may be a viable treatment option for both schizophrenic and other psychotic clients. Wilson and associates (1989) discuss the role of hypnosis and age regression as a means to reparent schizophrenics. They describe the treatment as a highly structured autohypnotic regression, though specific techniques used are not provided. Murray-Jobsis (1985, 1991) suggests that hypnosis might be used by the therapist, who may go into trance in order to increase empathy and understanding of the schizophrenic client.

Hypnosis to control a conversion catatonia in an apparent borderline personality disorder is reported by Jensen (1984). The catatonia seemed similar to psychomotor depression, although the apparent lack of control over the symptoms led Jensen to conceptualize the catatonia as a form of conversion.

Hypnosis was induced in the catatonic client by the therapist's offering to help the client relax, with permission being granted with an eye blink. The therapist subsequently began, in a slow monotone, describing the childhood experience of learning to write the alphabet. The therapist suggested that he was "speaking to the unconscious," which would hear the suggestion that the client's hand would imitate writing. When the client slowly started imitating this behavior, the suggestion was given for this ability to move from the client's hand to his mouth, enabling the client to speak. This allowed the therapist to engage the client with more active interventions (including posthypnotic suggestions).

Self-injurious behaviors, common among borderline clients, may be addressed with hypnosis (Malon and Berardi, 1987). These authors suggest that hypnosis be used to counter the depersonalization to the emotional arousal during the self-injurious behaviors. These should be done in order to maximize the client's perceived control over the anxiety and emotional arousal. Malon and Berardi suggest that breath counting and positive imagery preceding the negative behaviors may be used to distract them and to increase relaxation instead of acting out. Uncovering techniques and the affect bridge are used to facilitate working through traumatic memories. The authors also emphasize the importance of a strong and flexible relationship when working with these clients.

Sexual Trauma

There are a number of reports of hypnotherapy used in the context of sexual traumas. A few such cases have already been discussed, involving amnesia following a male rape and a dissociated incestuous relationship.

A technique for controlling excessive affect, previously discussed with respect to dissociative disorders, is illustrated through a thirty-year-old female client I saw, who first sought biofeedback for tension headaches. In the third session, the client volunteered a great detail of history of sexual and emotional abuse, which she reported having never discussed with anybody else. The client continued to relate these experiences over several subsequent sessions, despite attempts to get her to process her thoughts and feelings about the experiences more slowly and its impact on her current functioning.

One potential remedy for such situations involves a posthypnotic suggestion to regulate the flow of affect. This was done by repetitively amplifying the suggestion that "as you feel the pressure to release these emotions, picture the emotions in a sealed container with a pressure release valve on it. You will be able to control the valve, slowly releasing your feelings during the session, in order to discuss them in more depth during the sessions."

Several case studies in which hypnosis was used with victims of rape are presented by Ebert (1988). Techniques used in these cases include those fostering increased perceived power, control, and relaxation responses to stressful situations. The hypnotherapy needs to occur within a supportive psychotherapy relationship to work through trauma associated with the rape in a safe and comfortable environment.

One specific technique Ebert mentioned involved the suggestion that the client find the image that most represented strength to her; this client evoked the image of her grandmother (an early meaningful relationship). The therapist then directed the client to draw needed strength from the grandmother, store it inside her, and make it available when the client needed to feel strong. Additionally, imagery was used to counter the perceptual distortion of men being much larger and more powerful than the client. The imagery technique used allowed the client to perceive herself growing larger and the ominous figure shrinking whenever the client felt intimidated by this percept.

Treatment of a rape victim and her spouse by using conjoint hypnotherapy is reported by Somer (1990). Traditional regression techniques were used to help the woman abreact feelings stemming from the rape. The husband, who was also simultaneously regressed, was directed to assume a position near the scene as the wife described it (floating safely above it). Distance could be modulated depending on the needs of the husband and wife. The husband was given permission to choose between an observational or participational stance and engaged in both positions across sessions. This technique allows incorporation of family members into treatment, which may foster support for the rape victim, clarify misinformation, and allow therapeutic intervention with family members who may also have severe emotional reactions stemming from the rape.

Sleep Disorders

Several reports discuss the role of hypnotherapy in treating sleep disorders. Brown and Fromm (1987) suggest having the client visualize excessive cognitive activity on a screen and then dissociating the client from the somatic state as the therapist moves him to her toward falling asleep. For example:

> *Therapist:* Picture your thoughts moving across the screen. Notice several knobs beneath the screen, including a volume control and a knob controlling the size of the screen. As you feel disturbed by your thoughts as you try to sleep, you will find yourself able to adjust the knobs, allowing yourself to decrease the size of the screen and volume of the thoughts until they no longer disturb you.

Relaxation and tension reduction are also utilized.

The use of posthypnotic suggestions in the multimodal treatment of life-long nightmares is reported by Gorton (1988). The suggestion described here facilitates arousal from sleep upon onset of the nightmare. While under hypnosis, the therapist makes suggestions to the effect, "Just as you can open your eyes right now, so will you be able to open them whenever you want during a frightening dream." The therapist can lead the client to reexperience the dream while under hypnosis and practice the ability to be able to open the eyes and move away from the dream.

Other reports in the literature addressing sleep disorders include recurrent nightmares (Seif, 1985), sleepwalking (Nugent, Carden, and Montgomery, 1984), and cataplexy in a narcoleptic subject (Price, 1987). In the latter, metaphors used in suggestions centered around three themes. First, the therapist emphasized past ability to overcome problems through experiential learning. Second, the therapist emphasized the most efficient use of the solution. The third theme involved the ability of the unconscious to implement what the conscious had learned. These themes are intended to heighten expectation of success, foster an attention to detail in order to evoke solutions, and to autonomize training as it became unconsciously directed.

As an example, David, who experienced initial insomnia, was given suggestions to increase self-esteem and to promote confidence in his ability to come up with a solution. In the following session, David described racing thoughts that prevented sleep. During this and following sessions, David was given a number of suggestions and permission to implement his solutions. This might also be coupled with other techniques, such as television screen imaging.

Assorted Disorders and Applications

Family Problems

The integration of hypnosis into family therapy via an Ericksonian approach is discussed by Malarewicz (1988). The author suggests that group hypnosis can be used to change the way the family group communicates with the therapist, as well as developing alternate methods of communicating with each other. (Further discussion of Ericksonian approaches is found in chapter 5.)

Eating Disorders

Hypnosis has been used successfully with eating disorders (Brown and Fromm, 1987), not surprising given the empirical support that disorders like bulimia stem from an escape from self-awareness (Heatherton and Baumeister, 1991). (A detailed discussion of the clinical treatment of an eating disorder is found in chapter 7.)

Psychosomatic Disorder

The treatment of a psychosomatic disorder (in the context of family therapy and hypnotherapy) is described by Brink (1987). The client is instructed to imagine a warm (but not hot) blue flame at the base of the spine, which melts away tension and helps relaxation as it spreads throughout the body. The client is then asked to visualize the remaining tension and imagine it being placed in a sealed container. This might initially be done ambiguously, so that the client utilizes an image that is maximally effective for him or her. The therapist can subsequently ask the client to describe the image, for further use by the therapist. Changing the affect associated with this response pattern allows the client to develop more constructive ways of coping with distressing situations.

Mental Retardation

Werbel, Mulhern, and Dubi (1983) speculate that patients with mental retardation (MR) may be highly suggestible and easily hypnotized, though only hypnotherapeutic techniques that are within the cognitive grasp of the client should be used. They hypothesize that those with MR develop a "failure set," which could be changed, through hypnosis, to a "success set." For example, John, a twenty-five-year-old client who displays moderate retardation, was able to work in a structured environment, but his production has decreased to a level significantly below his apparent potential. Effective suggestions included enhancing self-esteem and self-efficacy, increasing motivation, and decreasing self-defeating thoughts.

Tourette Syndrome

Culbertson (1989) used a multimodal treatment for Tourette syndrome consisting of progressive relaxation, biofeedback, autohypnotic training, and imagery. Potential techniques include decreasing anxiety, increasing relaxation and control of tics, and mediating the effect of anxiety and stressful life events secondary to the tics.

Trichotillomania

There is some evidence that trichotillomania may be successfully treated with hypnotherapy and restricted environmental stimulation. Kovatsch (1987) employs a treatment approach to develop assertiveness and social skills training within group hypnotherapy and psychodrama techniques. These modalities are used to increase self-esteem and replace negative with positive and more adaptive self-messages and behaviors.

Overall Self-Techniques

The following techniques can be used generally to strengthen the individual's functioning. These are especially apropos for the psychological and habit control disorders.

Self-Perception Restructuring

The client's self-perception and self-esteem are critical components of his or her experience and behavior, with faulty self-perception and deficient self-support and esteem limiting behavioral effectiveness and magnifying perceived threat (van der Hart, Brown, and Turco, 1990; Friedrich, 1991). Often the most important focus of therapeutic work is on identifying and correcting the client's distorted self-perception, self-expectation, and self-esteem. These elements of experience are foundational, deriving from early learning and providing the assumptive support for other elements of the world as experienced.

Self-Strengthening

Particularly for clients whose self-perception is based on concepts of fragility, inability to cope with stress, a deficient sense of self, excessive dependency upon others, and so forth, the following type of strategy can be useful:

> *Therapist:* As you lie there deeply relaxed, you can let the words "calm and tranquil" repeat themselves in your mind, slowly, softly, soothingly, over and over . . . each repetition of those words feels like being stroked lightly with a feather . . . calm and tranquil . . . Now let the words "calm and tranquil" flow down, out of your mind and throughout your entire body, as if they are flowing in your bloodstream, to all parts of your body . . . and wherever those words flow, feeling a strengthening taking place, as if those words are being absorbed by every cell in your body . . . strengthening, nourishing, calming, soothing . . . feeling stronger and more confident with every passing moment, with every breath that you inhale, as the words "calm and tranquil" flow throughout your body, feeding and strengthening your body and your mind . . . and realizing within yourself that you are now using your own resources to strengthen yourself, enabling you to remain strong and calm even when under stress; all that I'm doing is helping you learn how to focus your concentration for your own benefit . . . And now that you are aware of your

> ability to strengthen and nourish yourself, this process will continue even when you are not aware of it, just as an underground river continues to flow, strong and sure, even when we are standing on the ground and are unaware of it; just as a flower continues to grow even though we can't see the growth from moment to moment . . . And the growth and strengthening within you will continue to develop . . .

Additional suggestions of increasing self-appreciation and acceptance, the freedom to be different than expected to be, and the opportunity for the future to be different from the past or present may be incorporated.

The therapeutic impact of this strategy is gradual and cumulative, requiring continued in-session and self-hypnosis practice for consolidation. This strategy can provide a good warmup for other utilization within the same session (for example, desensitization of phobia, part-self integration, behavior change), since it provides a generalized therapeutic orientation, which supports other purposes. Self-strengthening with self-hypnotic practice (see chapter 8) is also recommended.

Part-Self Integration

The client is often stuck in the attempt to resolve an ambivalence regarding a choice or is denying a particular aspect of the self (anger, fear, or something else). Hypnotic work can help identify the avoided self-aspect and can facilitate the resolution of ambivalence.

In the case of ambivalence, the therapist can suggest the experiencing of both sides of the internal conflict (both the angry and the fearful/guilty/ avoidant "parts of the self" in a relationship conflict), suggesting that within the next few days (or "whenever you are ready to resolve the problem") a solution will emerge within the client that will satisfy both "parts of the self."

In the case of a denied affect, the therapist can give "permission" for the denied aspect, suggest its functionality and nondanger, and suggest experiencing that which has been denied. When the client is complaining of distressing and unexplained affect, the therapist can suggest that the client remember a prior time when that same affect was experienced, exploring the meaning of the distress in that earlier context (affect bridge).

Script Revision

When the presenting problem appears related to early scripting (early, now-chronic self-verbalizations), the therapist can talk to the hypnotized client about the nature of scripts and their early survival value, suggesting the client's subconscious readiness to abandon the script in favor of self-determination. Using drama language (for example, refusing a "bit part in the family drama" in favor of a "starring role in your own play") can be metaphorically useful and vivid.

Ego Strengthening

More directive than the self-strengthening suggestions described, ego-strengthening suggestions can be chosen to fit the specific needs of the client, including increased alertness; "nerves" becoming "stronger and steadier"; increased calmness and confidence, decreased apprehension, depression, and upset; improved concentration and memory; and increased absorption in activities and decreased self-conscious preoccupation. These suggestions need to be reinforced by frequent and regular repetition and having the client practice them at home during self-hypnosis practice.

Hypnodiagnosis

A thoughtful and seminal general chapter on hypnodiagnosis is provided by Brownfain (1967), who discusses four uses of hypnosis in diagnostics. First, he suggests that hypnosis can be used as a projective technique, which facilitates an understanding of relevant interpersonal dynamics and personality functioning. For example, the reaction to the suggestion of hypnosis is gauged. A client who blindly accepts a foreign treatment modality might be demonstrating a dependent personality style. A client who becomes fixated over the perceived potential for loss of control while in trance may have paranoid personality features.

Second, hypnosis may be used to facilitate test administration by administering tests while the client is under hypnosis or by using posthypnotic suggestions to make the client less resistant and more comfortable with the testing procedures. Administration under hypnosis or following a posthypnotic suggestion to reduce anxiety can follow an administration without a posthypnotic suggestion as a gauge to measure the extent of the impact of the anxiety. Note, however, that the use of the latter technique must include consideration of the potential impact of the first administration of the test on the second.

The third use of hypnosis in diagnostics involves other assorted diagnostic techniques, such as age regression, to elicit diagnostically relevant information. Price (1987) discusses three cases with dissociative disorders in which hypnosis was used to elicit unconscious ego states (alters) that were controlling behaviors but were not otherwise readily accessible.

The final use of hypnosis in diagnostics is what Brownfain terms "clinical illustration," in which hypnosis is used to explore specific diagnostic hypotheses, such as sexual abuse, MPD (or other amnestic states), or the presence of denied affect. For example, intermittent amnesias might be a signal to consider MPD. Early traumatic or etiologically related events can be explored, lending support to clinical hypotheses.

Conclusion

Hypnosis is a viable tool to facilitate treatment of a variety of psychological dysfunctions, ranging from personality disorders to sleep and sexual dysfunctions. Certainly more empirical research is needed, but there is voluminous clinical support for the effectiveness of hypnotic techniques in a wide range of psychological disorders.

12

Applications in Pain Management and in Dentistry

And, after all, what is a lie?
'Tis but the truth in masquerade
—Lord Byron, "Don Juan"

The role of hypnosis in the systematic management of acute and chronic pain has been formally recorded for two hundred years. Franz Mesmer's "magnetic treatment" to open an "obstruction of the free flow of animal magnetism in the body" (Pattie, 1967, p. 15) was often intended to eliminate pain. The abbé Faria is said to be the first to use hypnosis specifically to insensitize an individual to the pain of surgery (Pattie, 1967).

The first scientific paper on hypnotism and pain was published in 1886 by Dr. Ambroise-Auguste Liebault. Liebault treated thousands of patients suffering from a variety of physical ailments that had not responded to standard medical treatment (Erickson, Hershman, and Secter, 1990).

The Nature of Pain

Pain is defined as "an unpleasant sensation caused by the stimulation of certain nerves, especially as a result of injury or illness; a distressing emotion" (*The New Lexicon Webster's Dictionary of the English Language*, 1987, p. 721). These two components of pain, physical and emotional, have given rise to the suggestion that pain exists on two dimensions: the sensory and the affective.

In 1965, Melzack and Wall proposed what has become a two-component theory known as the gate control theory. The sensory-discriminative system monitors data regarding the location and intensity of stimulation; the motivational-affective system is concerned with the suffering that pain causes. In this theory, modulation of pain is affected by impulses transmitted through the two systems. Neural impulses from the stimulated area can be modified at the sensory-discriminative level, the motivational-affective level, or both. The "pain" may be felt without affective interpretation, interpreted without "feeling" the sensory component,

218

felt on both levels, or the individual may not interpret, on either level, the stimuli at all (Hilgard and Hilgard, 1975).

Such phenomena are observed frequently. The phantom pain experienced by an amputee even when the neuromas at the end of the cut nerves are anesthetized; the soldier in the height of battle who does not "feel" a bullet wound except as a pressure; the mother who, unaware of all her own injuries from an accident, lifts a car off her child: in each case, one or both of the pain systems has been altered, at least for a period of time.

Hypnosis attempts to interrupt these systems in order to reduce pain or the affective sensation of pain. Shor (1967), from his review of the literature, asserted hypnosis primarily affected the emotional component of pain, and later theorists and researchers agree (Watkins and Watkins, 1990; Hammond, 1990). General findings are that physiological indicators such as galvanic skin response) remain unchanged between the waking and hypnotized states when painful stimuli are applied. However, the stimuli are not reported as painful in the hypnotized state though they are in the waking state. The subjective experience of pain is eliminated.

DeBenedittis and Panerai (1989) found significant increases of pain and distress tolerance during hypnosis compared to the waking state. They also found, in highly hypnotizable subjects, that distress was reduced more than pain. Thus, not only was the pain itself reduced, the individual was able to dissociate from the sensation of pain that remained. Miller, Barabasz, and Barabasz (1991) also found that high hypnotizability increases the analgesic suggestions and, in support of E. Hilgard's neo-dissociation theory, that relaxation was not necessary to gain an analgesic effect.

Theories of Pain Relief with Hypnosis

There have not been numerous well-controlled experimental studies regarding the physiological effects of hypnosis. Bishay and Lee (1984) found that vascular flow and bleeding may be influenced and controlled through the use of hypnosis. While some claim the flow of blood may be restricted hypnotically in a certain area or increased in another, others feel hypnosis simply increases heart rate and blood pressure through indirect influences to the autonomic nervous system. Overall, most believe that control of pain through hypnosis is primarily through the affective component of pain perception.

Malone, Kurtz, and Strube (1989) found hypnotic-analgesia suggestions were effective in altering subjects' perception of the intensity of pain without changing their perceptions of its unpleasantness. Hypnotic relaxation suggestions, on the other hand, reduced the unpleasantness but not the perceived intensity of the stimuli. Watkins and Watkins (1990) suggest that, under hypnosis, the pain one feels may be dissociated and displaced into another ego state, with possible undesirable consequences. Hilgard and Hilgard (1975) suggest the pain be displaced to other, smaller areas, where it may be more tolerable. In each of these instances, the affective component of pain is addressed.

The following case study introduces Ginny, whose case will be followed through the upcoming section on Hypnotic Techniques.

Ginny, a thirty-five-year-old woman, had suffered for months from pain resulting from a herniated disk. She had surgery twice in an attempt at fusion of the lower back. In each case, the pain had been reduced somewhat but not enough so that she could live in the way she would like. A lawyer and the mother of two young children, Ginny was unable to work or care for her family after the injury to her back. Pain medication made her drowsy and feel "out of it"; as a result, she preferred to take as little as possible. She began to feel hopeless about ever being able to lead a normal life again and became increasingly depressed. She was referred to a therapist to help her deal with this depression and to explore ways to manage her pain. Ginny's first visit consisted of an assessment of her psychological symptoms, focusing on her depression and its probable causes. Together, the therapist and Ginny agreed that her constant pain, as well as the associated changes in her life caused by it, contributed significantly to the depression. The possibility of hypnosis to reduce the pain was raised by Ginny, who was clearly hopeful that this technique might work where so many others had failed.

At the second session, the therapist talked further with Ginny about the nature of hypnotism. Ginny was then asked to sit as comfortably as possible and relax. As standard induction was used, and Ginny responded readily, entering a moderate trance state easily. Anesthesia of her hand (glove anesthesia) was then induced to deepen the trance and to introduce the idea of the mind's control over the body: "Ginny, you can now realize the power of your mind, your unconscious mind, has over your body. And as your mind was able to alter the sensation of pain or discomfort here, in your hand, so will your mind be able to alter the sensation of pain in the rest of your body."

Hypnotic Techniques

Several techniques are commonly used for the hypnotic management of pain. Barber (1986) provides a good overall schema consisting of five basic methods: analgesia or anesthesia, direct diminution, substitution, displacement, and dissociation.

Analgesia or Anesthesia

This is the perception by the client that the area where the pain was felt has been made numb to sensation. It is as if a local anesthetic had been injected into the afflicted area. Typically, the client is given a suggestion similar to the following:

> *Therapist*: Now your hand is beginning to feel as if an anesthetic had been injected into it. And you notice a tingling sensation. And gradually this tingling sensation gives way to no sensation at all. You have no feeling at all in your hand. And now I will poke the finger of this hand with this sharp point. Quite hard I'm poking it. But you have no sensation of pain or even pressure. You can see that I'm poking it, but you are not able to feel it.

Alternately, the hypnotherapist may suggest that the client visualize an image that suggests a blocking of pain, such as a numbing salve, a heavy glove over the hand, a heavy leather boot over the foot, or armor over other parts of the body. Hypnotic anesthesia may require a positive hallucinatory experience and may be difficult for some clients to achieve. When a client is able to achieve it, however, it may also serve as a means to deepen trance.

Direct Diminution of Pain

This is the suggestion that the client will perceive the pain as less intense. Such suggestions have reduced pain levels, which in turn allowed longer periods of intrusive and painful medical procedures, thus allowing more effective procedures (Weinstein and Au, 1991). Suggestions typically include an element of "turning down" the pain, such as turning down a thermostat, or turning down the "volume" of the pain. Another technique is to have the client, prior to hypnosis, rate the pain on a scale of one to ten, with one being the least amount of pain and ten being the most incredible pain that can be imagined. While in the hypnotic state, the therapist has the client reduce the number assigned to the pain, thus decreasing it:

> *Therapist*: And now you can see the number seven, the number you have given to your pain. And as you see this number, you see that it is slowly, slowly changing. Now the number is six. And as you look at that number, at the number six, you are aware that your discomfort has lessened. And a six is very

much like five. And as you watch, the six is changing into a five. And as you see the five, you begin to feel more comfortable. And a five is not much different from a four. Is only a little different from a four. And a four is very close to a three. The number is now a three. And with each change the number makes, each time the number changes into another number, your comfort becomes greater. And with only a small change, with very little effort, you can see the number three turn into a two. And as you see the two, as you experience the two, you are more and more comfortable.

Barber suggests that it may be helpful to the client to notice an increase in comfort rather than a diminution of the pain. Focusing on the increase in the comfort level rather than focusing on the pain is viewed as more positive. Additionally, by placing the focus on feeling good, the individual is more likely to "turn off" the pain and its affective components.

Substitution of Painful Sensation

Substitution or reinterpretation of sensation may also be suggested. For example, a dull, throbbing pressure may be substituted for a hot, stabbing pain. A burning sensation may become an itch. In each case, the substituted sensation may not be necessarily pleasant but is less uncomfortable. There are several advantages to sensory substitution. First, the client is still aware of the pain, so it may be monitored medically. Second, the fact that some discomfort remains may be more plausible to the client than attempting to eliminate all perception of pain. Third, if there are secondary gains the client receives because of the pain, these may still be obtained without the extreme discomfort of the original pain. Sensory substitution may be suggested in a fashion similar to the following manner:

Therapist: The sensation you described as a burning knife piercing your back can begin to change. And the knife feels less and less hot. And now the knife is warm. A warm knife. And now, interestingly enough, the knife itself begins to change, as if the knife is becoming less and less rigid. Less and less hard. It is almost as if a warm rubber knife is poking at you. Poking at you, a slight pressure that pushes against your back, not entirely pleasant, but so much different, so much of a relief from before.

Displacement of the Pain

Displacement of pain from one area to another is best accomplished when the pain is fairly well localized. Generally the pain is disabling to the individual because of the location of the pain or because of the affective component the client attaches to the location of the pain. The suggestion is made that the client is able to "move" the pain from one area to another:

Therapist: And you may notice that the discomfort has begun to move just a little. And you can notice that it has begun to move away from your abdomen. Moving gently and slowly. Down, down, moving from your abdomen toward your left leg. And you will notice that it continues to move, slowly, gently, through your thigh. Down past your knee, through your calf. And the discomfort seems to have moved down to your foot. And as you continue to notice the movement, you may become aware that the discomfort has traveled down to your toes, and seems to stay in the toes of your left foot.

Generally displacement of pain is more effective if the client is allowed to choose where he or she would prefer the pain to be and if the movement of the pain appears to have a kind of logic. Most clients respond to suggestions better if these suggestions make sense. A discussion of the interconnections of the nervous system may make the movement more plausible. Clients not sophisticated enough to understand neural impulses can be given visualizations of the nerves as a sort of train track; the pain can then be visualized as a train car that moves on this track to another location.

Dissociation

When the suggestion is effectively integrated so that the client becomes dissociated from the pain, he or she is able to describe the pain accurately but has no effective involvement with it. It is as if the pain were happening to someone else. This can be useful when an individual is immobilized or confined to bed. The client is taught to experience himself or herself in another place or time and not to be "in" the body that is experiencing the pain:

Therapist: Imagine yourself at your favorite place, on the beach. You can see the sun shining. You can feel the warmth of the sun and the soft breeze against your skin. You hear the gentle lapping of the water against the shore and the cry of the birds. You smell the tang of the salty air, and as you experience these things, as you are aware of them, you realize you can leave your body here, in this bed, and you can enjoy this favorite, restful, enjoyable place. You can take a vacation from the discomfort, from the routine things that must be done. Your mind can take you far away, where nothing can bother you.

Notice that in this suggestion various sensory modalities were employed; the senses of sight, touch, hearing, and smell all contribute to make the hallucinatory experience more real and vivid. This enables the client to enter more fully into the experience, increasing the dissociation.

Combination of Techniques

Often, given the particular client and the type of pain he or she is experiencing, a combination of these techniques may be employed. For example, hypnotic anesthesia may be used when painful hypodermic shots are given and diminution techniques employed for the general pain itself. A combination of sensory substitution and diminution may be used for individuals with widespread and chronic pain. The techniques and suggestions employed are a result of what seems appropriate, comfortable, and effective for client and therapist both. Most patients find the following technique to be comfortable and easy to follow.

Ginny was asked, prior to hypnosis, to rate her pain. On a scale of one to ten, she rated it as a nine. Now, deep in trance, she is asked to visualize the number.

Therapist: And now, Ginny, I want you to see the number that you gave your pain, the number nine. You can see it on a dial, a dial much like that on the volume control of a radio. You can reach out and touch that dial, grasp it, turn it with your hand. Slowly, you turn the dial and the nine disappears. An eight appears in its place. And as you see the eight you are aware that you have turned down your discomfort. You continue to turn the dial, and now you see a seven. You turn the dial again, and the seven becomes a six. Then a five. With each turn of the dial, with each new number, you are aware that you have lowered your discomfort. A four, three. Now you turn the dial again, and you see a two. You have turned down the intensity of your pain to where it is manageable, to where you can handle it and live with it. You know that you will continue to experience some discomfort, that you will be aware of it. It isn't reasonable to expect it to all go away entirely. But your mind has been able to lower the volume of your discomfort, and now you can do many more of the things that you did before your accident.

Precautions in Using Hypnotic Techniques

Therapists should be cautious when using the word *pain* within hypnotic suggestions. The word is loaded with negative affective meaning and may serve as a distraction or an inhibition to relaxation. More neutral words, such as *pressure, discomfort,* or *bothersome* are preferable, especially when attempting to diminish or eliminate the pain.

On occasion, it is not advisable to remove all of the patient's pain. While the negative affective component may be altered to a less noxious one, some sensation (pressure, dull throb, or something else) should be left. Pain functions as a warning that something is wrong. If all the pain is removed, any changes occurring in the individual's body may go unnoticed, with potentially negative consequences. There are exceptions. If the patient is in the hospital and is closely monitored by medical staff, the pain may be removed. Even in this case, it may be advisable to provide a posthypnotic suggestion that the patient will be aware of any sensations in the body different from the current ones and report those changes to the doctor.

There is another reason to "allow" the client to retain some of the pain. Many individuals derive some secondary gains from their pain and discomfort. To remove all the physical pain may result in increased psychological discomfort. It is more therapeutic to allow the client to retain whatever amount of discomfort is necessary to meet these secondary gains, at least in the short term. Other psychological interventions may then be employed to explore these secondary gains and further hypnotic pain reduction techniques used as those issues are resolved.

Extending a Relief from Pain

Although it is possible to help a client be relatively free from pain during the hypnotic session, this by itself is of limited usefulness. After all, people do not live in a trance. Posthypnotic suggestions offer a way of extending the benefits of hypnotic effects into the waking state. Generally the therapist will suggest a cue to the client that will enable him or her to reach the level of comfort acquired during the trance. Cues vary from client to client and are most effective if individualized for each case. Some individuals respond effectively to suggestions, such as, when relief from discomfort is needed, touching the thumb and forefinger together will enable them to "turn down" the pain or eliminate it entirely. Others may find that the experience of the pain itself provides the cue to pain relief. Still others may be provided with the suggestion that they relax when in discomfort, and this relaxation enters them into the hypnotic trance. With practice and with reinforcing hypnotic sessions, the therapist and client will be able to discover the most effective way for the client to obtain the needed relief.

Frequently, one of the components of the distress caused by chronic pain is the sense that the individual no longer has control over his or her own body. Teaching the client self-hypnosis not only provides the individual with a means to maintain control over the body but also allows provision of pain relief, relaxation, and a strengthening of the ego. By providing the client with a sense of control, anxiety may be relieved, thus reducing the physiological tension that exacerbates the pain. Additionally, use of self-hypnosis decreases the dependency the client may have on the therapist, reducing the need for follow-up appointments. The therapist needs to reassure the client that he or she is not "going it alone" and that help is available whenever it is needed. Occasionally a booster session may be needed, with the client then able to continue managing the pain independently. (Specific techniques employed in self-hypnosis may be found in chapter 8.)

We now close with the culmination of Ginny's case.

> Ginny has seen her therapist for six session. During that time a variety of hypnotic pain management techniques were used. Ginny found diminution of the pain to be generally the most useful technique for her. She has learned to cue herself to diminish the pain when she begins to feel uncomfortable. Additionally, she uses self-hypnosis and dissociation when she must have examinations of her back by her doctor. Because these examinations are in the doctor's office, she feels comfortable "leaving" her body for visits to a favorite place when these medical procedures must be done. While she continues to feel the discomfort in her back, she knows that these sensations are useful: they keep her from doing something that would further injure the area. She has been able to return to work part time and is again able to interact with her children and take part in their lives.

Managing Pain with Hypnosis

Screening Pain Clients

All individuals considered for hypnosis for the control of pain or for dental work should undergo a screening interview prior to the hypnosis. For certain individuals, including those suffering from active psychoses or depressed patients with suicidal ideation, hypnosis is probably contraindicated. Motivation for treatment must be evaluated. Symptomatology may be used to manipulate others or for their secondary gains. It is also important to assess whether the symptom is organic or psychogenic in origin. Hypnosis may be effective in either case, but the underlying causes should be known. A complete history of the client should also be obtained. This should include a brief exploration into the clients' value system, information that can be useful in the induction technique employed and in developing suggestions during the hypnotic trance. This initial interview provides the therapist an opportunity to discuss hypnosis with the client, correcting any misconceptions he or she may have.

Generally clients suffering from pain are highly motivated. By the time the hypnotherapist is called or the client is referred, more traditional medical treatments have been tried without success. These individuals are ready to try virtually anything to relieve their distress and are susceptible to induction techniques. Nevertheless, issues of malingering, secondary gain, and unconscious motivations need to be considered.

A complete description of the pain itself should be obtained: where the pain is located, the length of time the pain has been felt, and any fluctuations in its intensity. This information is helpful in tailoring the hypnotic techniques used to the specific client. A list of adjectives to describe the pain may also be given to the client if there appears to be any difficulty in adequately characterizing the sensation. Hammond (1990) suggests using a pencil and paper instrument such as the McGill Pain Questionnaire (Melzack, 1975). A detailed description of the pain is helpful in providing imagery to both client and therapist for use in diminution and sensory substitution.

Hypnosis and Headache Pain

Several headache pain or migraine can disrupt an individual's life and seem to prevent him or her from even being able to think. Many in the medical community believe one cause of chronic headache is stress and tension. Muscles in the head and neck are involuntarily and chronically tensed, and pain results. Hypnotic treatment would include suggestions for a focused relaxation:

Therapist: And as you move deeper and deeper into this calm, relaxed state, you find you are able to relax your muscles. Your shoulders become loose. You can relax those muscles in your shoulders and feel the warm feeling of relaxation there. The tension flows out of the muscles in your shoulders. And now the warmth of relaxation moves into your neck. The muscles feel warm, relaxed. And this relaxation moves into your head, into the base of your head, and up, up into your scalp. You feel the warm release of relaxation all through your head, through your neck, through your shoulders.

The sensation of coldness in the head is often effective in alleviating the pain of migraine. Migraine results primarily from the dilation of the arteries leading to the brain, so constriction of these arteries can reduce the pain of migraine headaches. Hypnotic suggestions could include feelings of coldness in the head:

> *Therapist*: You feel the winter air swirling around your face, around your head. And the snow is falling, falling on your hair, on your face, on your temples. The air is cold, crisp, and it feels so good, so refreshing, for this cold, this snowy breeze to blow around your head.

A more direct technique may be employed to reduce the pain of migraine. It may be suggested to the client to visualize the blood vessels in the head and "watch" them become narrower and more constricted (Anderson, Basker, and Dalton, 1990). This is most effective when the client has been given the medical explanation of the cause of migraine.

Hypnotic Pain Management with Painful, Life-Threatening Diseases

Hypnosis has been used with cancer patients to provide symptomatic relief to the pain of the disease and relief for the side effects of chemotherapy treatments. Additionally, hypnosis has been found helpful in treating other aspects of the disease and other similar diseases. (For further information on the uses of hypnosis with cancer patients, see chapter 14.)

Generally patients suffering from such severe disorders are good candidates for hypnosis. The life-threatening quality of their disease reduces the attractiveness of secondary gains and results in high motivation (Hammond, 1990). They are generally highly suggestible to hypnosis.

The focus in treatment may differ from one patient to another. Frequently the emotional reaction to the disease—uncertainty, depression, fear of death—may need to be dealt with before the physical one. Hypnosis forms a part of the overall treatment of the individual, both medically and psychologically.

It is unknown to what extent an individual, using hypnosis or any other physical approach, can effect changes in physiological healing. Use of hypnosis, however, focuses one's attention on an active healing process, giving the individual a sense of control over the body that had been taken away. Hammond (1990) suggests that the feelings of calm and tranquility achieved through hypnosis allow an individual's immune system to function at a maximal level. Auerbach (1990) and others suggest the client visualize the body's white cells attacking and destroying the diseased cells. He uses positive imagery, with the white cells being visualized as patrolling the body in a protective, loving way. Whether physiological changes occur may not be nearly as important (to the patients) as the sense that they are "monitoring" the disease. This releases them from the sense of "I am my disease" to a more distant "I have a disease."

Relaxed and contributing to the emotional aspects of severe disease is the actual pain that occurs from tissue damage or intrusion. Traditionally the only way to achieve pain relief has been through large amounts of medication. These pain medications (morphine, codeine, and others) tend to keep the patient in a drowsy, drugged state, unable to participate to the fullest extent in what time is left. This, too, can result in depression. Hypnosis can be used to relieve this pain, thereby allowing decreased use of medication with its side effects. Additionally, the pain often prevents the individual from being hungry or thirsty, preventing him or her from obtaining the nourishment that would be of benefit.

Whatever induction technique is comfortable for both therapist and client is used. During this induction phase, glove anesthesia is helpful. This only serves to reinforce the control of the unconscious mind over the body, it also is an elegant precursor to the pain control techniques that will follow.

The client is first encouraged to relax. Suggestions given by the therapist should include freedom from tension, tightness, stress and strain, relative freedom from discomfort, and that the individual will be relaxed and at ease (Crasilneck and Hall, 1985). Imagery can be employed to obtain this sense of ease and relaxation, utilizing whatever calm, peaceful image that is of value to that particular client. It can then be suggested:

Therapist: You have a feeling of well-being. You are calm and relaxed. You are relaxed now, and you can relax enough later to sleep peacefully, sleeping when you desire. You can eat well. You can be hungry at mealtime and can enjoy the food ordered for you. You will be relaxed and at ease. Your unconscious mind will allow you freedom from tension and any discomfort whenever you desire, just as you are now free from tension and discomfort.

These suggestions are repeated to the client and reinforced through self-hypnosis until a deep state of relaxation is reached.

The pain can then be approached. Glove anesthesia is induced, and the patient runs the anesthetized hand over the painful area of the body, "transferring" the numbness to that area:

Therapist: And you are aware that you are unable to feel anything in your hand. It is as if your hand is numb, without sensation, and you can take your hand and move it to where you feel discomfort, gently rubbing your hand over the uncomfortable area. And as you rub this numb hand, this hand without feeling, over the uncomfortable place, you are aware that the numbness is moving, is being transferred to that place, as if you were rubbing novocaine over the affected area, making the uncomfortable sensation cease.

Displacing the pain may provide relief. When the pain is in a part of the body (such as the abdomen) that is associated with a life-threatening disease, it may be suggested:

Therapist: Perhaps the discomfort is now in the back of the left hand. And perhaps it is the same discomfort that used to be in your abdomen. And, if you wish, this discomfort in your hand can occupy your attention so that it is the only discomfort you can feel, the only discomfort you are aware of.

This pain can then be reduced to where it is manageable using sensory substitution:

Therapist: And you notice that the discomfort you had described as a bright, white-hot burning is cooling, is fading, fading from white to red. Fading further and further. And you notice that the hotness is cooling. Now it is dimmer and dimmer, not bright at all now. Just a glow, a gentle glow, a dim orange glow.

The client should be asked, prior to hypnosis, to describe the pain, and that imagery may then be employed in the hypnotic session.

Hypnotic amnesia is another technique that may be employed. The client is asked, under hypnosis, to regress to a time when he or she was happy, comfortable, and peaceful. The client is asked to visualize a time and place where he or she felt relaxed, healthy, and at ease. Suggestions such as the following can then be made:

Therapist: You feel calm and content in this place. Happy and at peace. And if you want, you may again feel those feelings you now have, the calmness, the peacefulness, the happiness. And you may find that you do not remember. That you choose not to remember any physical sensation that may interfere with this sense of peace.

A posthypnotic suggestion can be made that whenever the client feels discomfort, he or she will be able to go back and feel that comfortable state and not remember the pain. This suggestion is most effective for the discomfort, nausea, and pain experience following surgery, chemotherapy, or radiation treatment.

It is often desirable not to remove the sensation of pain entirely, as it may provide clues to the patient and physicians as to the progress of the disease. In these cases, a diminution technique may be utilized, rating the pain on a scale of one to ten, with ten being unendurable. It is then suggested that the pain diminish to a level of two or three and that, although the discomfort will be noticeable, it will not interfere in any way with the client's life. In this way, proper precautions and monitoring of the disease can be carried out (Crasilneck and Hall, 1985).

Self-hypnosis can be an integral part of such treatments. In this way, patients are able to maintain control over their own bodies, providing themselves with pain relief, relaxation, anxiety reduction, and a strengthening of their ego. Many of these patients, when using self-hypnosis in combination with therapist-assisted hypnosis, are thus able to live out the remainder of their lives in relative comfort, with a reduction of anxiety and depression.

Carl's case demonstrates how a therapist can apply some of the prior techniques in a cancer case.

Carl, age sixty-two, was diagnosed with bone cancer. Chemotherapy had left him weak and in much pain. The cancer itself caused him a great deal of physical distress. A man who had been active all his life, Carl was depressed not only about the disease and the poor prognosis for recovery but by the limitations placed on his busy life-style. The depression, nausea from the chemotherapy, and the pain of the disease had caused him to refuse food. At the time he was seen by the therapist, more aggressive means of providing him nutrition were being considered. Additionally, pain medication had proved unsatisfactory; in order to provide relief, large, powerful dosages were required. This kept him in a drugged state, a fact Carl was most upset about. Hypnosis was suggested to Carl as a means of managing much of the pain that resulted both from the disease and the treatment. Carl was ready to try anything.

A hypnotic induction technique including relaxation was performed. It was then suggested the sensory perception of his pain would be altered; instead of a throbbing, searing pain, Carl would feel a slight ache in the affected areas. It was also suggested that by eating what was provided to him, he was actively helping his body fight the cancer cells. Because Carl had been a football player in his younger years and actively followed his college football team, he was given the imagery of his healthy cells being a part of the "offensive team," battling against an opponent (his least favorite team): "You can imagine these cells, these healthy cells, battling against the unhealthy ones, much the way your college offensive team battles their rivals, knocking them over, weakening the defensive line, taking them out of the game."

Intake of food and drink was linked with providing "his" team with better training and greater strength than the "opposing" team (the cancer). Carl took readily to this imagery, which gave him a sense of control over his body and provided him with the psychological lift that he was doing something constructive and was active in his treatment. Posthypnotic suggestions were provided to give him the ability to relax against the pain and nausea chemotherapy caused, as well as to reduce the pain of the treatments themselves. Training in self-hypnosis as well as posthypnotic suggestion allowed him to enter a trance and provide himself with hypnotic anesthesia when painful medical examinations were required.

Carl was seen on an outpatient basis by his therapist for booster sessions after his release from the hospital. Pain medication was necessary only occasionally; when it was required, dosages were considerably lower than they had been prior to hypnotism. Carl lived for approximately six months following his initial hypnotherapy session. He was relatively pain free during this time and was able to be awake, alert, and involved with his family. Just prior to his death, he said, with a laugh, that although his football team nearly always beat their rivals, occasionally the underdogs managed to get lucky.

Hypnotic Pain Management and Burn Treatment

In burn injuries, the pain of the burn itself is only one component that must be addressed. Even more painful is the treatment necessary for healing. Debridement (the removal of dead tissue from the burn area), dressing changes, and skin grafts create acute discomfort for the client. Pharmacologic interventions, in dosages high enough to be effective, may increase the risk of respiratory failure, as well as reduce client responsiveness. Other potential problems are the loss of appetite, contracture resulting from failure to exercise the injured area because of pain, and severe depression and negativism. Hypnosis has been shown to help in the management of all these components.

Patterson, Questad, and de Lateur (1989) found evidence that hypnosis offers an efficient and effective method for controlling the severe pain of burn debridement. In this study, subjects were given the suggestion that the area being debrided would become "heavy and numb" and that they would be comfortable and relaxed throughout the procedure. These subjects showed reductions on pain rating scores relative to their own baseline and also showed reduced pain rating scores compared to a historical control group. Although there are threats to validity in this study, it provides encouraging empirical support for the clinical literature.

Ewin (1990) reports a clinical case using hypnosis not only to relax a burn victim in the emergency room of the hospital but to decrease the blood supply to the injured area. The theory is that inflammation is mediated by the release of a bradykinin-like substance released during the first two hours of a burn. This inflammation damages the deeper dermal layers of the skin. Ewin reports that hypnotic suggestion can block the release of the substance, thus reducing the severity of the burn. Suggestions are made to the client that the burned area is feeling cool and comfortable. These suggestions, according to Ewin, are anti-inflammatory; once these ideas are accepted by the client, the area cannot logically be hot and painful. Blood flow to the area is likely reduced and inflammation limited. Ewin also reports that reduction of inflammation prevents the edema that results from burn injuries, decreasing the risk of shock and kidney shutdown. Although there is little empirical evidence for Ewin's claims, clinical reports support him. From a practical viewpoint, incorporating suggestions that the burn area is cool and comfortable into hypnosis provides pain relief and increases relaxation. If prevention of additional injury also occurs, that is a bonus.

After induction, the client is given the suggestion to relax into a deeper and sounder level. Glove anesthesia can then be suggested. When this occurs, the patients can be told that he or she can realize the power of the mind over the body:

Therapist: You can imagine a safe, peaceful place. This place can be wherever or whatever you want it to be. You can go to this special place whenever you want, as often as you'd like, and you'll be able to ignore all the irritating things that are done and anything negative that may occur. And because of the power your mind has over your body, you will be able to increase your food intake. This food will help you get well. The food will taste good to you, and with each bite you eat, you are improving your physical and mental state. Because exercise is important to your recovery, you can and will exercise the way and as often as your doctor tells you.

Further suggestions may include sensory substitution during wound debridement, with the client substituting a feel of pressure for pain. Hypnotic anesthesia or amnesia may also be suggested when the client must undergo other various medical procedures as part of treatment.

It may also be suggested that the client focus on his or her strengths and assets. Frequently disfiguration and physical limitations can result from severe burn injuries. When these occur, the client's attention is naturally focused there, possibly contributing to a feeling of hopelessness and inadequacy. By suggesting to the client, during trance, that he or she focus on the strengths and inner resources retained, the sense of despair is lessened—for example: "You will find that your attention is focused less and less on your disabilities, the changes in your appearance, and more and more on your assets, your self-control, your abilities, your inner strength." Other suggestions to improve self-esteem, tailored to the specific client, may be offered.

Kevin's case demonstrates an application of some of the prior concepts relevant to burn victims.

Kevin, age twenty-three, suffered third-degree burns on his hands, arms, and the side of his face during an industrial accident. Medication had been effective in controlling his pain, but medical staff were concerned that he was becoming addicted. Additionally, it was felt that Kevin was using the medication, which kept him in a semiawake state, to avoid dealing emotionally with the extent of the injuries he had sustained. In fact, one of his primary concerns was that no woman would ever look at him or desire him again—that he was now a "monster" who would scare people away. Therefore, it was desirable to reduce his pain medication.

Partly because of his apathetic depression and partly because of the pain from his injuries, Kevin seldom ate much of the high-nutrition meals prescribed for him. He refused to do his physical therapy exercises. When debridement of the burned area was necessary, Kevin screamed in pain. To help him handle the pain of both the injury and the necessary treatment and to help him come to terms with the disfiguring aspects of his injury, a hypnotherapist was called in.

During the first session with the therapist, Kevin was suspicious and somewhat hostile. He expressed anger that "something else was going to be done" to him, without his control or permission. The nature of hypnotism was explained to him, with much emphasis on the fact that hypnosis is something an individual does himself. He was reassured that at no time would he be asked to do something he did not want to and that he was in complete control of the process.

A nondirective induction procedure was used, emphasizing relaxation. At no time were the words *trance* or *hypnosis* used, as it was felt this would be counterproductive. Kevin was encouraged to relax:

Therapist: Deeper and deeper. Sinking deeper and deeper into a profound state of relaxation. And paying attention to your breathing, you may find that with each inhalation you are able to breathe in relaxation. And with each exhalation, you are able to let go a little more, releasing a little more of your tension. But it is your body, and your relaxation, and your tension, and you are able to control it as you would like.

And you may find that it is so comfortable, so easy, so nice, to just relax and let the feelings of calmness and well-being surround you. And you may find, if you wish, that you are so relaxed that what is happening with your body is unimportant at this moment to you. You may find that it is so nice, so relaxing, to just lay back and be comfortable, that you are able to turn down any discomfort you may feel. You may choose to imagine a little dial, a little dial like that on a radio, and you may choose to turn that dial way down, just like turning down the volume of a radio. And when you turn that dial down, you may find you are able to turn down the discomfort. Wouldn't that be nice? To just decide to turn down any sensation in your body that is uncomfortable or bothersome? And because it is your body and your mind, you may do that whenever you wish. You may choose to do that whenever you feel discomfort.

In making these suggestions, Kevin's therapist gave the control of the diminution of pain to Kevin, providing him also with a way to control what was happening to him.

Therapist: And because it is your body, of course you want to have a part in the healing process. You know, Kevin, one of the best ways to help yourself heal is to eat, to provide your body with the good things that will help it repair itself. You know that, so you may find that you are interested in your meals, and you may find that you are hungry. And you may choose, if you'd like, to help yourself, to have some control over what is happening, by eating and drinking all that is offered to you, all that your doctors give you. The control over this is yours, you may choose. And you may also choose to do the exercises you've been given. Exercises that will allow you to strengthen your hands. This is up to you. This is your choice. You may find that you want to do the exercises the way you've been instructed. But the choice is up to you. You are in charge of your body.

Subsequent sessions built on the suggestions of the first session, strengthening them and continuing to emphasize Kevin's active role in the healing process. Kevin was taught self-hypnosis, which furthered his sense of control and allowed him to utilize diminution techniques to manage his pain and discomfort. He was given suggestions in imagery, chosen by him, to allow him to dissociate during debridement procedures. Additionally, nonhypnosis sessions dealt with Kevin's fears about facial scarring. Positive, self-esteem-enhancing imagery was introduced into hypnosis.

Through the combination of hypnosis and regular therapy, Kevin was better able to help himself and deal with the changes that had occurred in his life. He was able to manage the pain from both the wounds and from the necessary treatment. He was able to begin to view himself in a more positive manner, improving his outlook and enhancing his recovery.

Hypnosis and Dentistry

Hypnosis is used in dentistry not only to reduce anxiety and to relieve pain but also to help in the healing and recovery process.

Hypnosis and Dental Anxiety

It is common for people to be afraid to visit the dentist. When this anxiety becomes intense, needed dental treatment may be avoided, resulting in increased dental problems. Hypnosis can be used to reduce this anxiety. Suggestions rely largely on relaxation and reassurance. The client can be instructed to tense and relax various muscle groups, experiencing the difference between the tension and relaxation. Once the individual is in a state of relaxation, the anxiety that has been experienced can be reframed: "Anxiety consists of many components, and some of these are quite positive—excitement, energy, challenge. Life would be boring without these things and you may find you can enjoy these feelings, this excitement and energy. And you may find that everything becomes easier" (Murray-Jobsis, 1990).

Generally simple relaxation technique and reframing are effective in reducing the typical fear of dentists. Where the anxiety appears to have a deeper cause, the dentist should refer the patient to a therapist who may explore the underlying reasons for the fear.

Hypnotic Analgesia and Dentistry

Hypnotism is often used as a substitute for, or along with, chemoanalgesia. Because of the wide range and availability of local anesthetics, hypnotism is generally used as an adjunct to those anesthetics. In certain high-risk patients, the use of chemoanalgesia may be contraindicated, and hypnosis may be used instead. Hypnotic suggestions for anesthetizing these patients is similar to those used in other medical and surgical areas (see chapters 13 and 14). Dissociation may also be used; the patient may simply "leave" the body during the dental procedure, allowing the pain to occur to the body without "being present." Less dramatic is the hypnotic anesthetizing of the mouth and gums. After induction, glove anesthesia is developed. Then the patient transfers the numbness from the hand to the appropriate area by rubbing the finger over the gum and tooth area.

Temporomandibular Joint Syndrome and Bruxism

Temporomandibular joint syndrome (TMJ) and bruxism (grinding of the teeth) may be treated with hypnosis (Clarke & Reynolds, 1991; Rodolfa, Kraft & Reilley 1990). Since stress seems to be at least a prominent contributing variable in both TMJ and bruxism, hypnotic suggestions and training in self-hypnosis to reduce stress and anxiety may provide lasting relief. An explanation may be given that grinding of the teeth or clenching the jaw is one way people respond to stress. Symptom substitution can then be suggested: "And you may find that flicking your fingernail, flicking your nail, helps ease the stress, helps reduce the tension much better than clenching your jaw. Is much more effective." Clarke and Reynolds (1991) found that suggestions to the effect of keeping the lips relaxed, with the teeth relaxed and apart, along with suggestions "like having a hot, pleasant steamy towel on your face," successfully reduced the symptoms in eight clients with bruxism.

Most instances of bruxism and jaw clenching occur during sleep. It can be suggested that the individual will awaken when this occurs. It is also suggested that if the individual wants a full night's sleep, the subconscious will "control the conscious" to keep the mouth slightly open. This suggestion to keep the mouth slightly open, wide enough to place the tongue between the back teeth, is generally the most effective. It is paired with the suggestion that placing the tongue between the teeth will serve as a cue to relaxation of the facial muscles (Neiburger, 1990): "Whenever you feel your teeth clench together, when you feel your teeth grinding, you will want to open your mouth slightly, enough to place your tongue between your back teeth. And you will feel the muscles in your face and mouth becoming loose, becoming relaxed, becoming more and more comfortable. The longer your tongue stays between your teeth, the more your muscles will become loose and relaxed."

Exaggerated Gag Reflex

An exaggerated gag reflex, the abnormal response of mouth and throat muscles to a psychological or physiological stimulus, may interfere with the performance of dental work. This reflex is often a result of a fear of choking or being unable to breathe. Hypnotic suggestions typically involve relaxation of the mouth and throat, followed by transfer of glove anesthesia to the entire inside of the mouth. Clarke and Persichetti (1990) suggest the use of imagery involving breathing through an opening in the neck. This allows the patient to focus on breathing, bypassing the gagging area of the throat. Clients who are disturbed by this imagery may concentrate on the feeling of air going in and out of the nose, bypassing the mouth. Another image dentists use is thinking of the touches of the dental equipment as food (Heron, 1990): "When you place food in your mouth it touches your tongue, the roof of your mouth. You swallow it, it touches your throat. This feels pleasant. You enjoy eating and drinking. The feeling of food and drink in your mouth. And when I place this instrument in your mouth, when you feel it touching your mouth, your tongue, you will be reminded of your favorite food. Your mouth will relax. Your throat will relax. You may think of those touches as food."

Tooth Extraction

Once the client is in a state of trance, fully relaxed, glove anesthesia can be introduced and transferred to the area of the mouth that will be worked on. It should not be assumed that anesthesia is present; this should be tested prior to actual work on the teeth. Kroger (1990) suggests the tooth that is to be extracted to be depressed in the socket and that it be suggested that the area is getting more and more numb, losing all feeling. By associating pressure with numbness, the actual extraction of the tooth will serve to deepen the anesthesia. Kroger suggests testing for numbness in the area by using a sharp dental instrument to press the area before any work is done.

Once the tooth is removed, suggestions for healing can be given:

Therapist: You can let the socket fill with blood. The place where the tooth was will fill with blood and clot normally. You will feel refreshed. You feel no discomfort. You can be aware of the area we worked on today, aware of any changes that may occur after you leave the office. And you can also be aware that the area will heal normally, without discomfort.

In cases in which a posthypnotic suggestion for anesthesia has been given, it is recommended that it be time limited, so the patient will be aware of any unusual changes that may signal an abscess.

Control of Bleeding

Control of bleeding in hemophiliacs is a special problem in dental surgery. Generally transfusions of whole blood or plasma are necessary prior to dental extractions. The control of bleeding through hypnosis has been reported by Hilgard and Hilgard (1975), though it is not understood how this works; perhaps it may be related to the control of vasomotor responses.

Sally's case demonstrates an approach that can be useful with most dentistry patients.

Sally, a thirty-three-year-old woman, has not been to the dentist since she was a child. She remembers dental procedures as painful and frightening, with little or no attention paid to her fears and discomfort. Her parents had reinforced her fear by telling her that all dental work hurts and she would just have to "grin and bear it." Instead Sally avoided going to a dentist.

For the past few weeks, though, Sally has experienced severe pain from one of her molars. Finally, she has realized she must have the tooth attend to. On the advice of a friend, Sally made an appointment with a dentist who utilizes hypnosis to help patients manage the fear and any pain involved in dental work.

Sally was obviously frightened when she entered the dental office. Her respiration was rapid, and she was pale and sweating. Sally's history was obtained, and hypnosis was discussed. Hypnosis was then induced, using progressive relaxation. As each muscle group was relaxed, Sally's ability to let go of tension was reinforced.

Therapist: You can feel yourself becoming more and more relaxed, and this is so nice, so peaceful. You are really doing well. You are really able to just let go and let the tension run out of you, replacing it with peaceful relaxation. You can feel each breath. And with each inhalation you breathe in relaxation and exhale tension. You are doing so well, Sally. You are very good at relaxing.

After Sally had reached a deep level of trance, the dentist introduced glove anesthesia and had Sally transfer the "numbness" from her hand to her mouth and cheek. The examination then began:

Therapist: And now, you may find that you are ready to open your mouth. You are so relaxed. You have no sense of discomfort in your mouth, around the tooth, in your cheek. You feel a slight pressure, a pressure around your gum. And as you feel this pressure you can use it as a signal for your mouth to become more and more numb. No feeling, no discomfort, and more and more relaxed, calm, without fear.

In order to make this as positive an experience for Sally as possible and because he did not know her well or how deeply in trance she was likely to remain, the dentist opted to use chemoanalgesia in conjunction with hypnosis. The hypnotic anesthesia sufficiently numbed the area surrounding the affected tooth for the dentist to inject the medication. Work on the tooth then proceeded, with the dentist continually reassuring Sally of her ability to remain in trance and how pleasant it must feel to be so relaxed. After the treatment, a posthypnotic suggestion was given to maximize comfort. A suggestion was also given to increase Sally's ability to relax on subsequent visits to the dentist's office.

Sally has since had several dental procedures done with hypnosis as the sole anesthesia, with a minimum of discomfort and without fear. Although she states that a visit to the dentist is not her favorite activity, she no longer is afraid.

Summary

The use of a formal hypnotic procedure on pain has been around at least since the days of Mesmer and his "animal magnetism." While there is still less than a full understanding of how and why hypnosis can relieve pain, clinical reports have consistently indicated success with its use. Empirical research runs into ethical problems: one cannot assign individuals suffering from chronic pain to a waiting list control group. Therefore, most of the research has been conducted on induced pain in the laboratory. While helpful in understanding some of the mechanisms involved, induced pain is temporary in nature and cannot be reliably compared to chronic pain.

Hypnotic techniques for pain reduction include relaxation, anesthesia and analgesia, diminution of the pain, dissociation of the pain, and displacement. Posthypnotic suggestions provide a means to extend the benefits of pain management. Hypnosis for the management of pain should not be viewed as a therapy in and of itself. It is, rather, a technique used as a part of the total therapeutic picture.

13

Hypnotherapy and Medical Disorders, I

> One Soviet woman went to an American doctor and tried to strike
> up a conversation about Toulouse-Lautrec. . . . [The doctor] had no
> idea who he was. Our doctor typically would've known all about
> Toulouse-Lautrec, though he'd have only a vague idea
> where her liver is.
> —Tatyana Tolstaya

There is evidence that medical practitioners and patients are showing a growing interest in and acceptance of hypnosis. In one of their studies, McIntosh and Hawney (1983) reported that 80 percent of their questionnaire sample of prospective patients had heard of hypnosis, 36.6 percent would accept hypnotherapy if recommended by their doctor, 5.5 percent would refuse treatment by hypnosis, and almost all of the remainder of the sample would request further information before making a decision. Forty-one percent of the study participants were unaware of any medical indications for hypnosis.

Over and above its uses as a primary or adjunct treatment for symptoms, hypnosis allows for a strengthening of constructive forces within the patient to assist in managing illness, and it facilitates an active participation of the patient in treatment. The strengthening of constructive forces is seen most clearly in the area of immunology of and the treatment of cancer with hypnosis. Since hypnosis is becoming more widely accepted within the medical field, it is reasonable that not only physicians but also related health professionals are interested in how to incorporate hypnotherapy into their treatment programs.

This chapter addresses first the practical application of hypnotic techniques in the medical treatment of intractable respiratory and cardiovascular dysfunctions and then the use of hypnosis in surgery. With regard to the former, the term *intractable* is used to denote disorders that are resistant to organic-based treatments, due to either the presence of a psychological component or the absence of an effective cure for the disorder. Hypnotic treatment can be a useful adjunct therapy in both instances.

The major use of hypnosis with psychophysiological disorders can be

241

thetic (SNS) and parasympathetic nervous system (PNS). Variations on this theme are used to achieve changes in a variety of physiological states, including but not limited to:

- Relaxation.
- Vasoconstriction or dilation.
- Expansion of bronchial passageways.
- Changes in heart rate.
- Changes in blood pressure.
- Control of bleeding.
- Control of temperature.
- Reduction in muscular tension.

By stimulating one of the processes controlled by the PNS, the arousal becomes generalized to the other processes mediated by that system. For example, tachycardia can be addressed by stimulating the PNS through deep breathing, suggestions for peripheral warmth, progressive muscular relaxation, or any number of other channels. If an individual demonstrates a particular aptitude for controlling one of these channels, then this can be used to her or his advantage in treatment.

Individual control over autonomic arousal can be achieved through hetero- and self-hypnosis. In many ways, it is similar to biofeedback, which has been used for years as an adjunct therapy. Hypnosis, however, has the advantages of being more flexible in addressing individual differences in its application, more easily lends itself to out-of-session practice, and does not require expensive instrumentation. Some subjects respond to visual or kinesthetic imagery, some to direct suggestion, and some to verbal biofeedback from the hypnotist; these individual differences can be more readily addressed in hypnosis than in biofeedback.

Control over autonomic arousal is not the only application of hypnosis. When a trance state has been achieved, imagery and suggestion can be used to address both psychological and medical issues such as:

- Noncompliance.
- Anxiety and panic.
- Cognitive restructuring and relabeling experiences.
- Self-efficacy and enhancement.
- Acute and chronic pain control.
- Habit control.
- Autoimmune enhancement.
- Nausea and vomiting.

A number of these topics are dealt with elsewhere in this book, but before the focus shifts to dealing with specific disorders, several generic issues in dealing with psychophysiological disorders should be addressed. As the name implies, there are both psychological and physiological components to the dysfunction. To address one and not the other is to treat only part of the problem, and it can, in fact, do more harm than good. For example, administering medicines with harmful side effects (such as addiction) to problems that may be primarily psychological is inappropriate. So is expecting a patient to change what we perceive as psychological symptoms that may, in reality, have primarily an organic etiology. Any attempt at treating a disorder with a psychophysiological component needs to make a thorough assessment of the relative contributions of both organic and psychological factors in causing and maintaining the disorder. Then, with this information, treatment is designed to address both components rather than one, and more realistic goals can be set.

Respiratory Dysfunction

The psychogenic aspects of asthma and related disorders received much attention from both early researchers (Dunbar, 1938; Turnbull, 1962; Freeman et al., 1964) and in recent research and case study presentation as well (Collison, 1975; Jencks, 1978; Frankel, 1987; Acousta-Austan, 1991). While the diversity of hypnotic and hypnoanalytic techniques makes cross-study comparison difficult, it would appear that, as with so many other areas, at some point in various cases, some techniques are useful with some subjects. Advantages (targets) to the use of hypnosis in the treatment of asthma include the following:

- Reduction in the frequency, duration, and intensity of wheezing spells.
- Reduction in the amount or elimination of corticosteroids in treatment.
- Reduction in the need for inhalers to ameliorate symptomatology.
- Increase in self-confidence, assertiveness, self-esteem, self-reliance, and ability to produce relaxation, especially in light of data that suggests that personality traits of shyness and inhibition predispose one to allergic responses (Kagan et al., 1991)

The asthmatic patient often comes first to the pediatrician, as the onset of this disorder typically occurs in childhood and early adolescence. In the situation where a child or adolescent patient presents with the asthmatic symptoms, several variables need to be considered: the distinction between extrinsic asthma, with an identified allergen or group of allergens, and intrinsic asthma, with no allergens identified. This distinction is theoretically important in that patients who present the same asthmatic symptoms without an identified organic etiology would presumably be more susceptible to psychological intervention. But this distinction has not received much research attention, so it is not clear if there is a different affect.

Some attention has been directed toward comparing asthmatics to nonasthmatics and, in particular, intrinsic asthmatics to nonasthmatics. While to date there has been little success in establishing a distinct personality profile for those who suffer from asthma (the so-called asthmatic personality), there is some research that pertains to personality variables. In reviewing this research, several things become evident. The intrinsic asthmatics tend to be seen as being more passive, dependent, and anxious, more often placing hopes for treatment in medication, and seeing hospitalization as the preferred vehicle for receiving that treatment. In any case, the degree of benefit gained by the asthmatic patient is positively correlated with the degree of hypnotizability and the depth of trance achieved by the patient (Gardner and Olness, 1981; Collison, 1975).

Consistent with systems theory, it has been shown that many of these patients' symptoms are tied in with sources of secondary gain within the family structure. Patients may, at least on occasion, use their symptoms as an escape from a dysfunctional setting or may draw attention to themselves as the identified patient in order to redirect parents away from their own marital conflict. If such is the case, then it is unlikely that hypnotic techniques alone will help to ameliorate the individual's symptomatology; they would have to be combined with some form of systemic family therapy.

Several techniques have been associated with improvement in children and adults suffering from asthma. The relevant outcome research has shown, with a few exceptions, that hypnosis, regardless of the techniques used, produces fairly reliable and significant symptom reduction.

Several points need to be made regarding this research in general. Most of these studies involved hypnosis in combination with other therapeutic techniques (systematic sensitization, progressive relaxation, steroid therapy, psychoanalysis, structural family therapy and the like), due to methodological flaws, the effects of the hypnosis are often confounded with the other treatment effects.

Second, due to the idiosyncratic nature of both relevant personal imagery and the types of suggestions that are responded to by subjects, between-groups comparisons may not be the best way to measure the impact of these techniques. Almost invariably, however, this is the form of experimental research that is conducted rather than the more appropriate single-subject designs (multiple baseline). Many of the reports are not even experimental research; they are simply the documented progress of a group of patients, with no control group. Further, many of the studies did not covary symptom severity or depth of trance with measures of improvement, and so it is difficult to assess the role these important factors may have had in improvement. In sum, there has been little true empirical research in this area.

Some patients can employ a posthypnotic suggestion to use their own asthmatic symptoms as a cue to trigger reinduction. The goal is for them to return to a relaxed state, where they will be aware of their surroundings and able to interact but will feel the same sense of physical calm and control that they felt during deep hypnosis. This can be enhanced by utilizing the client's own imagery to personalize the script. A prototypical case illustrates the technique.

Sam, a thirty-four-year-old male insurance salesman with a long history of asthmatic symptoms, presented with wheezing, coughing, and feelings of choking. He complained of allergies to pollen, and his recent move to the Ohio River Valley area (with its generally high pollen count) had produced a recent exacerbation of his condition. His asthma had responded minimally to corticosteroid therapy, and his frequent attacks were producing significant impairment in his ability to work.

He was induced via progressive muscular relaxation and deepened with imagery involving descending a staircase and the timed breathing approach (Watkins, 1986) into a somnambulistic state. Several sessions were spent in promoting relaxation and helping him achieve mastery over both his respiratory rate and his level of autonomic arousal. His relaxation was then keyed to an image drawn from his own descriptions of seeing himself sitting on the beach, breathing clean, cool, crisp air, feeling a cool relaxing sensation in his lungs with every breath that allowed him to breathe freely and to feel more and more relaxed. This imagery facilitated his relaxation, and he was able to breathe freely after a relatively brief time in trance.

After he demonstrated the ability to control his breathing and remaining asymptomatic while in trance, the focus shifted to his ability to control his breathing when not in hypnosis. This was addressed with posthypnotic suggestion. While Sam was in trance, he was given a direct suggestion that when he sensed any signs of an oncoming asthmatic episode (wheezing, coughing) while out of trance, he would interpret them as cues that could allow him to trigger autohypnosis or reinduction; the ocean beach image would return, and he would reexperience the same relaxation and control that he felt while under hypnosis at the clinic. This allowed him, with some self-hypnosis training and three follow-up sessions, to resume his work.

Often patients respond to one perceptual set of hypnosis suggestions better than another. In the example, the content of the suggestions was oriented toward change in physical sensations. With other patients, it may be more useful to utilize suggestions based on feelings of self-efficacy and mastery, vivid visual images, or even abstract idiosyncratic patient-generated content.

One creative example presented in Gardner and Olness (1981) illustrates the application of vivid visual imagery in the treatment of an asthmatic seven year old. After the induction, the child was asked what color his lungs were, to which he replied, "Green." When asked what color the air was today, he replied, "Orange." His therapist then utilized guided imagery to help the child visualize the process of free breathing; as the child "watched" the orange air flow into the green lungs, they changed to orange as all of the rich oxygen was absorbed. As he breathed out, the lungs turned back to green as all of the orange air was expelled. This example shows how the creative hypnotherapist can use the strengths of the patient to enhance the meaningfulness of suggestions used in the treatment.

Other researchers have used combinations of techniques to produce similar outcomes. In a study by Diamond (1959), hypnoanalysis was used on fifty-five intrinsic asthma patients to achieve age regression to the time of the first asthma attack. Then insight-oriented techniques were used, including positive recapitulation of the family experience, to aid in the children's understanding of how they used the asthmatic symptoms to gain parental attention. Other researchers (Jencks, 1978) focus on combining the hypnotic stage with breathing exercises that serve to counter the asthmatic's normal pattern of large inspirations and short expirations.

Cardiovascular Dysfunction

Migraine Headache

Hypnotherapy can be a useful subject to other forms of therapy in treating migraine headaches. Several research studies demonstrate the clinical effectiveness of the technique. A long-term study by Friedman and Taub (1984, 1985) compared six treatment groups and a waiting list control group on several outcome measures. The six treatment groups contained four hypnosis groups (two groups each of high and low hypnotizability), one biofeedback group, and one relaxation training group. Of the two groups each in high- and low-susceptibility subjects, one group received training aimed at thermal regulation. This group focused on regulation of peripheral temperature. The other hypnotic group received more general training, including progressive relaxation and direct suggestions that the specific headache symptoms would disappear. While all treatment groups showed benefit over the waiting list control group, highly susceptible subjects showed greater change than the other groups, and there was no difference between the two hypnosis protocols on dependent measures of headache rating scales or the amount of additional medication required. The difference in headache monitoring was maintained at a one-year follow-up, and the reduction of medication was maintained at one-year and three-year follow-ups. Similar results have been obtained by Singh (1989).

Once physical causes (such as brain tumors, damage to the facial nerves, and the like) have been ruled out, treatment with hypnotherapy can take a number of different forms. One set of techniques is designed to reduce the blood flow to the brain, with the emphasis of removing the throbbing sensations that are often experienced during migraine headaches. Examples of techniques in this category include direct suggestions of warmth in the peripheral parts of the body, with blood being shunted away from the core and to the periphery. Equally effective in some of these cases are direct suggestions that blood is being shunted to another part of the body. The following sample script may be used in such a case, beginning with the induction.

Therapist: As you sit in the chair, I want you to focus on the sensations that you are feeling in your body. As you are able to focus your visual attention, you are also able to focus your kinesthetic attention and pay attention to the sensations that you feel in the muscles of your body. I want you to focus on the tension that you feel in the muscles of your hands. Squeeze your hands into fists now, and feel how the tension in the muscles increases. Feel how the tightness and the tension increase as you squeeze tighter and tighter. Hold that tension in the hands. Be aware of the sensations that are there in the hands. Then release the fist and feel how the tension runs out of the hands and the hands become relaxed and warm and so very much more comfortable than before. As you relax the hands, notice how the fingers seem warmer and the muscles in the hand seem more relaxed and the hand feels much more comfortable . . . and after you enjoy that sensation for a moment, I want you to focus on the muscles of your arms, feeling the tension that is currently in the arms, now increasing the tension by flexing the arms and hands tightly. Flexing as hard as you can. Feeling the tightness and discomfort holding that in the arms and hands . . . then relaxing. Feeling the tension leave the arms and hands, and feeling the sensation of warmth and comfort and relaxation and heaviness returning to the hands and arms. Feeling the sensation of warmth spreading from the hands through the arms and bringing with it a sense of relaxation and feeling of pride and accomplishment that you are so easily able to control the amount of tension and relaxation that you feel in the muscles in your body.

The procedure is repeated with regard to the muscles of the head and neck, the chest and abdomen, the legs, thighs and buttocks, and the feet, each time adding the corresponding muscle group to all of the others, so that at the end, the client is tensing and relaxing the entire body. Including in this process are ego-strengthening suggestions that the client is perhaps surprised and pleased at being able to exercise such control over muscular tension and relaxation. Then a deepening technique is used:

Therapist: As you are so able to direct your attention internally to the perception of your relaxation, I want you now to attend to your breathing. Feeling your lungs fill with life-giving oxygen each time you breathe in, and as you breathe out, feeling yourself go deeper and deeper into relaxation. As you breathe in, I want you to become ever so slightly more alert, letting yourself come up a little, and as you breathe out, I want you to go deeper and deeper into relaxation. As you breathe in, come up a little, and as you breathe out go deeper and deeper and deeper into relaxation . . . up a little, and deeper and deeper and deeper into a state of relaxation and comfort and warmth . . . up, and down, deeper and deeper, more and more relaxed.

The hypnotist should increase the volume and length of the "deeper . . . down . . . more relaxed" expiration phases so as to match the pattern of breathing and decrease the volume and shorten the length of the phrases used in the inspiration phase, as it is not necessary to accentuate the entire length of the inspiration. The procedure is continued until an adequate level of trance has been achieved. The level of depth of trance desired is dependent on both the type of suggestion utilized and the orientation of the hypnotist, but a very deep trance is not a prerequisite for producing change. Then one or more of the following therapeutic suggestions can be utilized to facilitate change.

Therapist: As you are sitting there in your relaxed state, I want you to imagine that you are wrapped in a soft, warm cotton blanket, one that is thick and fluffy and warm. It can be colored or white, whatever you would like, but it feels warm and comfortable and cozy. While wrapped in this blanket, your body feels warm and comfortable and relaxed, not too warm, but just warm enough to be comfortable and relaxed.

Signal me when you are imagining this scene by raising your index finger slightly so that I can see it . . . as you see yourself in your blanket, feeling warm and comfortable, notice how the pulsing in your head has disappeared, and the pain from your headache has vanished as your body has become warm and comfortable.

A suggestion can be made to link this state of warmth and relaxation to the early warning signs of an upcoming migraine (obtained through interview, as there is interindividual variation) through an autohypnotic suggestion technique. Alternately, a suggestion can be made to use the early symptoms of the attack as a signal to find a place to practice relaxation, with the image being linked with the relaxation:

Therapist: Resting there in your blanket, you feel pleased and excited knowing that you can create this feeling of relaxation at any time, by yourself, simply by remembering this image, and feeling that wonderful feeling of warmth and relaxation return to you instantaneously. And you feel good about yourself having learned this wonderful way of using your mind to help yourself feel so comfortable. In the future, when you are feeling that a migraine headache is coming on because of [reliable symptom], this symptom will be a cue for you to practice your relaxation . . . Should you choose to do so, the image of the blanket will return to you, and you will feel the same sense of warmth and comfort and relaxation that you are feeling right now. And you will also feel the confidence of knowing that your headache will not cause you any trouble . . . that you can eliminate your headache at any time simply by practicing your relaxation.

This suggestion can be repeated and reinforced as long as necessary before bringing the client out of the trance. Practice can be promoted by making a posthypnotic suggestion that the client practice relaxation several times a day, with or without a headache.

Another set of techniques is focused on treating the pain that results from the migraine headache rather than the headache itself. Techniques such as the glove anesthesia technique and allowing the analgesic effects to spread to the head and face are commonly used to control the pain signal without affecting the etiology of the headache. Alternatively, the hypnotist could adapt the image of a suit of plate armor to enable the client to facilitate the spread of the glove anesthesia over the entire body. The hypnotist can begin the glove anesthesia with the image of a steel gauntlet, rather than the traditional electrician's glove, and then allow the subject to don the rest of the armor as the sensation of protection from pain spreads.

This allows the advantages of having an easily visualized image and a logical extension of the "armor" over the head as a helmet so that there is no pain in the head either.

Still another technique focuses on treating the nausea and kinesthetic imbalances and dizziness that result from the headache, primarily through direct suggestion. (The section on prenatal care in chapter 14 provides more specific techniques associated with the management of nausea.)

These techniques are not mutually exclusive; it may be appropriate to apply all of them with a client. In the case of a disorder like a migraine headache, with a multimodal set of symptoms, it would be ideal to conduct research in a single-subject format, with a multiple baseline design, targeting different components of the disorder—for example, focusing the treatment on relief from pain, without addressing the throbbing in the head or the nausea.

Further, like any other disorder that contains a psychophysiological component, the client cannot be perceived or treated in a vacuum. In addition to ruling out any organic etiology, the hypnotist is advised to obtain a full psychological profile prior to the administration of hypnotic techniques. This is useful both to assess possible secondary gain from the symptoms and in general to understand the client better. If the client's symptomatology proves resistant to treatment, despite being able to achieve a deep level of trance, there may be other internal or external factors that are sabotaging the client's success. For example, if a client has had a history of severely disabling migraine headaches and then finds that it was "all in his mind," there may be resistance from the client in giving up the symptoms. If the presence of these symptoms ensures the attention and concern from an otherwise distant spouse, this secondary gain would impede progress even further. The resistance to giving up the symptoms can be dealt with during trance by asking how long the client feels that he or she will need to effect the rehabilitation and then use direct suggestion to suggest that the symptoms will gradually disappear over the next few days (weeks, months) and be completely gone at the end of the time period suggested by the client. In the second problem, the client could be taught to manage the symptom in the hypnotic sessions and encouraged to bring in the spouse, for nonhypnotic couples' therapy to address the interpersonal issues exacerbating the client's condition.

Essential Hypertension

Hypnosis can lessen the effects of chronic hypertension by lowering peripheral resistance in the blood vessels and reducing cardiac output. Cardiac output is composed of stroke volume and heart rate. Consistent success has been demonstrated in the control of heart rate through hypnosis, but reduction of mean blood pressure measured over time has often been more elusive. Yet some researchers (Jana, 1967; Deabler et al., 1973) have reported consistent success in their ability to reduce both systolic and diastolic blood pressures through hypnosis. Their techniques involved direct suggestions of deeper breathing, relaxation, heaviness in the limbs, and imagery of descending down a flight of stairs. These researchers taught their patients to practice these techniques through self-hypnosis and report to have maintained benefit past the termination of formal therapy. However, other research (Case, Fogel, and Pollack, 1980) has found variable progress in the status of hypertension but found that all patients reported that they experienced an improvement in mood and demeanor.

There are several ways to assist clients in practicing self-hypnosis. Posthypnotic suggestions such as the following can be used directly: "You will practice your self-hypnosis at least six times daily," or "Your symptoms will serve as a reminder for you to stop and practice your self-hypnosis." Or they can be used indirectly: "When you experience [symptoms] you will remember how well you were able to control them in the session and how much better you felt after you took control of yourself and made [symptom] go away."

When addressing the problem of reducing heart rate, many different techniques can apparently achieve success. The hypnotist could decide to focus on the heart rate through direct suggestion and suggest that the heart will beat slower and slower:

Therapist: As you focus on the sensations in your body, you begin to feel the rhythmic pulsing of your heart as it pumps blood through your body, carrying life-giving oxygen and nutrients to all of the parts of your body, and you know that as your heart beats so rapidly, it is impaired in its ability to adequately supply your body with what it needs, so you begin to concentrate on your heart rate, and as your concentration increases, so does your control over the rate with which your heart beats, and just by concentrating on it you are able to slow your heart rate. Relaxing your heart so that it can work better . . . slower and slower . . . your heart rate is slowing and you feel good being able to exercise such control over your body and deal with what you used to think was such an insurmountable problem.

Another approach could involve biofeedback in the hypnotic state; the client, in trance, would utilize the biofeedback to assist in monitoring progress. The hypnotist may instead use an external stimulus like a metronome and suggest that the subject concentrate on synchronizing the heart rate with the beat of the metronome.

Any technique that produces peripheral thermal increase will serve to dilate the blood vessels and, subsequently, reduce peripheral resistance. Imagery can be used to facilitate relaxation—for example, imagining resting in a hot bath, nestling under a comforter by a fire, or lying in the sun on the beach. Direct suggestion can be used to increase peripheral temperature:

Therapist: As you begin to relax, you can feel sensations in your body that you were unable to perceive before, the rhythm of your breathing, the beating of your heart, the pulsing of the blood through your veins, bringing warm blood from your heart to your arms and legs . . . hands and feet . . . fingers and toes. Feel the blood pulsing through your fingers and toes, warming them, and as they become warmer, feel the veins and capillaries dilating, allowing even more warm blood through, making your hands become warmer and heavier . . . your fingers, warmer and heavier . . . your hands and fingers are becoming warm and heavy.

Indirect suggestion of relaxation will similarly effect vasodilation and also reduce peripheral resistance to blood flow.

Brady et al. (1974) reported that they were able to induce significant reductions in blood pressure through a technique that involves a thirty-minute period when the individual listens to direct suggestions to "let go" and "relax" the muscles. The suggestions are presented so that they are paced with the beat of a metronome set at sixty beats per minute.

Other applications of hypnotherapy include addressing the personality structure and coping mechanisms of the individuals suffering from hypertension. Some therapists have used posthypnotic suggestions in attempts to get patients to "stop worrying and take time out and relax." Research examining the Anger-in hypothesis and type A behavior has suggested that some persons' inability to express anger directly contributes to the elevation of their blood pressure. In such individuals, the opportunity to cathart under hypnosis and process their inability to do so during a normal waking state may prove invaluable in attempts to allow them a more stress-free life.

Cardiac Arrhythmias, Tachycardia, and Extrasystoles

A case study by Wain, Ahmen, and Oetgen (1983) showed that through implementation of dissociative techniques, it is possible to correct cardiac arrhythmias in some patients. With this patient, the hypnotist suggested that the client imagine that his chest was separated from the rest of his body and was completely relaxed. Some of the advantages reported in this case were fewer extrasystoles, an increased tolerance to exercise, and an increase in the patient's perceived self-control and self-efficacy. A disadvantage of this particular treatment was the later dissociation of awareness of the arrhythmia, both in the trance state and out of trance. Previously this client was able to sense when his heart "skipped a beat." The later dissociation obviously presents a risk to the client in that he may tend to stress himself too much and not be aware of the increased risk that he is in.

Another technique that could be used is a combination of psychoeducational techniques and imagery. The hypnotist explains the process through which the stimulation of the heart muscle occurs, including the conduction of the neural impulses, the nodal systems, and the propagation of the muscular contraction. Then the particular abnormality of the individual's heart is explained to the patient. Following this, imagery is used to strengthen the understanding of appropriate heart function in general and the particulars of the inappropriate functioning in this case. Then the hypnotist instructs the client to turn her or his attention inward, to assist perception of the aberrant occurrence, and the hypnotist can instruct the client to imagine the heart functioning without arrhythmia. After some success has been independently monitored, the hypnotherapist can use this as a reinforcer to show clients that they can control their arrhythmia.

Other researchers have implemented hypnotic techniques in correcting arrhythmias caused in childhood by rheumatic fever. In these cases, the technique involves age regression to a point before the heart was damaged by the disease, reexperiencing the sensations associated with the appropriate heartbeat, and giving direct and posthypnotic suggestions that the heartbeat will conform to those earlier parameters. Neither of these treatments has been evaluated through controlled research to date, but they show enough promise to be useful clinically.

Angina Pectoris

Techniques for the treatment of angina pectoris typically involve hypnotic relaxation and imagery of warmth in the chest and around the heart. In one case, the therapist aided the patient in warming his hand through enhancing the circulation and instructed the patient to place his hand over his heart and allow the transfer of warmth and relaxation to occur, thus improving the associated constricted pericardial and coronary circulation (Kroger and Fezler, 1976). Like many other approaches involving the cardiovascular system, this one combines relaxation, psychoeducational imagery, and thermal regulation.

Another approach to treating angina involves pain management. Although it is often unwise to mask the signal qualities of pain, particularly in the case of angina, the pain can be reduced to a tolerable level. Techniques like glove anesthesia, where the anesthesia is allowed to spread to the affected areas, can be modified to suit this purpose. In the following example, the client has been through induction and is at a sufficiently deep level to perform glove anesthesia.

Therapist: Your hand is beginning to feel numb and tingly, just as if your hand has fallen asleep. Your ability to feel pain in your hand has been reduced to where your hand can feel only enough pain to know that there is some pain. It is similar to when you have been to the dentist's office, and the novocaine is beginning to wear off; you can feel some pain, but only very little . . . [testing the anesthesia here]. Most of what you feel is pressure, a strange sensation of pressure, along with a little bit of pain . . . not enough to bother you, but just enough to alert you to the fact that there is pain in your hand. This sensation of tingly numbness is now spreading to your forearm, and along with it is this upper limit to the amount of pain that you are able to perceive in your forearm. Regardless of how much pain is afflicting this forearm, you will only feel a minute fraction of it . . . just enough to let you know whether the pain that is afflicting your arm or hand is dangerous to you. This sensation is spreading, spreading now to your shoulder and chest area, to the places where you feel the pain of your angina when it afflicts you . . . When it afflicts you, your mind will still be conscious of the relative severity of the pain and be able to make appropriate decisions about what to do, but there will be only a minimal sensation of pain, and mostly this numb, tingly, novocaine-like feeling that you are feeling now. After that minimal pain alerts you to the presence of pain in your arm, chest, or hand, your intellectual experience of the pain will be as if you were watching a pressure gauge. This gauge will have it on a red zone, and when the level of pain reaches the red zone, you will take the appropriate measures to deal with your angina . . . whether to take your nitroglycerin, or to stop exerting yourself and practice your relaxation, or to call your doctor or an ambulance for help. Your mind will remain clear, and you will be able to make the decision that will best provide you the care that you need to deal with the angina . . . and you will feel good that you can manage the pain from your angina, and be able to make clear and appropriate decisions, and take such an active part in ensuring that you get the medical care that you need and deserve.

If the client lacks the intellectual ability to make informed decisions about medical status, a particular response, such as calling the doctor and relaxing, can be keyed in rather than the more open-ended scenario described.

Postmyocardial Infarction Syndrome and Sexual Activity

There are a number of potential applications for patients recovering from myocardial infarction, among them pain control, relaxation, habit management for cases where obesity, poor nutrition, smoking, drinking, and other bad habits are factors, anxiety reduction, and self-efficacy enhancement. The majority of these are presented in depth in other chapters in this book, but a prototypical case example here indicates how they might be combined to facilitate the recovery of a patient subsequent to myocardial infarction.

> Joseph, a fifty-three-year-old morbidly obese black male, had a history of two previous myocardial infarctions and chronic hypertension. He smoked up to one pack of cigarettes per day, which was a reduction from the two to three packs per day that he had smoked prior to his first heart attack. His first heart attack had forced him into early retirement from his position as a dock supervisor, and his second had followed three months later when he was gardening at home. He prided himself on being a man of great physical strength in his youth and had suffered severe blows to his self-esteem as a result of the restrictions now placed upon his life-style secondary to his physical limitations. Joseph had come to our clinic in an attempt to receive help in quitting smoking and in losing weight. He previously had limited success with various dieting strategies and felt that while his reduction in smoking was positive, he wanted to quit completely.
>
> Treatment planning for Joseph identified several problems: two within the domain of habit management (weight loss and smoking cessation), essential hypertension, low self-esteem, and low self-efficacy. Attempting to address the self-efficacy first, Joseph was instructed on how to perform self-monitoring on his smoking and eating behaviors, and he was taught how to monitor his blood pressure. After a week of baseline data collection, hypnosis sessions were begun, focusing on relaxation training and self-efficacy building. The content of the suggestions demonstrated to Joseph that he could induce relaxation merely by concentrating on his own self-hypnosis and that by producing this state of relaxation (and peripheral temperature increase), he could have a direct effect on his blood pressure. By learning to internalize his locus of control and to relax in the hypnosis sessions, he became well motivated to practice his self-hypnosis on the outside. He quickly learned how to self-induce a state of deep relaxation and by the third week had shown a significant decrease in

his mean blood pressure levels, which he had been measuring three times daily since the first session.

The next phase of the intervention was to address his smoking behavior and obesity. Three sessions were dedicated half to didactic instruction about exercise, nutrition, weight loss, and smoking and half to establishing and reinforcing posthypnotic suggestions. The purpose of the suggestions was to identify his tension states (hunger, nicotine craving, anxiety) and to use them as cues for him to utilize his self-hypnosis. Initially the tension situations were to trigger the suggestion to practice, and this was later changed to trigger autohypnosis, with a different specific imagery for each tension situation. During the seventh week, he had stopped smoking entirely but had, unfortunately, gained five pounds by increasing his eating dramatically. However, by the tenth week, he had remained without cigarettes, and his weight gain had leveled off at a net increase of eleven pounds. His mood was markedly improved, and he reported feeling much better about himself and his ability to produce changes in his life-style. He was seen an additional six sessions, during which the focus was on his weight loss and his hypertension. He had managed enough control over this hypertension to achieve a substantial decrease in the medication required for maintenance but achieved only a minimal weight loss, recovering his baseline weight. At six-month and one-year follow-ups, he had maintained the progress with his hypertension and had remained without cigarettes but had not lost an appreciable amount of weight.

An important but seldom addressed side effect of heart attack is diminished sexual drive, at times resulting in psychosexual dysfunction and/or fear of dying during intercourse. Even after verbal reassurance that sexual intercourse is as safe as any other mild to moderate exercise, many patients still suffer from this fear and avoidance. This is readily amenable to treatment with hypnosis (Gibson and Heap, 1991). After induction, the patient can be instructed to imagine himself or herself engaging in the various stages leading up to his or her usual pattern of sexual intercourse, in the style of covert sensitization. While doing so, the therapist suggests to the patient a state of relaxation and control and pairs relaxation with the sexual arousal in a counterconditioning paradigm.

In almost all of the applications associated with cardiology, the emphasis is on decreasing anxiety and increasing mastery over autonomic arousal. Even in disorders of circulation like Reynaud's disease and Buerger's disease, the techniques employed typically involve relaxation, warmth imagery, and control of autonomic arousal, including thermal regulation.

Metabolic and Blood Disorders

Insulin-Dependent Diabetes Mellitus

This disorder is difficult for anyone and is especially problematic for children. They face the daily reality of the shot(s) and diets and other restrictions required to keep them alive and asymptomatic. Noncompliance and frequent hospitalization are often the sequelae to diagnosis with this disorder at a young age. Hypnotic treatment, whether of adults or children, tends to focus on three general areas: facilitating compliance, increasing body awareness, and pain control.

Pain control as a potential benefit should not be underestimated when considering individuals who require daily or even more frequent intramuscular injections. Particularly with younger children, the ability to control this pain can dramatically change their attitude toward the entire process required of diabetics. Body awareness is also important due to the diabetic's increased chance of infection and other immune-related problems. This can be addressed in hypnosis by helping the diabetic patient conduct a "body check," a guided imagery survey of all parts of the body on a mission of self-diagnosis. Facilitating compliance involves a number of variables that are amenable to treatment with hypnosis, including the following:

- Self-efficacy enhancement and internalizing the locus of control.
- Habit management, in the form of strict dieting and weight control, and the daily use of medication.
- Addressing possible sources of secondary gain influencing noncompliance.

Hemophilia

This disease is characterized by uncontrolled bleeding. The bleeding typically occurs in the joint cavities, and the treatment used to be transfusing whole blood to get the benefit of the clotting agents. Today, patients use self-administered doses of clotting factors to reduce the amount of internal bleeding, but this is an extremely expensive treatment and does not completely stop the bleeding. There are three types of hemophilia distinguished by the absence of different clotting agents. Hemophilia A patients are missing factor VIII, hemophilia B patients are missing factor IX, and the third group, labeled hemophilia A inhibitors, is missing factor VIII but has developed antibodies that prevent the functioning of infused doses of this agent and they are treated instead with factor IX. These last patients require greater quantities of factor infused and receive reduced efficacy.

Internal bleeding can result from external trauma, such as injury, or from minor wear and tear on the joints from walking. It also can occur spontaneously (without an identifiable external trauma). These spontaneous bleeds are reported by patients with hemophilia following emotional stress, such as fear, anxiety, anger, and even after positive emotional stress, like holidays and vacations. This spontaneous bleeding in the joints eventually produces a severe form of arthritis that can be extremely painful. In addition, by requiring frequent transfusions of factor VIII, these patients are at a greater risk of developing hepatitis and acquired immunodeficiency syndrome (AIDS) than are the general public, particularly since the blood from many thousands of donors may be used in preparing a single lot of the concentrated clotting agent.

The focus of hypnotic intervention can be directed toward five areas:

1. Management of emotional stressors to reduced the frequency of spontaneous bleeds, either through relaxation or using hypnotherapy to address underlying personality structures.
2. Control over peripheral vascular constriction, to reduce the severity of the bleed, either through direct suggestion to stop the bleeding and/or to constrict the blood vessels or through indirect suggestions of cold and/or the use of creative imagery.
3. Suggestions aimed at increasing self-confidence and promoting the practice of other techniques.
4. Psychoeducational and imagery approaches designed to increase the hemophiliac's production of the necessary factor.
5. Pain control techniques designed to treat the pain from the arthritis and the injections.

Several studies have documented the effectiveness of these hypnotic treatments, although, as is so often the case, the hypnotic treatments are confounded with other treatments, and it is difficult to tease out the effect of the hypnosis alone. LaBaw (1975) successfully used hypnosis to control spontaneous internal bleeding, as measured by decreases in the amount of blood transfusions needed. Swirsky-Sacchetti and Margolis (1986) produced a similar effect, as measured by the amount of concentrated clotting factor required by the patients.

Von Willebrand's Disease

Von Willebrand's disease has been treated effectively with hypnosis. In this disorder, the bleeding usually occurs from the skin and the mucous membranes rather than in the joints, as in hemophilia. Several case reports have indicated that suggestions of relaxation and use of relaxing imagery during periods of emotional tension can result in shortened duration and severity of bleeding (Fung and Lazar, 1983).

Surgical Applications

Hypnosis has been documented as being used in surgical procedures as early as 1829; Gravitz (1988) provides an excellent review of these applications. Hypnosis has been shown reliably to produce a number of beneficial effects over and above anesthesia and analgesia (Blankfield, 1991; Watkins, 1986). Hypnotic suggestion is used in the surgical process preoperatively to:

1. Reduce anxiety.
2. Induce relaxation.
3. Educate the patient about the operative protocol.
4. Improve the patient's self-confidence.

Hypnosis is used intraoperatively to:

1. Induce hypnoanesthesia in patients where traditional chemoanesthesia is contraindicated (some forms of neurosurgery, with patients who are allergic to anesthesia, or patients with heart conditions).
2. Reduce the quantity of any required chemoanesthesia.
3. Give the patient suggestions to assist in staunching bleeding or other actions that the patient can take to assist the surgery.
4. Give posthypnotic suggestions to forget anything that was recalled in the surgery that may prove traumatic to the patient.
5. Give posthypnotic suggestions of postoperative comfort, relaxation, and lack of pain.

Hypnosis is used postoperatively to:

1. Facilitate recovery through direct suggestions of compliance with treatment and relaxation, increasing the patient's active involvement in recovery and perceived self-efficacy.
2. Manage postoperative pain and avoid extensive use of chemical analgesics.
3. Manage anxiety and boredom and affective disturbances through creative use of relaxation imagery.
4. Supplement the functioning of the immune system through psychoeducational techniques and direct suggestion, thereby reducing the possibility of postoperative iatrogenic complications, such as infection and secondary illnesses.

Preoperative Procedures

Many researchers and clinicians have reported the advantages of preoperative hypnosis in the preparation of patients for the surgical process. Anderson and Masur (1983) conducted a fairly comprehensive critical review of these procedures. Despite methodological flaws in their study, they found that psychological preparation preoperatively has shown a number of consistent beneficial effects.

One of the most frequently commented upon techniques is Schultz's preoperative rehearsal technique for hypnoanesthesia (Schultz 1954; Finer, 1980). This technique involves inducing a hypnotic trance and then, through guided imagery, taking the patient through the entire surgery from preoperative preparation through postoperative care. This technique has been associated with a wide variety of benefits, such as decreased anxiety, decreased affective disturbance, fewer units of blood transfused during surgery, reduction in required sedative, antianxiety, and analgesic medications, and shorter postoperative stays in the hospital. The research on this technique has not included attention control groups, and thus the contribution of the hypnotic trance itself is not yet clearly demonstrated. Further, if unexpected complications occur, the patient can become agitated and may require additional anesthesia and/or antianxiety medications. Even so, the technique has received such widespread approval that it has become a standard in many settings.

Hypnoanesthesia and Analgesia in Operative Protocol

Distraction Techniques. Distraction can be used as a means of pain control and serves to occupy the individual's attention on some event or sensation other than the pain. For example, following induction into an appropriately deep level of trance, the hypnotist could help the client to form a pleasant, pain-free image and enhance the image by helping the client focus on the sensory cues he or she is experiencing in the image. Or the client may imagine the face of a loved one, and the hypnotist could help the client focus on all of the positive feelings that the image evokes. Alternatively, the client could attempt to relax a different part of the body from the one being operated on.

Temperature Metaphors. These can be used to control the pain sensations, primarily through direct suggestion and somatosensory imagery. For example, after an appropriate induction the following script could be used:

Therapist: I want you to form an image of a wintry lake scene, with a small lake and pier extending out into it. Visualize yourself out on the pier . . . How are you dressed? . . . it is very cold . . . there is snow on the ground. You brush the snow off a small area of the pier and sit down and take your left boot off, and take your left sock off as well . . . Right away your foot begins to become cold and numb in the cold air. You place your foot into the water, and it becomes cold and numb . . . so numb that you can reach down and touch your leg and you can't feel anything at all . . . no pain, no sensation at all, just coldness and numbness.

Glove Anesthesia and Direct Suggestion. Glove anesthesia can be used to produce either localized or a generalized control over pain. The section on migraines explained how glove anesthesia is achieved in the hand and extended over the body.

Dissociation and Symptom Substitution. The hypnotist can induce a state of dissociation so that either the client dissociates from the body or the pain is dissociated from or relabeled for the client. In the former case the script may sound as follows:

> *Therapist*: As you lie there in your relaxed state, you begin to feel an unusual sensation of lightness . . . you are conscious of yourself leaving your body like a ghost . . . floating up into the air . . . high above your body . . . free from the sensations that your body feels, because you have left it behind in the care of your doctor . . . as you travel away from it and tour a special place.

In the case of symptom substitution, the hypnotist can cause the pain to be relabeled for the client as less severe or as a different sensation, have it fade away into nothingness, or have it expelled from the body with each breath.

Suggestions Given with Regular Anesthesia

Some surgeries require extensively invasive procedures, and questions have been raised as to whether the patients recall this trauma, and if so, what effect it has on the patient's recovery and psychological state. For example, in corrective spinal surgery for scoliosis, patients experience surgical procedures that often extend for eight to ten hours and may involve exposing the entire length of the spine, possibly from both posterior and anterior approaches. In addition, one facet of this procedure, referred to as the wake-up test, involves the actual return to partial consciousness of the patient, who is then asked to perform various movements to check the functioning of the motor pathways of the spinal cord. It is reasonable to investigate whether patients recall this trauma; so far the results seem to indicate that postoperatively, if asked in a nontrance state, they do not. This does not, however, mean that the experience cannot be recalled at some other level.

One way to address this issue would be to use posthypnotic direct suggestions intraoperatively for the patient to forget the experience and to test for recall in postoperative trance sessions. If the intraoperative suggestions were not effective, the hypnotist could explore the impact of the experience on the client and make appropriate decisions regarding treatment. If the experience was recalled and distressing to the patient, the hypnotherapist could do several things. One approach would be to attempt to reframe the meaning of the experience from a state where the patient was cut open to a healing process that the patient endured with great courage and strength in order to assist the surgeons in their task. Another approach could be to reinforce the direct suggestion of forgetting and accompany this with a sensation of satisfaction and pride that the patient went through the session without difficulty. If this approach is utilized, it would be important to make sure that the patient did not manifest some later symptom substitution.

Postoperative Applications

There are a number of useful postoperative applications for hypnosis. Use of hypnotic suggestions in postoperative recovery has been associated with shorter hospital stays, fewer pain medications, less overall discomfort, and fewer secondary infections (Blankfield, 1991; Watkins, 1986) (Enhancement of the immune system is addressed in the next chapter covering cancer; readers are referred there for the benefits that result from these procedures.) When assessing the other potential benefits from postoperative use of hypnosis, several things become evident. Noncompliance with rehabilitative therapies is a major cause of longer hospitalization. Patients who actively participate in their treatment tend to recover faster. Compliance can be reinforced in a number of ways, including directly suggesting compliance with medications and therapies; by an indirect focus on how compliance will shorten the hospital stay; and by self-efficacy building suggestions that reinforce clients' control over their own recovery. Similarly, by reinforcing the practice of self-hypnosis, clients can rely more on themselves, and less on medications, to produce relaxation and pain control. Even after the hospital stay is over, there are often rehabilitative therapies that the patient is prescribed, and compliance with these is equally important for full recovery. A sample script addresses these issues:

Therapist: As you practice your self-hypnosis during the days ahead you will feel good about yourself that you are able to help yourself feel better without medications that are addictive . . . that you can relax without Valium, that you can control your pain with the power of your mind rather than a dangerous narcotic . . . and this sensation of power will make you want to practice your hypnosis even more so that you can achieve this comfort instantaneously . . . and it feels so good to know that you are playing such a large part in your own recovery . . . speeding up your return to health and helping yourself in the ways that you know how, that you will want to participate actively in all of your therapies . . . working hard to make your recovery 100 percent of what it should be . . . knowing that each time you engage in some part of your therapy it will leave you feeling good about yourself . . . feeling good that you take such good care of your body and your mind, and knowing that by working hard, you will recover faster and more fully.

By looking at the examples and recognizing the wide variety of settings and disorders that hypnotherapeutic techniques have been effective in, it should become clear that we are just beginning to scratch the surface of the benefits that can be reaped.

14

Hypnotherapy and Medical Disorders, II

> I don't want to achieve immortality through my work.
> I want to achieve immortality through not dying.
> —Woody Allen

Obstetrics and Gynecology

Obstetrics

Since ancient times, attempts have been made to alleviate the pain associated with childbirth (Stampone, 1990). Many types of methods have been used, from herbal remedies to prevent the formation of memories of the birthing experience to the current use of anesthetics. In 1831, Foissac was the first to use hypnosis for obstetrical medicine (Stampone, 1990). He mentioned that obstetric analgesia was induced using "magnetic" influence, based on Mesmer's theory of animal magnetism.

The reaction against Mesmer and his followers led to a decline in the use of hypnosis in obstetrics until the middle of the next century. In 1943, Kroger and Delee were the first to report anesthesia and amnesia in a woman during labor without the use of drugs but through the use of hypnosis (Stampone, 1990). Delee (1955) was a strong advocate for the use of hypnosis to produce anesthesia during childbirth. He asserted that the only anesthetic that is without danger during childbirth is hypnotism, chiding his colleagues who neglected to use "this harmless and potent remedy." During the 1950s, the use of hypnosis increased but then declined.

There has been a revival of the use of hypnosis in obstetrics (Harmon, Hynan, and Tyre, 1990). Between 1982 and 1985, there was a sharp increase in the number of articles published on hypnosis, and all indications are that this trend has not abated (Nash et al., 1988).

Advantages and Disadvantages of the Use of Hypnosis in Obstetrics. The revival of the use of hypnosis has prompted many individuals to question whether its use for obstetric care is safe and beneficial. All indications are that it is. Indeed, there is evidence that hypnosis in obstetric care

264

- May be maintained for a long period of time.
- Allows the mother to be fully conscious and cooperative with the physician.
- Allows the mother to speed up or slow down her labor, and premature labor may be prevented by hypnotic suggestion.
- Reduces chemoanalgesia and anesthesia or completely eliminates them.
- Reduces postoperative nausea, vomiting, anoxia, and other side effects of chemical anesthetics.
- Unlike medication, places no extra stress on the circulatory, respiratory, hepatic, or renal system.
- Reduces or eradicates fear, tension, and pain before and during labor.
- Provides resistance to fatigue.
- Controls painful uterine contractions.
- Shortens labor time by approximately three hours in primiparae women and approximately two hours in multiparae women.
- Eases delivery, episiotomy, and suturing of the perineum.
- Eases transfer of hypnotic rapport to an intern or nurse.
- Requires no elaborate education.
- Allows for quicker healing since many anesthetics slow the healing process (Stampone, 1990; Harmon, Hynan, and Tyre, 1990; Kroger, 1977).

It is noteworthy that Rock, Shipley, and Campule (cited by Crasilneck and Hall, 1985) reported that only twenty minutes was necessary to induce hypnosis for patients in active labor. (They might be a bit overconfident.)

There are some disadvantages to hypnosis during childbirth. Despite a high percentage of people susceptible to hypnosis, maximal relief of pain and discomfort can be achieved for only one out of four women, and not all women (or men for that matter) are good hypnotic subjects. Furthermore, hypnotic induction can be affected by other psychological factors. For example, a few "well-prepared" hypnotic subjects "fall apart" when they hear other women screaming during labor or they are eventually talked out of using hypnosis by friends and family. Among the disadvantages of the use of hypnosis in obstetrics are the following:

- Time is required to establish rapport and achieve the depth of hypnotic trance needed for operative procedures.
- It can require a number of conditioning visits, and such a large investment of the therapist's time may be expensive or impossible.
- A trained hypnotherapist must be available throughout the entire labor and delivery unless the woman can use autohypnosis.
- Lay misconceptions of hypnosis disrupt its use.
- Hypnosis should not be used with deeply disturbed persons, such as psychotic or borderline individuals.
- A faulty interpersonal relationship between a woman and her hypno-

therapist may damage her relationship to all medical caregivers. (Crasilneck & Hall, 1985; Kroger, 1977).

When to Begin Treatment. If a woman requests hypnotic anesthesia for
childbirth, the hypnotherapist should first explore her reason for choosing
this form of anesthesia. Both personality type and her responsiveness to
hypnotic suggestions should be considered. If the hypnotherapist decides to
treat the woman, then when to begin treatment must be decided.

One approach suggests beginning hypnosis in the first trimester of pregnancy. The woman should be seen weekly during the first month and every
three weeks until one month before her estimated delivery date. At this time,
hypnosis should resume a weekly schedule. The hypnotherapist should be
called immediately after the obstetrician has instructed the woman to report
to the hospital. Once the woman has begun labor, hypnosis should be
induced.

Another approach at any point in the pregnancy by offering a complete
orientation on the subject of hypnosis. Any misconceptions about hypnoanesthesia are corrected. In a group, a counting technique is used to relax the
woman and induce a trance state. This counting technique includes counting backward from one hundred to zero. From one hundred to eighty is
counted in increments of one, and from eighty to zero is counted in increments of five. At each twenty-count increment, suggestions are given to help
deepen the trance state. Next, the women are instructed to dissociate from
themselves and picture themselves doing something especially enjoyable. At
this point, the women are taught a method of self-hypnosis. Hypnosis during labor and delivery begins when the woman is completely dilated.

Finally, hypnotherapy may begin in the third or fourth month of pregnancy. If anesthesia is not obtained after ten hypnotic sessions, the prognosis for effective hypnoanesthesia is poor (Kroger, 1977).

Treatment Techniques. Although the time when treatment begins varies
with hypnotists, the hypnotic techniques are similar (Crasilneck and Hall,
1985; Kroger, 1977). First, the woman, while in the waking state, is shown
the area in which analgesia is to be induced. When the woman is in a
hypnotic trance, hypnotic suggestions may be given:

Therapist: You will sense pressure building, but you will feel secure,
relaxed, and at ease. You feel free from tension, tightness,
stress, and strain. The area of your body that we discussed
will simply be anesthetized. It will feel numb or may have no
feeling at all. You will have no discomfort. You are so relaxed and calm, your baby will be delivered with comfort.

Following these suggestions, hypnoanesthesia is induced in one finger or
the entire hand, producing glove anesthesia:

Therapist: And now you will go into a deep, hypnotic state, way down, deeper and deeper. You are going to produce a loss of feeling in your hand, much as a glove might fit over your hand to close off the feeling. As I stroke this hand, it is going to get numb, heavy and woodenlike.

The reality of the anesthesia is demonstrated to the woman by vigorously stimulating the tip of her anesthetized finger, or her hand, with the point of a moderately sharp object like a nail file.

Next, the anesthetized feeling is transferred to the face and abdomen:

Therapist: With every movement of your hand toward your face, it will get more numb and woodenlike. When your hand touches your face, press your palm firmly against your face. Make certain that your hand is pressed closely to your face. Let the numbness in your hand flow from it to your face. You are getting deeper and deeper relaxed as your hand presses against your face and numbs it. You can feel the numbness being transferred from your hand to your face. That's fine. Good. When you feel the numbness leave your hand and numb your face, drop your arm and your hand. Your hand will not feel numb or woodenlike, but your face will be anesthetized.

After the face becomes numb, the woman is then similarly instructed to transfer the numbness to her abdomen.

Finally, the following suggestions (Chiasson, 1984) are provided:

Therapist: The remaining part of your pregnancy will be easier. Your labor will be shorter, easier, and safer. Your delivery will be so much easier and pleasant, and your stay in the hospital so much more comfortable. When you are in labor and when you are in the hospital, you can use your contractions as a signal to get more and more relaxed and make all the muscles in your pelvis very numb, loose, and relaxed.

When labor begins, the woman can go into hypnosis by herself, by the idea of a written note from a nurse, or over the telephone by her doctor.

Hyperemesis. Hyperemesis, or vomiting, is often a problem during pregnancy. It usually occurs during the first trimester of pregnancy and may progress to the point of dehydration, hospitalization, and loss of the fetus. Hypnosis has been used to address this problem (Chiasson, 1984). Several hypnotic script suggestions may be helpful: cessation of a dirty or metallic taste, which is replaced by a pleasant taste just like that of the woman's favorite chewing gum or toothpaste; or the idea that the esophagus will stop contracting and reversing and have smooth, rhythmic waves, taking the food down to the stomach where the digestive juices will start to digest it, the food will go into the small bowel, and the peristaltic waves will propel it along in a normal fashion, allowing digestion to be completed and the food to be absorbed.

The following hypnotic suggestions may be used for the treatment of hyperemesis:

> *Treatment*: The thought and taste of food will not be discomforting. You will not become sick to your stomach or nauseous. Imagine the smell of your favorite food. When you can imagine the smell of your favorite food, let me know by slightly raising your forefinger. Good. The food smells pleasant and satisfying. You notice your mouth begins to water. You want to eat this food. Imagine yourself sitting at a table, with the food on a plate in front of you. When you have an image of this, let me know by raising your forefinger. Fine. You begin to eat. You are able to eat your food, and you do not feel nauseous or queasy. You take in the food easily. It tastes good. You realize that the food will give you the strength necessary to adjust well to your pregnancy and to give you and your baby the strength you both need.

Cesarean Childbirth. Hypnosis may be used to achieve anesthesia for a birth by cesarean. During each session, time is taken to help the woman attain deep hypnosis. Hypnotic suggestions are given to produce glove anesthesia and transfer the anesthesia to the jaw, back to the hand, from the hand to the abdomen, and in some cases from the hand to the breast. The transfer of anesthesia to the breast is used to show the woman that even in this very sensitive area, the numbness can last as long as necessary for a given time. The woman is taught to spread the level of numbness up to two inches above the umbilicus, and if she is familiar with spinal anesthesia, she can be asked to stimulate this without any of the side effects or complications of spinal anesthesia.

The suggestions are repeated on each visit. The woman is tested for the depth of her trance and the extent of anesthesia. Finally, she is given the suggestions that her postoperative recovery will be smooth and uneventful. Her muscles will stay relaxed, the blood circulation will be improved, and healing will be better and faster. The woman is asked about her experience of the hypnosis, and any misconceptions about the technique are clarified. The woman is usually admitted to the hospital the night before the procedure. A rehearsal, with stimulating preparatory noises and conditions, should be performed (Chiasson, 1984; Stampone, 1990).

The following case illustrates the use of hypnosis in obstetrics. The case combines hypnotic suggestions traditionally used, in combination with my own suggestions.

> Olivia, a thirty-four-year-old Caucasian female, came to her gynecologist with complaints of nausea, dizziness, intolerance for food, and a missed menstrual cycle. She was several weeks past the expected commencement of her period. A pregnancy test was positive. As her pregnancy progressed, she developed severe hyperemesis and consequently missed several days of work. Again, she requested the assistance of her gynecologist to alleviate her vomiting. Her gynecologist, reluctant to administer medications during the pregnancy, suggested that Olivia visited a noted hypnotherapist to help her with her problem. Olivia agreed.
>
> After an initial interview to determine why Olivia requested the use of hypnosis and to assess Olivia's motivation to engage in hypnotherapy, the hypnotic induction was administered, using a technique similar to those provided in chapter 3. After she was sufficiently relaxed, a deepening technique was used. Olivia imagined she was in an elevator on the tenth floor. She was asked to focus on the floor number panel and watch as the lighted numbers moved from ten to one. As the numbers decreased, Olivia was told: "You are becoming more and more relaxed. You do not feel any tension in your body. You feel at rest and at ease. You are comfortable, relaxed and peaceful. You feel very calm with no worries or fears."
>
> Once in a moderate to deep trance, the following hypnotic script was used:

Therapist: Now that you are completely relaxed and at ease, you will be able to imagine the thought and taste of food. It will not be discomforting but will be quite pleasant. You will not experience a queasiness in your stomach. You imagine the smell and aroma of the food filling the room. It is appealing, and you wish to eat some of the food. When you are able to imagine the smell of your favorite food, let me know by slightly raising your forefinger. Good. Now continue to relax and imagine the smell of your favorite food. You do not feel queasy or nauseated.

Now, imagine a movie screen in front of you. On the screen you can see yourself sitting at a table with a dinner plate in front of you. Let me know when you can visualize this image by slightly raising your forefinger. Good. You continue to remain relaxed and at ease. You do not feel queasy or nauseated. You begin to eat the food, and it tastes good. Your stomach remains very relaxed. You continue to eat the food. You have finished all the food on the plate. You still feel relaxed and at ease. You have no sensations of nausea or queasiness. You feel satisfied. You realize you have successfully fed yourself and your baby. You feel happy that your baby will grow strong and be healthy. Whenever you begin to feel nauseated or queasy, you will be able to achieve this comfortable and relaxed state on your own.

The success of hypnosis to decrease the hyperemesis led Olivia to request the use of hypnosis during the remainder of her pregnancy and as an analgesia during her labor and delivery. Since she had responded well, the hypnotherapist agreed.

Olivia was instructed on how to develop glove anesthesia. Once she successfully mastered the ability, subsequent sessions focused on transferring the anesthesia to her abdomen. The following hypnotic script was used:

Therapist: When you are sure your hand is numb, you will then transfer this numbness to your stomach. With every movement of your hand toward your stomach, your hand will become more and more woodenlike. Press the palm of your hand on your stomach. You can feel the numbness in your hand leave, and as it does, your stomach begins to feel numb. Your stomach is relaxed and numb. When your labor begins, you will be able to transfer this numb feeling to other parts of your body. You will feel the numbness in your stomach flow to other parts of your body. The numbness will flow across your pelvic area. Your inner thighs will feel numb, as well as the entire area between your legs. You will be able to feel this numbness for a long period of time.

When labor begins you will feel an ache in the smallness of your back. This ache will move around to your belly. This is a positive feeling. When you feel this ache, you will be able to use hypnosis and become very relaxed. You will become relaxed and feel the numbness in your stomach and feel it flowing and spreading through your pelvic region and to the entire area between your legs. You will stay relaxed and at ease. As you stay relaxed, you will hear sounds and voices, and they are comforting. You hear yourself moan and groan and maybe scream. You will feel your labor contractions, stronger and stronger, but you know these feelings are a good sign. You know you are progressing through your labor. You know your labor contractions are present, but they do not hurt. You know that you can ask for medication to help you. You will not feel guilty for asking. You will feel pressure between your legs. You know this pressure is a positive sign because your baby will soon be born. You continue to feel relaxed and at ease. You know that if you want, you can ask for medication to help you. You will not feel guilty for asking. You hear your baby cry, and you feel tired but relaxed. You feel comfortable and at rest. The numbness begins to leave your stomach. The numbness leaves your pelvic area and the entire area between your legs. You do not feel ill after your baby is born. You feel tired but comfortable. You are able to sleep when you want as much as you want. You are relaxed, calm, and feel peaceful.

Olivia met with the hypnotherapist once every three weeks until the seventh month of her pregnancy, when she moved to weekly hypnotic sessions. When labor began, Olivia was able to use hypnosis successfully throughout her labor and deliver without the use of medication.

Research with Obstetric Patients. Despite the disadvantages, hypnosis appears to be an effective treatment for problems associated with pregnancy and for inducing anesthesia during childbirth. Hypnosis seems to be effective in significantly increasing the ease and speed of labor and in decreasing the anxiety and discomfort associated with labor and delivery (Harmon, Hynan, and Tyre, 1990). A literature review reported that hypnosis successfully reduced nausea and vomiting in pregnant women, as well as for anorexic women, and for cancer patients experiencing the side effects of chemotherapy treatments (Frankl, 1987). Successful delivery of full-term babies for forty of forty-four women who were at risk for premature labor has been documented (Mehl and Lewis, 1988). During their pregnancies, the women received hypnosis and body awareness techniques designed to decrease autonomic reactivity and muscle tension. Group hypnotherapy appears to offer virtually all of the advantages of individual hypnotherapy, plus the supportive atmosphere of the group.

Gynecology

Such gynecological difficulties as menstrual irregularities, menopause, pseudocytosis ("false pregnancy"), pain relief, and infertility have been successfully treated with hypnosis. Hypnosis also has been used in the controversial treatment of breast enhancement. From another perspective, given the increasing reports of problematic side effects from breast implants, hypnosis offers even more merits. Through the use of hypnotic suggestions, women are instructed to engorge their breasts with blood, which may be a significant factor in reported increases in breast measurements (Cransilneck and Hall, 1985) though this could also be an "eye of the beholder" phenomenon.

The more common menstrual irregularities are amenorrhea (absence of periods), dysmenorrhea (painful menstruation) menometrorrhagia (bleeding at abnormal times during the cycle), and mittelschmerz (pain associated with the time between menstrual cycles when the ovum is released).

Emotional upset and worry may produce such irregularities, so a careful review by the clinician of potential psychological factors underlying the disorder is recommended. The review should explore the woman's childhood training about sex and menstrual functioning; a survey of dating and sexual relationships; an inquiry into the current state of the woman's marriage or significant emotional relationships; the woman's attitudes about sex; the attitudes of other individuals in her life toward sex; and possibly an inquiry into her dream and fantasy life. Any or all of these factors may contribute to the stress, which is likely producing the menstrual irregularity.

With all of the menstrual irregularities, the following hypnotic suggestion, a variation on a theme generated by Crasilneck and Hall (1985), may be employed:

> *Therapist*: Fears and tension can bring on alterations in your body's chemistry and hormones. The powerful dynamic forces of your unconscious may reverse or slow such activity. You will now become extremely relaxed. As you relax, you feel your body changing. This change is good. It signals a return of normal physiological and psychological menstrual activity. The anxieties, the tensions, and the fears that may have prevented you from [add the appropriate menstrual irregularity, such as menstruating, conceiving, painful menstruation] are leaving your body. Your body is relaxed and returning to normal function.

Amenorrhea. For the treatment of amenorrhea, the initial interview should explore physical changes the woman may have experienced during menstrual cycles prior to the onset of amenorrhea, addressing such issues as breast tenderness, low back pain, anxiety, moodiness, irritability, depression, and pain, possibly associated with blood flow. Answers to these questions should be incorporated into the hypnotic suggestions.

An example of a hypnotic script to use with an amenorrheic woman follows:

Therapist: In two weeks you will begin to feel some tenderness in your breasts. You will feel bloated and experience an uncomfortableness in your stomach. You will not be concerned about these feelings. You will be glad because they are a good sign. At times, you will feel uneasy, tense, anxious, and depressed. You will have a dull ache in your back. You will experience these feelings in about two weeks, and they will last for a few days. You will then feel some discomfort and cramps. You will stay relaxed when you feel the cramps. You will know the cramps are a positive sign because your period will soon begin.

A similar procedure, with some variations, may be followed to treat menometrorrhagia (bleeding at abnormal times during the cycle).

Dysmenorrhea. For dysmenorrhea (painful menstruation), the woman may be instructed to follow suggestions similar to those used for the treatment of immunological dysfunctions, detailed later in this chapter. Briefly, for dysmenorrhea, the woman may be told:

Therapist: You have eaten a sweet substance that will lower the level of prostaglandin in your body. Prostaglandin, a hormone which causes smooth muscle contraction, causes the discomfort, bloating, and irritability you feel each month. Imagine yourself doing something enjoyable. After your hypnosis, you will have a period without discomfort.

For the relief of pain associated with menstruation or metastatic tumors, the techniques outlined in chapter 12, which address general pain management, are beneficial.

Menopause. Menopausal symptoms are typically associated with estrogen deficiency. The symptoms are varied and include vasomotor instability ("hot and cold flashes"), profuse sweating, and faintness. As with other gynecological problems, emotional factors may be a contributing and/or necessary component to address in alleviating the symptoms of menopause. An extensive interview should be conducted to explore these issues. The answers from the interview may be incorporated into a hypnotic script similar to the script presented to treat amenorrhea.

Infertility. Hypnosis may help women who experience infertility. Not only does it help with evaluation, but as with other gynecological problems, psychological factors and emotions stress may affect a woman's ability to conceive. Hypnosis may help remove psychological blocks to the consummation of coitus, reduce tension, and aid in the normalization of ovarian cycles. The following script may be used to treat an infertile woman:

> *Therapist*: You will be relaxed and at ease. The tensions and stresses that have kept you from conceiving will come under control. You will be able to relax when you want. Your unconscious mind is very powerful. The unconscious power will help you to conceive. Your body will respond to your relaxed state and will become increasingly accepting of the growth of a child within it. You will eventually conceive and carry your baby successfully.

Peusdocyesis. Pseudocyesis, or false pregnancy, is a delusion of pregnancy. It may cause the woman to protrude her abdomen in such a way as to appear several months pregnant. Menses may even cease. It is crucial to define the mental conflict that led to this particular delusion, which may be treated with psychotherapy and hypnotic suggestion.

Immunology

The immune system operates to defend the body from a number of insults, such as bacteria, viruses, and other pathogens. Traditionally, the immune system was thought to operate autonomously without central nervous system involvement. However, given numerous clinical observations suggesting that psychological and emotional factors alter resistance to the disease process, this view is outmoded (Halley, 1991; Vollhardt, 1991; Spiegel et al., 1989). Vollhardt's (1991) important review of this area leads to the conclusion that one can psychologically intervene in the immune system in three dimensions.

1. *Immunosuppression.* The suppression of the immune system increases susceptibility to infections (such as mononucleosis and tuberculosis), psychocutaneous disease (such as inflammatory dermatoses), respiratory illness (such as asthma), AIDS and AIDS-related complex, neoplastic diseases (such as cancer), allergies, and autoimmune disorders (such as rheumatoid arthritis, psoriasis, and myasthenia gravis). Trauma, irradiation, malnutrition, drug and alcohol use, temperature, and aging are some environmental factors associated with immunosuppression. Stress, coping mechanisms (including psychological vulnerability, lack of control, and introversion), emotional distress (such as anxiety, depression, and helplessness), and bereavement also have deleterious effects on the immune system and the ability to fight off infectious, neoplastic, and autoimmune diseases.

2. *Mediating factors.* Stress sets off a chain of biological, especially endocrine, responses that activate the organism and decrease immunological efficiency. Stress is perceived and processed, and the limbic system relays this emotional information; the hypothalamus releases neuropeptides; then adrenocorticotropic hormones are released, then corticosteroids and then catecholamines, which decrease immunological efficiency, which in turn increase disease susceptibility. In terms of specialization of brain function and the immune system, "the left hemisphere of the brain is involved in the processing of positive emotions as well as in the stimulation of the immune system, while the right side of the brain is responsible for processing negative emotions and for suppressing the immune system—either directly or by inhibiting the activity of the left brain" (Vollhardt, 1991, p. 43). Research with animals has demonstrated these physiological connections through such experimental manipulations as classical conditioning (such as pairing saccharin water with an immunosuppressive drug) and brain lesions (such as in the hypothalamus).

3. *Immunoenhancement.* The notion that one can increase the immune system's ability to fight off disease rests on the premise that one can reduce environmental, emotional, and behavioral stressors that lead to disease susceptibility in the first place. Such interventions as psychosocial treatment, hypnosis, and social interaction have reduced pain and anxiety and increased longevity in women with metastatic breast cancer.

Certain medical journals have dismissed the relationship between psychological and physical health as folklore. However, empirical studies with both humans and animals have substantially supported psychoimmunology as an area for further study. The area of psychoimmunology has responded enthusiastically to the use of hypnotic treatment in the area of treating cancer patients. At an experimental level, the immune system of unstressed mice has been shown to contain the growth of experimentally implanted lymphoscarcoma cancer cells partially or totally. When the animals were experimentally stressed, tumor growth occurred (Riley, 1981). Longer survival rates for humans suffering from cancer have been associated with decreased stress using hypnosis (Newton, 1982–1983); Spiegel et al., 1989).

Cancer

Hypnosis has been helpful in assisting individuals diagnosed with cancer to accept the diagnosis, facilitate surgery and postoperative recovery, relieve pain without excessive narcotics, and decrease side effects, such as severe nausea and vomiting from chemotherapy and radiotherapy. Additionally, hypnosis has been used as a treatment in and of itself, with a focus on strengthening the patient's immune system to attack and destroy the cancerous cells.

Several therapists have developed programs to use hypnosis and allied techniques to develop immunological control and to treat diseases like cancer directly. Carl Simonton, a radiation oncologist, and Stephanie Matthews-Simonton, a psychotherapist, have developed the most well-known imagery program for treating cancer. They suggested eight features of imagery treatment, which they assert are important in altering the course of cancer (see Hall, 1984):

1. The cancer cells are imagined as weak, confused, soft, and easily broken down. The authors indicate that imagining the cancer cells as hamburger meat or fish eggs works well during the hypnotic treatment.
2. Treatment is presented as "strong and powerful," and the treatment can interact with and destroy the cancer cells.
3. During imagery, the healthy cells can repair any damage to themselves from chemotherapy or radiation therapy. The cancer cells are not able to repair themselves; they die.
4. The white blood cells are seen as greatly outnumbering and overwhelming the cancer cells.
5. The white blood cells are viewed as aggressive and eager to destroy cancer cells.
6. The dead and destroyed cancer cells are viewed as flushed out of the body.
7. The patients view themselves as healthy and disease free.
8. Patients imagine future life goals.

An alternative imagery program (Hall, 1984) recommends providing a technique linking an activity yielding a physiological response to a sensory imagination, such as tension in the body flowing out of the body and floating like a balloon. The trance-deepening stage should be linked with self-control. Guided imagery should be used for deepening and to induce local anesthesia. Time distortions, such as remembrance of an enjoyable activity or event, should also be included. Motivation and ego strengthening suggestions should be provided and instructions for self-hypnosis given. Finally, reorientation by bringing the individual to the present moment should not be neglected. (Chapter 12 also describes a technique for coping with the pain and the process of life-threatening diseases.)

Terminal Patients

Hypnosis can be helpful in a terminal case if the patient is anxious to avoid medication or has a fear that medication will cloud consciousness, wants to control pain without the side effects of narcotic drugs, needs help psychologically to face the end of his or her life as normally as possible, and needs help in maintaining adequate food intake and delay cachexia.

The hypnotic script should always include the ideas of freedom from tension, tightness, stress, and strain; of being relaxed and at ease; and of the body as relatively free from discomfort:

> *Therapist*: You will have a minimum of discomfort. You feel relaxed and at ease. You feel your muscles relax. The tension and tightness in your muscles lessens and flows out of your body. You feel a sense of well-being. You will be able to sleep when you desire. You will be able to reinforce these suggestions yourself. As frequently as you desire, you will be able to reinforce these suggestions. You will be able to relax yourself and remind yourself of these suggestions. You can eat well and enjoy the food the doctor has ordered for you. Discomfort, anxiety, and tension will be minimized and be under control most of the time. You will be relaxed and at ease. You rest well, secure in the knowledge that your unconscious mind will allow you to be free of excessive tension and any physical of psychological discomfort.

A case of an individual diagnosed with cancer may demonstrate the use of hypnosis to treat emesis associated with chemotherapy. Additionally, the use of hypnosis to strengthen and help fight the cancer was incorporated into the individual's treatment. The hypnotic suggestions encompass the areas recommended by Simonton and Simonton (Hall, 1984) and use traditional suggestions and my own.

> Charlie, a fifty-five-year-old black male, was diagnosed with a cancerous tumor in his stomach. The tumor was surgically removed, and Charlie received radiotherapy. Following the radiotherapy, Charlie began a program of five chemotherapy treatments weekly. This was expected to last approximately five months.
>
> Approximately three months after resection and irradiation treatments, Charlie was referred to the psychology department. Reportedly, he was unable to sleep the night prior to his chemotherapy treatment, evidenced severe nausea and frequent vomiting at home prior to and following treatment, and was rarely able to eat dinner on nights prior to his chemotherapy.
>
> The focus of intervention was twofold: to treat Charlie's anxiety, insomnia, and emesis and to focus on providing suggestions to combat and extinguish any possible remaining cancerous cells. The following hypnotic script was used:

Therapist: Time will go by rapidly, your anxiety and fears will be much less. You will be unafraid with little anxiety and tension. You can sleep for long periods of time. You will sleep as often as you wish and sleep easily. When you awake, you will feel calm and refreshed. You will eat as much as you wish, and you will enjoy your food. You will not feel nausea, and you will feel only a minimal need to vomit, but if you do have to vomit, you can. Should you be asleep when you need to vomit, you can awaken, vomit, and immediately go back to a deep, restful, peaceful sleep. Time will pass by quickly, hours will seem like minutes, there will be little discomfort, and vomiting will grow less with each treatment. Your body will respond maximally to treatment. During the day, you will be able to have a period of time in which you are very relaxed. You will feel at ease, peaceful, and virtually free of pain.

You will be able to have an image of your immune system as powerful and strong. You know your powerful immune system can attack and destroy any cancer cells. You will be able to see the cells of your body. Observe that the cancer cells look confused, weak, and powerless. You can see the powerful and strong healthy cells in your body. You can see the chemotherapy enter your body. It looks like tiny bullets of energy. You see the energy bullets attack the weak, confused, and powerless cancer cells. The healthy cells are affected by the chemotherapy, but they are able to recover. You see the healthy white blood cells and the energy bullets of the chemotherapy attack the cancer cells. The cancer cells are surrounded. The cancer cells are powerless and confused. The cancer cells cannot escape from the healthy white blood cells. See the weak, confused, and powerless cancer cells die, and the healthy white blood cells carrying the dead cancer cells away. You see your blood. Your blood flowing through your body. It is flowing effortlessly and swiftly. In your blood, you see the dead and powerless cancer cells being flushed away. The dead and powerless cancer cells are flushed through your kidneys and out of your body. You feel alive and strong. You feel relaxed but full of energy. Every day you will feel a greater feeling of personal well being, a greater feeling of personal safety and security. Enjoy this feeling of complete relaxation and calm. You will get stronger and better, and gradually recover and get well.

Children with Cancer

Children with cancer present special problems for the staff treating the child and for the parents. Children often do not understand the nature of their disease and the meaning of the painful procedures, such as bone marrow transplants. Chapter 15 provides information on how to tailor hypnotic treatment to use with children, but imagery scripts such as the one above can be developed for children as well.

Research with Cancer Patients

Hypnotherapy contributes to the alleviation of pain, reduction of side effects associated with chemotherapy, and longer survival rates for cancer patients (Spiegel et al., 1989; Newton, 1982–1983). Cancer patients in Newton's study who received adequate treatment, defined as a minimum of ten one-hour hypnosis sessions over a three-month period, had a better survival rate than individuals who received less hypnosis or none at all. In another group, intervention consisted of weekly group meetings with a psychiatrist, with discussion focused on physical problems, side effects of chemotherapy or radiotherapy, and the teaching of a self-hypnosis strategy for pain control (Spiegel et al., 1989). Those in the group showed higher survival rates.

Furthermore, success has been documented with respect to the alleviation of pain associated with cancer (Spiegel and Bloom, 1983). The use of hypnosis for the treatment of cancer pain is similar to the treatment used for general pain management.

Finally, the effectiveness in treating pre- and postchemotherapy emesis with hypnosis has been documented (Redd, Rosenberger, and Hendler, 1982–1983). More recently, the successful reduction of nausea and vomiting in reaction to chemotherapy in the case of an eleven-year-old boy treated with hypnosis was reported (Kaufman, Tarnowski, and Olsen, 1989). Training in cue-controlled relaxation, guided imagery, instruction in self-hypnosis, and parental instruction on using these techniques was provided. During the imagery, the therapist suggested that the child notice an increased sense of coolness and tension in the abdominal region, and cues for nausea and emesis were provided. In response, the child was asked to increase the warmth in the area and reduce muscle tension. The goal of the treatment was to help the child recognize bodily cues associated with nausea and vomiting and then use relaxation and imagery techniques to mitigate the discomfort.

Rehabilitation

The rehabilitation of individuals with traumatic brain injuries, strokes, and other calamities is one of the fastest growing areas in the health industry, and hypnosis lends itself well to the rehabilitation setting (Blankfield, 1991). It aids in differential diagnosis of functional and organic problems; maximizing functional ability even in cases when full recovery is not possible; diminishing pain and improving the patient's ability to tolerate the discomforts of illness; and increasing motivation for rehabilitation.

Many people in a rehabilitation facility are elderly and may by physically impaired by the normal changes of aging. They may display impaired visual and auditory abilities and memory loss. Additionally, stroke victims may be especially difficult to treat. Often they are emotionally labile and anxious, express negativism toward the rehabilitation exercises, lack motivation, and are depressed, possibly showing a "death instinct," a nonverbalized apparent desire not to survive. Nonetheless, hypnosis remains a legitimate adjunct to the treatment of stroke and other physical disabilities.

The usual induction procedure of progressive relaxation with eye closure is usually acceptable to most elderly patients. Then modifications are incorporated into the hypnotic script for working with rehabilitation patients; therapists should speak slowly, use simple vocabulary, increase the repetitions given for each suggestion, and persevere in continuing to visit the patient in spite of minimal response or apparent negative response.

The following case example will demonstrate how hypnosis may be used in a rehabilitation setting. The case incorporates my work with suggestions from various sources (Bowen, 1989; Manganiello, 1986).

Rodney, a seventy-eight-year-old Caucasian right-handed male, was the restrained unintoxicated driver involved in a motor vehicle accident. He incurred multiple injuries and suffered a pulmonary arrest. At the hospital, he was placed on a ventilator. A computed tomography scan revealed a left cerebrovascular accident. It appeared he suffered a stroke, lost control of his car, and crashed. During the course of Rodney's treatment, an attempt was made to wean him from the ventilator. He developed a bronchial mucous plug and consequently was reintubated. Rodney was treated for several weeks in the hospital, and then he was transferred to a rehabilitation facility. Prior to his transfer, another attempt was made to wean him from the ventilator. Rodney's concern about developing another mucous plug led to severe anxiety, and he did not sleep for three days. Again, he was reintubated. At the time of his transfer, he remained ventilator dependent, and he was hemiplegic on the right side.

Rodney received his rehabilitation therapies in bed. His therapists reported improvement; however, they were limited in the scope of his treatment because of his reliance on the ventilator. Staff approached Rodney about the possibility of weaning him from the ventilator, but he remained resistant. After referral and then an extensive interview, the use of hypnosis seemed appropriate, and Rodney agreed to participate.

Rodney was given a relaxation induction session similar to those outlined in chapter 3. After a trance state was induced, Rodney was given hypnotic suggestions:

Therapist: You are relaxed and at ease. You feel comfortable and full of energy. You are going to have therapy for your lungs just as you have therapy for your arms and legs. You will be off the ventilator a few hours each day. You will be off the ventilator so you can exercise your lungs and respiratory muscles. You will be comfortable and relaxed when you are off the ventilator. When you are off the ventilator, you will feel your respiratory muscles and lungs getting stronger. Your lungs are strong, and they are working on their own. You feel good because your lungs are getting stronger. You will get well and not need the ventilator.

Rodney was instructed on how to use self-hypnotic techniques and encouraged to perform the self-hypnosis daily. Additionally, he was seen by the hypnotherapist daily for two weeks. At the end of the two weeks, Rodney was successfully weaned from the ventilator. Rodney enjoyed working with hypnosis and asked to continue in hypnosis. It was decided that the hypnotherapy would continue and focus on increasing his arm and leg strength in his affected right side.

During the remaining sessions, with the use of age regression techniques similar to those outlined in chapter 7, Rodney was regressed to the age of fifteen years old. When Rodney was fifteen, he was an avid tennis player and was on the school tennis team. He continued to enjoy playing this sport throughout his life but quit playing the game approximately ten years previously. The following hypnotic script was used:

Therapist: You are fully relaxed, but you are not tired. You are full of energy and feel like you felt when you were fifteen years old. You can ride a bike, run, and play tennis very well. You enjoy playing tennis very much. You will remain in a trance and be able to show me some tennis positions.

At this time, a deepening technique was used. After Rodney was in a deep trance, the following hypnotic script was given:

Therapist: You are on a tennis court. Just like the court you played your championship game on in high school. You are relaxed and full of energy. You will be able to open your eyes when I tell you, but you will stay in a trance. When you open your eyes, you will show me some tennis positions. You will feel no pain when your arm is in the position. You will be relaxed and calm. Now open your eyes. Show me how to hold the racket for a forehand swing. Good. You are still very relaxed. Now show me how to hold the racket for a backhand swing. Very good. Now put your arm in the air like you were at the top of the arc on your serve. Your arm does not hurt.

Now relax your legs. Your legs feel relaxed, but with much tone and energy. You feel like you want to trun. Your legs have so much energy. You will stay in a trance and feel relaxed, but you will be able to show me how to stand when you receive a serve. You will not feel tense or anxious when you show me. You will feel relaxed. You will not feel guilty about asking me for support if you need to rest or lean on me. You will be able to show me how to stand. Now stand as if you were receiving a serve. Good. You can see some tennis balls in the corner of the court. You walk over to get the balls. You do not feel any pain. Your legs are full of tone and energy. You can lean on me if you need to, but you are able to walk to the balls. You will not feel guilty if you lean on me for support.

Again, Rodney was instructed on how to use self-hypnosis techniques and encouraged to use the self-hypnosis daily. Within several weeks, Rodney was walking with the aid of a quad-based cane. His strength was increasing in his arm and leg, and he continued to improve.

Stroke Victims

Hypnosis has proved successful in treating stroke victims. The use of hypnosis accompanied by electrical stimulation to improve and influence movement in hemiparetic individuals has been examined (Radil et al., 1988). The extent of movements of the hemiparetic upper extremity considerably improved during and immediately following hypnosis.

In a case study, Manganiello (1986) reported that an individual who suffered a left cerebrovascular accident with subsequent right-sided hemiparesis regained full function of his leg and arm movements within five weeks following his stroke. The patient began hypnosis treatment within two months following his stroke. The hypnosis treatment continued for five weekly sessions. The treatment consisted of using a counting technique to induce a trance state. Guided imagery was used to deepen the trance. Suggestions were given that the patient's speech would become clearer and his hearing would improve. Suggestions also were given that concentrated on digit and gait control. Manganiello noted that this subject was highly susceptible to hypnosis, evidenced by the patient's ability to open his eyes while in trance. It is very possible similar treatment results would not be found with less susceptible subjects.

In another case study, Holroyd and Hill (1987) reported improvement in the arm movements of a patient who suffered a left cerebrovascular accident. The patient began physical therapy five days after her stroke and hypnotherapy six months following her stroke. The authors commented that this patient improved in her ability to raise her arm approximately three feet higher than prior to hypnosis and was able to arise from a chair unassisted. Interestingly, this patient scored in the low range on the Stanford Hypnotic Susceptibility Scale, Form C.

Amputation

Hypnosis can be used to help with amputation and the after-effects of the surgery (Blankfield, 1991). When addressing the surgery and pain involved in an amputation, it is useful to utilize those techniques outlined in chapters 15 and 13 on anesthesia in surgery and pain management, respectively. A case study discusses the beneficial effects of hypnosis for treating an individual suffering from hyperhidrosis—increased sweating at the site of the amputation (Minichiello, 1987).

> The patient's leg was amputated, and he was fitted with a prosthesis three months following surgery. He experienced no sweating in the stump area until six years later, after he had a revision surgery. The sweating occurred only when he wore his prosthesis and was so severe that ulcerations formed on his stump. The hypnotic trance was induced as an electric fan blew on his stump. Suggestions such as, "In days ahead your stump will feel drier and cooler, you will feel as if a cool breeze from a fan is blowing on your stump, and this feeling will continue throughout the day, and you will develop the power to cool and dry your stump," were given. After two and one-half weeks, the patient reported healing of his stump ulcers and significantly decreased sweating.

Other Rehabilitation Disorders

Hypnosis has been used with neurological, musculoskeletal, and hematologic disorders sometimes seen in the rehabilitation setting. These disorders include multiple sclerosis, alateral sclerosis, Bell's palsy, cerebral palsy, arthritis, rheumatism, and Raynaud's disease. Finally hypnosis may be used to help set bone fractures and in surgeries requiring hip pinning or spinal fusion.

Other Medical Conditions

The creative health professional can apply hypnosis to virtually any type of medical condition (Blankfield, 1991; Frankl, 1987). Once a patient is instructed on simple relaxation techniques, the deepening procedure and hypnotic suggestions are tailored to the specific condition, as modeled throughout this chapter and the prior one. The verbiage of the script incorporates vocabulary associated with the medical condition. Other medical conditions treated with the help of hypnosis are cardiovascular, pulmonary, gastrointestinal, endocrine and metabolic, neuropsychiatric including migraines and tension headaches, and dermatologic disorders.

Cardiovascular Conditions

Cardiac conditions to which hypnosis can make a positive treatment contribution include hypertension, arrhythmias, angina, congestive heart failure, and coronary heart disease. Weinstein and Au (1991) used hypnosis to extend the time a patient could tolerate the angioplasty procedure, thus making for a more effective result. In most cardiovascular procedures, the imagery focus is on the walls of the heart, arteries and veins, and the rhythm of the heartbeat (Hunter, 1987). For example, in the case of an individual who has experienced coronary heart failure, suggestions may include:

> *Therapist*: You are able to see in your mind's eye the walls of your heart healing and recovering. You see a scar on your heart. This is where your heart was once weak. It is now becoming stronger and is able to work and beat with the rest of the heart muscle. The scar is not worrisome. It acts as a strong bridge that reaches to the rest of your heart and gathers strength. It receives oxygen from the body and is strong. Your veins and arteries leading to and from your heart are clear. They are long, open, hollow tubes. The blood flows freely through them. There are not obstacles in the way of the blood. It is able to flow, and your heart works effortlessly to keep your blood moving.

Pulmonary Conditions

The pulmonary disorders most often treated with hypnosis are the hyperventilation syndrome and asthma. Other disorders may respond positively as well. Acosta-Austan (1991) successfully treated chronic dyspnea using hypnosis and supportive-educational techniques. Usually when treating an asthma disorder, the individual is a child. (Reference to chapter 15 is recommended). The general approach to working with asthma sufferers is to ask the individual to simulate an asthma attack. The hypnotic script involves asking the child to imagine a field of flowers, having a picnic in a field, running fast, or some other activity specific to the child that precipitates an asthma attack (Hunter, 1987).

When the child begins to wheeze, he or she is congratulated on performing the hypnosis well and told to return to normal. Generally the child will spontaneously release the bronchial tension and return to normal. This event shows them they can control their asthma by relying on bodily cues and reacting appropriately. It is mandatory that when performing hypnosis and stimulating an asthma attack that a physician be immediately available in the event of a serious attack.

Gastrointestinal Conditions

Gastrointestinal conditions involve dysphagia (swallowing difficulties), vomiting, ulcers, diarrhea, constipation, and colitis (inflammation of the colon). Dysphagia and vomiting conditions may be treated in the same manner as hyperemesis experienced during pregnancy. For treating stomach and intestinal conditions with hypnosis, the hypnotic script should focus on relieving anxiety and tension and suggest smooth and normal functioning of the musculature and acid-producing cells of the stomach and a calm and normal digestive process. For example, in the case of an individual with ulcerative colitis, the following suggestions may be used:

Therapist: You are able to relax. You can feel the tension and anxiety in your body subside. You feel more relaxed, and the anxiety you once felt is flowing out of your body. You are no longer tense but very calm and relaxed. You are able to imagine the walls of your stomach and intestine. You are able to imagine the areas of your intestine that need more lubrication to help prevent painful ulcers. As you find these areas in your intestine, you are able to imagine the mucous lining of your intestine becoming richer and thicker. You feel the healing begin and realize the delicate lining in your intestine is beginning to be protected. You can see the smooth, well-lubricated lining on the walls of your intestine. You feel the smooth, pulsating rhythm of your intestine, digesting your food. You are able to digest your food successfully. Your stomach and intestine is protected from harm.

Endocrine and Metabolic Conditions

Many of the endocrine conditions involve disorders of the ovarian function, such as menstrual irregularities, infertility, and menopause. An earlier section of this chapter discussed these conditions and treatment suggestions.

Dermatologic Conditions

Dermatological conditions traditionally treated with hypnosis include warts, acne, psoriasis, and eczema. Spanos, Williams, and Gwynn (1990) compared hypnotic treatment of wart sufferers to topical salicylic acid, a placebo group, and a no-treatment control group. Although the three treatment groups were measured to have equal expectation of success, at six-week follow-up, only the hypnotic subjects had lost significantly more warts than the no-treatment controls.

Hypnotic scripts for dermatological conditions involve messages that focus on tension reduction and relaxation, which is believed to cause many of the blemishes. Furthermore, the blemish may be visualized to disappear. For example, in the case of severe acne:

> *Therapist*: Close your eyes and imagine your face. You see your face with many unflattering marks and blemishes. You know your mind is powerful, and you can visualize the blemishes leaving your face. The marks are powerless and weak against your powerful mind. Slowly, you see the red marks fade. Your face and skin is becoming clearer and smoother. There are a few rough spots on your cheeks, but they will not become red or inflamed. Your face will clear of major blemishes.

Ophthalmology

Ophthalmological conditions amenable to hypnosis include amblyopia (uncoordinated eyes, which affect proper focusing) visual acuity, glaucoma, adjustment to contact lenses, eye surgery, and blepharospasm (involuntary eye blinks). For disorders that involve visual acuity, one should include obvious suggestions of clarity, pinpoint vision, and strength in ability to focus successfully in the hypnotic script. For the use of hypnosis in eye surgery, the chapters that address pain management and anesthesia for surgery are recommended.

The treatment of glaucoma addresses the tension and anxiety that exacerbates the condition. Individuals with glaucoma are often elderly and are experiencing many life-style changes, such as worry about financial difficulties and other health issues. Often blurred vision, itching, and a throbbing sensation intensify when individuals with glaucoma become upset. Treatment involves addressing tension reduction and providing relaxation techniques for the individual to use. Decreasing anxiety about other issues helps alleviate some of the discomfort associated with the glaucoma.

A common problem associated with ophthalmological care is treating individuals who wear contact lenses. They often experience difficulty inserting the lenses into the eyes or cannot tolerate the initial discomfort of the lenses. It has been recommended to use a distraction technique to help with lens insertion (Kroger, 1977):

> *Therapist*: As you move your finger toward your eye, concentrate on the pressure of your feet on the floor. You feel the floor as solid and hard. Your finger is moving closer toward your eye. As your finger gets closer to your eye, you are able to feel the pressure of the floor under your feet more intensely. Your finger with the contact touches your eyeball; the floor is hard and solid, and it is comforting. The contact is in your eye, and your eye is sensitive. The contact feels tight, but you blink, and the contact becomes more comfortable. You are able to tolerate the initial discomfort of the contact lenses. Each day you will be able to tolerate the lenses for a longer period of time. You will be able to notice increased discomfort if soot or grit enters your eye. If the lens feels extremely uncomfortable, you will not feel guilty for taking it out of your eye. You will be able to insert the lens again. Your eye will continue to be sensitive to important changes in how your eye feels and also vision changes. But your tolerance for discomfort from wearing will lessen each day you wear the lenses and every minute they are on your eyes.

Complete anesthesia of the eyeball is not indicated, and the individual should be specifically directed to retain some sensitivity in the eyeball. This will allow the contact lens wearer to be able to notice ill-fitting lenses or foreign objects, such as grit or an eyelash, in the eye. Furthermore, a hypnotic technique that addresses increased relaxation and focus of the sensation of the contact lenses on the eyeball could also be used instead of the distraction technique.

Summary

The use of hypnosis in medicine is an interesting and intriguing area. Research has documented successful outcomes of the use of hypnosis in many medical areas.

In obstetrics, hypnosis has helped in alleviating vomiting during pregnancy, with childbirth, including cesarean sections, and with menstrual irregularities. The area of immunology, especially care of cancer patients, has responded earnestly to the use of hypnosis to help patients accept their diagnosis, adjust to various treatments such as chemotherapy and radiotherapy, and even live longer and possibly recover from the cancer. Successful outcomes for rehabilitation patients and individuals experiencing various internal medical disorders, such as cardiovascular disorders, pulmonary distress, gastrointestinal, dermatological, and ophthalmological complaints have been shown.

While self-hypnosis seems to be becoming more widely accepted by practitioners and patients, it still has not achieved its deserved level of recognition as an alternative or adjunct treatment. However, over 50 percent of a questionnaire sample of medical practitioners requested training in the area of hypnosis (Hadley, 1988). At least 36 percent of a questionnaire sample of prospective patients indicated they would accept hypnotherapy if recommended by their doctor (McIntosh & Hawney, 1983). Yet, 41 percent of the sample were unaware of any medical indications for hypnosis. It's clear that increased education is needed in order for hypnosis to become successfully incorporated into the medical arena.

15
Hypnosis with Children

> The term "child actor" is redundant.
> He should not be further incited.
> —Fran Lebowitz, *Social Studies* (1981)

The modern history of the use of hypnosis with children appears to begin with Franz Mesmer (1734–1815) (Gardner & Olness, 1988). Mesmer reported the successful use of his animal magnetism in curing several child and adolescent patients. One of his first "hypnosis" patients was a seventeen-year-old girl whose sight was restored by the treatment.

In 1784 the Franklin Commission conducted an experiment with a twelve-year-old boy in order to test the underlying theory of the existence of magnetic fluid. They concluded that the real cause was the subject's imagination rather than any sort of magnetism. This led to considerable controversy, with professionals choosing sides either in support of or in opposition to the findings. The noted hypnotist John Elliotson (1791–1868) defended the theory of animal magnetism and reported many successful treatments of children using mesmeric passes. On the other side of the debate, Jean-Martin Charcot (1835–1893) considered hypnosis to be a pathological state that was a form of hysterical neurosis; he believed that children were not susceptible to it.

Auguste Liebault (1823–1904), together with Hippolyte Bernheim (1840–1919), found that children were good hypnotic subjects, provided that the child was able to pay attention and understand instructions. Liebault conducted normative studies and found that in a sample of persons ranging in age from infancy to old age, the highest percentage of somnambules occurred in the seven- to fourteen-year-old age range.

J. Milne Bramwell published *Hypnotism: Its History, Practice, and Theory* in 1903. This widely used text reported the successful use of hypnotherapy with children aged three to nineteen, on such childhood disorders as behavior problems, chorea, eczema, enuresis, nail biting, night terrors, seizures, and stammering.

Based on the number of publications during the first half of this century involving pediatric hypnosis, interest in the area appeared to wane. However, interest in the use of hypnosis with children was renewed with the publication in 1956 of Ambrose's book *Hypnotherapy with Children*, which argues the successful use of hypnosis in treating a wide variety of childhood problems.

Current Research

Are Children Hypnotizable?

The studies by Liebault in the late nineteeth century found that children respond well to hypnotic suggestions. These findings remain largely undisputed, with recent researchers in almost complete agreement that children are excellent hypnotic subjects Plotnick, Payne, and O'Grady, 1991; Friedrich, 1990; Gardner and Olness, 1988; London, 1965).

Appropriate Ages for Hypnosis and Hypnotherapy

At what age may hypnosis be used with children? The answer appears to lie in how hypnosis is defined. Often hypnosis is considered to be something that occurs as a result of a specific induction technique, a technique that is usually verbal in nature. But this definition limits the use of hypnosis to children with an appropriate level of verbal skill and comprehension, often thought to be around the age of five to seven (Plotnick, Payne, and O'Grady, 1991). Yet the data are clear that younger children are more responsive to suggestion in general (Hulse-Trotter and Tubbs, 1991; Sanders, Copeland, and Elkins, 1987).

Research attempting to verify at what age hypnosis is possible is often restricted by the limitations of the instruments used. For instance, measures of hypnotic susceptibility for children, such as the Children's Hypnotic Susceptibilty Scale (London, 1963) and the Stanford Hypnotic Clinical Scale for Children (Morgan and Hilgard, 1979), are frequently used in studies designed to determine at what ages children are easily hypnotized. However, these measures are verbal in nature, which assumes that they are reliable only when used with children possessing appropriate verbal skills.

Although this issue of instrument reliability seems obvious, research indicates otherwise. Normative studies utilizing measures of hypnotic susceptibility for children have found that hypnotizability is limited in young children (ages five and six), increases and peaks during middle childhood (ages seven to fourteen), and then declines slightly in adolescence (London, 1963; Morgan and Hilgard, 1979). However, although these scales are not able to be administered to children younger than age five (due to limitations in childrens' verbal skills below this age), researchers generally assume that younger children would score even lower on these measures. From these findings, though the evidence is that they are suggestible in a general sense (Hulse-Trotter and Tubbs, 1991), it is often concluded that hypnosis is not appropriate for preschool-aged children (below age five or six).

Another limitation of the research addressing the question of age is that some researchers assume that items on children and adult hypnotic susceptibility scales tap identical phenomena. However, from early on, there were indications that this was not so. London and Cooper (1969) reported on the difficulty of items on hypnotic susceptibility scales for children compared to adults. Interestingly, eye closure was one of the easier items for adults but the most difficult one for children. Thus, on an eye closure task a child would be expected to score much lower than an adult, implying that the child is less susceptible to hypnosis. Of course, it may be that children merely find it difficult to keep their eyes closed, an indication of their curious nature and short attention span rather than an implication of their ability to experience hypnoticlike states. Thus, although the tasks on adult and child hypnotic susceptibility scales are similar in appearance, they probably are tapping two different phenomena.

Given the problems, a different definition of hypnosis appears to be in order. Gardner (1977) suggests that the criteria of hypnotizability shift from scale scores or verbal reports of one's hypnotic experience to the presence of certain behaviors associated with the hypnotic state in both adults and children. That is, children should be considered hypnotized if they exhibit one or more of the following behaviors:

1) Quiet, wakeful behavior, which may or may not lead to sleep, following soothing repetitive stimulation which is a primary characteristic of most formal induction procedures, 2) involvement in vivid imagery during induction in children beyond infancy, 3) heightened attention to a narrow focus with concomitant alterations in awareness, 4) capacity to follow post-hypnotic suggestions as evidenced by behavior which deviates from what is known to be the child's usual behavior in a particular situation. (Gardner, 1977, pp. 158–159)

Based on these criteria, it seems quite likely that very young children experience hypnotic states. In support of this is a growing body of literature that details the effectiveness of hypnotherapy with preschool children on a variety of problems, including easing induction of anesthesia, pain reduction, and control of enuresis and encopresis.

Differences in the Hypnotizability of Adults and Children

Are children more responsive to hypnosis than adults? Research investigating this issue is limited. However, studies by London (1965) and London and Cooper (1969) found that children are more easily hypnotized than adults. This greater response to hypnosis may be due to a number of factors unique to children, according to Gardner (1974):

1. The ability to concentrate intensely, to focus attention on a limited stimulus field, and to become fully absorbed in the immediate present.

2. A tendency toward concrete, literal thinking.
3. A decrease in reality testing, a fascination with magic, and a readiness to shift back and forth between reality and fantasy.
4. A propensity to feel intensely, often in an all-or-nothing way.
5. A willingness to accept new ideas and to enjoy new experiences in a context of felt safety and trust.

General Recommendations for Child Hypnotherapy

Parental Involvement

Parents must both formally and genuinely agree to the use of hypnotherapy for the child before the intervention may begin. As in other therapeutic interventions with children, a covertly resistant parent can subvert the effectiveness of the procedure. Therefore, it is most important for the parent to understand the therapist's rationale for the use of hypnosis for the child. The therapist should meet with the child's parents and explain and demystify hypnosis. A useful illustration is to explain to the parents that people experience different levels of consciousness, of which the hypnotic state is one. An everyday example is a parent who may awaken at the slightest sound made by a child but who sleeps through much louder noises.

The boundaries of parental involvement should be established from the outset. For instance, if a child is taught self-hypnosis, as is often the case in habit disorders (such as enuresis), it may prove therapeutic to restrict parents from reminding their children to practice self-hypnosis. The child should be informed of any such rules in the presence of his or her parents to establish that the child is in control of any gains that are made.

Preinduction Interview

During the preinduction interview with the child, the therapist discusses the reasons for using hypnosis, gains an understanding of the child's views about hypnosis, clarifies misconceptions, and educates the child about the procedure. It is also important for the therapist to gain information about the child's likes and dislikes, fears, and hopes, so that the therapist does not unwittingly mention an image that is frightening to the child (for example, soft, fluffy puppies may be an enjoyable image to most children but not to a child who recently received stitches because of a dog bite). It is often worthwhile to state to the child that the hypnosis experience will be "our secret" (from friends and school chums and from parents if that is contractually clarified ahead of time). They may not always keep the secret but they will appreciate hearing that the therapist will keep it secret.

Differences in the Hypnotic State for Children

Children shift quickly from fantasy to reality, and vice versea (Plotnick, Payne, and O'Grady, 1991; Valente, 1990). This makes a child's hypnotic experience different from an adult's in several ways. First, because of this ability to shift from reality to fantasy, children may go into hypnosis without a formal induction. Second, the deepening phase is often shorter for children than for adults because children are able to shift quickly to the hypnotic state. Third, because of their ability to shift quickly from fantasy to reality, children may come out of a trance state quickly. One way to prepare for this possibility is to use a less structured dehypnotization procedure for children than is often used for adults: "Enjoy this a little bit longer; then when you're ready, just slowly and comfortably open your eyes." The child can signal the therapist as to when he or she is finished with the trance experience and is ready to return to a normal state. This gives the child the control of returning to a normal state of awareness and avoids the surprise to the therapist of the child's popping out of trance before the therapist was prepared.

Compared to adults, children are more physically active, more likely to open their eyes or refuse to shut them, and more likely to speak spontaneously during hypnotic inductions. Some clinicians view these behaviors as indicating that the child is not experiencing a hypnotic state, because it is commonly thought that a person must have closed eyes in order to experience a hypnotic state. However, it is possible to induce an active, alert hypnosis when the subject is involved in physical activity. Thus, children may accomplish a hypnotherapeutic goal while engaging in play activity (Gardner and Olness, 1988).

The therapist should not insist that children close their eyes for hypnosis. Eye closure for children may trigger negative attitudes about sleep. It is best merely to suggest to the child that it may be easier to concentrate with eyes closed, but that the decision is the child's.

Induction techniques should be altered in order to accommodate children's short attention spans (compared to adults) and accompanying restlessness and boredom (Rhue and Lynn, 1991). The monotonous, repetitive inductions such as standard "adult" relaxation suggestions should be avoided in favor of more interesting inductions by using moving stimuli (a swinging pendulum or moving mobile), avoiding long pauses, during which a child's attention may stray, and keeping the child engaged in the procedure at all times. A relatively constant stream of verbal patter and suggestion may prove useful.

The Language of Hypnotherapy with Children

Choice of words is important. Words like *sleepy, tired,* and *drowsy* should be avoided because many children have negative attitudes about sleep and going to bed. Also, children may equate the terms with a favorite pet who has been "put to sleep." Words like *try* imply the possibility of failure.

The therapist must use language and images that the child understands. In the preinduction interview, the therapist should gain information about the child's favorite activities, places, toys, and so on and refer to these specific images in the hypnosis procedures rather than making general statements—for example, rather than saying, "Think of a special place," say "Think of the pond on your grandmother's farm where you said you like to be."

Younger children love magic words or magic objects, which can be used during the hypnotic process. If the child creates the image, he or she has a sense of control over the problem. For example, a boy who was recently involved in a serious car accident is now afraid to travel in an automobile. When asked what would make him feel safe, he replied, "Being able to just rub my elbow and have an invisible force field go up all around me and the car. Like they have in space ships. That way nobody could smash into us." Hypnotherapeutic work would then center on pairing the rubbing of the elbow with accompanying feelings of safety and security.

The therapist should not make sudden changes in the tone or content of the suggestions. This could make the child anxious. Smooth transitions are better—for example, "In a few moments I am going to ask you to imagine yourself playing your favorite game, baseball. I'm just going to ask you to imagine yourself doing that, imagine playing baseball like you do so often, imagine the fun you have doing this. Are you beginning to see yourself doing this?"

Rather than supplying the child with many of the minute details of the activity of interest, the child can use his or her very active imagination to do this—for example, rather than, "See that silvery colored cloud floating slowly through the sky?" say, "See that cloud? I wonder what color it is ? Is it moving?"

It is helpful on occasion to provide immediate praise or reward of some type for the child who achieves goals or expends much effort on the requested task. For example, a child reporting on a ride on a magic carpet is praised for this participation: "You're really doing a good job riding the carpet. What a wonderful magic carpet ride."

Authoritarian methods and the use of challenges, such as "You will not be able to move your arms, no matter how hard you try" (Gardner and Olness, 1988), should be avoided, based on the belief that the goal of hypnotherapy (and any other therapy) is to increase a child's sense of control of the targeted behavior or feeling. An induction that emphasizes loss of control is viewed as countertherapeutic.

Children, like adults, may resist giving up their symptoms in general, and specifically via hypnosis, for various reasons:

- Their symptomatology is acting in some fashion to maintain family stability.
- There is some other direct secondary gain, for example, abetting a school refusal pattern.
- The symptom provides attention or a sense of identity.
- Hypnosis is perceived as a loss of control.
- The hypnotic state is equated to death or nonbeing or, alternately, freedom from symptoms is equated with death.

Considerations for Preschool-Aged Children

For children under six years of age, it's usually inadvisable for the therapist to attempt to get the child to remove himself or herself from a situation through fantasy. Hilgard and Morgan (1978) suggest that the young child is more responsive to a type of protohypnosis or external distraction. That is, preschool-aged children are more easily distracted by listening to a story or participating in a verbal game. The content of the story or game is gradually altered so that the child eventually achieves control of the situation. This protohypnosis is also useful for any child who, for various reasons, is unable to use formal hypnosis. For children older than six years of age, there appears to be little difference in the effectiveness of relaxation and distraction techniques.

For example, a four-year-old girl has identified her favorite story as Jack and the Beanstalk. While the medical personnel begin preparations to perform a painful medical procedure on the girl, the therapist begins telling the story to shift the girl's attention away from their activities. "Mistakes" in the storytelling may be made in order to invite the girl's participation in the story: "Soon the pumpkin seeds sprouted and spread across the ground . . . What? You mean they were bean seeds?" Items or people in the room may be incorporated into the story to alleviate some of the anxiety that they may arouse: "Jack saw the giant counting all of his shiny treasure, shiny just like the things laying on that table over there."

Limits and Cautions

The contraindications for hypnosis with children are similar to those for adults:

- Expectations are too high or too low.
- The child and/or parents are resistant.
- There is a direct organic disorder that cannot be pinned down.
- The parents are hoping to use the hypnosis as a behavior control procedure.
- Physical endangerment or aggravation of emotional problems is a risk.

- From the available literature, hypnotherapy is not considered the most effective treatment.
- Immediate medical or surgical treatment or another form of psychotherapeutic management takes precedence.
- The symptom provides significant secondary gain for the child, which he or she is clearly unwilling to give up.

General Techniques

Children's abilities vary widely at any given chronological age. When ages are used in this chapter, they are only a rough guide as to the general expectations associated with a given chronological age. Children develop emotionally and cognitively at widely varying rates, yet hypnotherapeutic techniques should be chosen with the developmental level of the individual child in mind. At all ages, the techniques should be implemented by repetition, by rehearsal, or by role playing (Sanders, Copeland, and Elkin, 1987).

Concerning general hypnotic techniques, children of different ages appear to respond favorably to different techniques. Gardner and Olness (1988) have provided an outline for induction techniques for various age groups of children. A sample of these techniques follows. (Since there is no clear distinction between induction and therapeutic work, these techniques are useful in all aspects of hypnotherapy.)

Preverbal: Up to Two Years

Children of this age naturally develop ways to comfort themselves, including rocking or verbalizing rhythmically. Kinesthetic stimulation such as rocking or moving an infant's arm back and forth is effective in soothing and quieting an infant (outcomes associated with hypnosis). Also effective are tactile stimulation, such as rubbing or patting the infant, auditory stimulation, such as the sound of a vacuum cleaner or playing music, and visual stimulation, provided by moving objects such as mobiles.

Early Verbal: Two to Four

Effective induction techniques for this age group include storytelling of made-up stories or familiar stories with real-life characters substituted for the original characters, such as "Nurse Burridge Ate the porridge." Although some people may consider storytelling to be more of a distraction than a hypnotic technique, children often respond with a narrowed focus of attention and altered sensation, which are characteristic of the hypnotic state.

Also effective is to find out the child's favorite activity and ask the child to imagine doing it—for example, "Diane, just picture in your mind that you are doing your favorite thing, building with your Lego toys. Where is your favorite place to play with your Legos? O.K. Picture in your mind that you are sitting out in your yard, and all around you are your colorful Lego toys. What kind of fun things are you building?" Children sometimes respond by acting as if they are participating in the activity, such as making gestures as they would do when building with their blocks.

Use of a stereoscopic viewer with a picture known to be enjoyable to the child may be effective: "Do you see the cute little puppy? What is he doing? What color is he?"

A puppet, teddy bear, Raggedy Ann doll can serve as a model for behavior. The therapist can have the puppet as teacher, or middleman, for the specific techniques being employed. Conversely, I have found it effective to have the child teach the puppet the technique, which in turn makes the child much more receptive to the technique.

Preschool and Early School: Four to Six Years

An especially effective technique is to have children imagine they are watching their favorite television show or movie:

Therapist: Just sit back and get comfortable and imagine that you are getting ready to watch your favorite show. Picture in your mind that you are all snuggled up and comfortable on the sofa and are really feeling quite nice. You may have the remote control in your hand so that you can remain all comfortable while you watch your show. Imagine that you turn on the TV, and you adjust the sound until it's just right for you, not too loud and not too soft. Now just picture that you are flipping through the channels until you find your favorite show, feeling a little bit more relaxed as each channel goes by. Let me know when you have found your show. Now you're so comfortable and relaxed and you're just enjoying watching your favorite program.

At this point different therapeutic avenues may be undertaken. For instance, if the child has refused to take medication, the hypnotic suggestion is made that the heroine in the television show is glad to take her medicine that will help her get better.

An ideomotor technique such as the might oak tree (or redwood for West Coast therapists) is useful when the therapist wishes to convey to the child a sense of being able to control physical responses (such as pain) that the child thought were beyond his or her control. The mighty oak tree is also useful for groups or for children who have difficulty sitting still:

Therapist: You know those big trees in the park that look so big and strong and stretch way up toward the sky? Stand up and be one of those trees. Stand up really straight and tall, as tall as you can be, and stretch your arms out toward the sky like branches on that big oak tree. Stretch, stretch your branches far out. Now, those big trees have long, deep roots that keep them from falling over. Feel your feet go down, down through the floor, just like roots on the big, strong oak tree. Feel how strong you are, how very, very strong you are. Now, when you're ready and feel just like that oak tree, powerful and strong, I'll try to lift you.

Another useful method is to have the child imagine that he or she is a bouncing ball and can go anywhere:

Therapist: Have you ever seen one of those balls that can bounce really high, like the ones you use to play kickball? Just picture in your mind that you are one of those balls. You can bounce and bounce and bounce wherever you wish to go. You can bounce down the sidewalk, bouncing over all of the people who are walking on the sidewalk. You can bounce over all of the cars to get to the other side of the street. Bounce and bounce; you can bounce over buildings, over this hospital building if you like. You can bounce through the park, bounce over the trees, or bounce up a tree to the very top. If you are worried about anything, you can just let that thing bounce right off you. Just keep bouncing until you find a place that is just right for you to stop. Let me know when you have found this place.

Not surprisingly, hyperactive children often relate well to this technique.

Early school children as well as middle childhood children may respond to the use of pets, similar to the description of the use of puppets as a go-between for early verbal children.

Middle Childhood: Seven to Eleven Years

At this age, children usually can easily imagine that they are flying on a magic blanket. They board the blanket and fly to a very special place of their choosing:

Therapist: Imagine that you are having a picnic in the park, and are sitting on a blanket. But this is not just any blanket. It is a magic, flying blanket. And you are the only person who knows how to fly this blanket, so you are in complete control. You can fly really low to the ground, just barely skimming over the top of the grass. Or you can fly over the tops of the trees or do loop the loops in the air. You can fly this blanket to the most special place you know. When you are ready, why don't you fly to that very special place. Let me know when you get there.

Another effective technique is to have the child imagine some beautiful clouds, watching how they change into the child's favorite colors and into different shapes. This can easily be adapted to either diagnostic or therapeutic purposes.

Children of this age usually respond well to the coin drop technique. They are asked to hold a coin out between two fingers and to focus on the sensations they experience from the surface of the coin, feeling that it is gradually sliding out of their fingers, and that when it drops, they are ready to go off to their favorite place and/or "sink into a state of deep relaxation."

An ideomotor technique useful when the therapist's objective is to instill a sense of control over physical responses is the balloon levitation technique:

Therapist: Imagine that you have a large helium balloon, one that rises up on its own. You're sitting outside in a very comfortable spot, and there is just a little breeze blowing. Imagine that you tie the balloon to your wrist to keep it from blowing away in the breeze. As you let go of the balloon, you watch it slowly, lazily drift upward in the breeze. Pretty soon you feel your arm begin to rise a little bit as the balloon gently pulls it upward. As you watch the balloon go up and up, your arm floats up a bit more. And the higher the arm goes, the lighter it feels. You can just let the arm float in the gentle breeze, or if you want, you can imagine that you let some of the helium out of the balloon and let that hand slowly, gently float down onto your lap again.

Adolescence: Twelve to Eighteen Years

Virtually any adult induction is effective at this age, but arm catalepsy and deep breathing techniques are usually those most easily accepted. Immersions into imagined sports activities are useful where there is a problem with attention to the hypnotic process and/or with some hyperactive children.

Applications of Hypnotherapeutic Techniques

Developmental Disorders

Mental Retardation. Some success in the use of hypnosis with relatively mildly retarded children (IQ 50–70) who have medical or psychological problems amenable to hypnosis has been reported. Researchers suggest the use of techniques appropriate for the child's mental rather than chronological age. Children with more severe mental retardation respond poorly, if at all, to hypnotic inductions. "Even if they do respond to induction, they usually do not benefit from hypnotherapeutic suggestions, probably because of limited conceptualization, memory, and language skills" (Gardner and Olness, 1988, p. 78).

Learning Disabilities. The therapist must be careful to distinguish between emotional problems (such as self-esteem issues or anxiety), which may impede a child's learning, and a true learning disability. Hypnotherapeutic techniques are appropriate for the former but not the latter. This is not to say that self-esteem issues may not coexist with a learning disability; however, it is the issue of self-esteem that is appropriate for hypnotherapy, not the learning disability.

The specific learning disability should be considered when selecting an induction technique. Jampolsky (1975) suggests that since children with developmental reading disorders have difficulty visualizing images in their mind, they may be more responsive when asked to imagine how things feel rather than how they look. An example is the feeling of the balloon tugging on the child's arm.

Useful hypnotic suggestions include increased enjoyment of the task (such as reading or writing), increased ability to perform the task, confidence in being able to perform the task, increased comprehension, and the improved coordination among the child's eyes, brain, and memory. Imagery techniques may also be beneficial, with the child picturing himself or herself successfully performing the task.

Attention Deficit Hyperactivity Disorder. Although hypnotherapy may be of use in the treatment of attention deficit hyperactivity disorder (ADHD), it is seldom appropriate as the primary treatment. Where hypnotherapy may prove beneficial is in addressing the secondary problems of the disorder, such as low self-esteem and negative attitudes toward school and learning. Other areas that may be addressed by hypnotherapy include lowering anxiety, increasing the child's ability to recognize his or her emotional lability, and developing strategies for controlling behavior.

Since these children by definition are highly active and have short attention spans, induction methods that involve movement (either movement imagery, such as the flying blanket induction or ideomotor techniques such as the mighty oak tree induction) are often the most effective. Group induction techniques are likely to prove ineffective due to the disruptiveness of the subjects when placed together.

An example follows of the use of hypnotherapy in addressing self-esteem issues with an eight-year-old boy with ADHD. The focus is on having the child image himself as being confident and in control. Before the induction, the therapist needs an idea of the type of the behavior the child would like to be able to do, or thinks other people would like him or her to do, such as staying in his or her seat, not speaking out in class, or focusing on homework. Jeremy identified that he would like to be able to sit still in his chair at school.

> Jeremy is induced using the flying blanket technique. Once he has reached his special place on his magic blanket, suggestions are made:

> *Therapist*: Jeremy, picture yourself in your classroom at school. Imagine yourself feeling calm and comfortable . . . you don't even want to move around much or get out of your chair. You just feel so calm and comfortable. Picture how good you feel for being able to do this, how proud you are of yourself for being able to sit in your chair without being told by anyone to do it. Imagine how pleased everyone will be when they see you do this.

> Jeremy is also told that "by just thinking of this special place you will be able to relax and control your behavior, just as you are doing now." Jeremy is instructed to practice being relaxed and in control by thinking of his special place four times a day, in addition to times when his teacher points out that his behavior is not appropriate.

Anxiety Disorders

Academic Performance. The clenched-fist technique (discussed in chapter 16) has brought about improvement in examination performance in high school students with high levels of test anxiety (Stanton, 1988). For younger children, a similar but less complex technique may be used (Ambrose, 1956). To cope effectively with anxiety, the child is told (amplified from the present, rather terse presentation): "Make a fist. Now inside that fist are all of the things that are worrying you. Count to five, and when you get to five open up your fist. Watch all of those problems and worries just afloat away into the air. Now notice how good and confident you feel." The posthypnotic suggestion is made that "you can feel this good and confident whenever you want to, just by making a fist, counting to five, and letting go of all your worries."

Separation Anxiety. Hypnotic techniques may prove useful in uncovering the underlying source of anxiety that is triggered when separation from the attachment figure occurs.

> Nine-year-old Jessica refused to go to school, would go to sleep only with her mother present, and clung to her mother whenever parting was imminent. During regression, Jessica was asked to go back in time to when she first began to fear that something bad would happen to her mother. Jessica revealed that she had watched a television show in which a woman broke off a romantic relationship with a boyfriend and was subsequently murdered by the man. Jessica's mother had recently ended a romantic relationship, and Jessica expressed fear that something terrible would happen to her mother if she let her mother out of sight.
>
> Suggestions were made while Jessica was in the hypnotic-like state, such as "[Ex-boyfriend] does not want to hurt Mommy. He is not like the man on TV. And Mommy is a strong adult who can take care of herself. You do not need to worry about protecting her because she can take care of herself even when you are away." Clarification of the misbelief then ensued in the waking state, including discussion on the differences between what is real and make believe and receiving comfort from her mother.

Tic Disorders. Hypnotic techniques have been used successfully in the reduction of tic behavior in children with Tourette syndrome. An effective technique is to have the child, in a trance state, develop an image of a pleasant place that is calm, peaceful, and quiet (Culbertson, 1989). For instance, the child may have the image of a calm, quiet bay near the ocean where the water is so still that there are no waves or ripples on the water's surface. The child is then instructed to transfer this image to the portion of the body where the ticcing behavior occurs. The child is further instructed that he or she may experience this calm feeling whenever desired, and instruction in self-hypnosis is given.

Hypnotic techniques may be used in implementing other therapeutic interventions. Young and Montano (1988) used hypnosis to help children identify the subjective urge that precedes their tic behavior. For instance, Jay's ticcing behavior was jaw thrusting. While in a hypnotic state, the child was asked to visualize a time when this behavior occurred. Jay then identified the sensory cue of a feeling of discomfort in his jaws, which made him think his mouth was hanging open.

The next step in Young and Montano's treatment method is for the child, while in the hypnotic state, to select one of two procedures (habit reversal or response prevention) that he or she would like to use to help decrease the tic behavior. Self-hypnosis is taught in which the child visualizes applying the chosen technique and the accompanying decrease in tic behavior. Jay chose response prevention and then imagined a situation in which the time between the urge to tic and the tic behavior was prolonged.

Elimination Disorders. Before beginning treatment, the therapist must determine the words the child uses for urination and defecation and use these terms when addressing the disorder. Nocturnal enuresis may be addressed using the following format (Friedrich, 1990).

In a joint meeting with the parents and child, the therapist explains the physiological aspects of voiding. Charts and pictures for the child to take home are helpful. Then the therapist explains that the bladder "talks" with the child and the child "talks" with the bladder throughout the day. The child and bladder need to keep talking to one another at night. Explanations may take the form, "Sometimes at night you don't hear your bladder talking to you. It's saying, 'I've got to pee, get me to the bathroom.' " The hypnosis is a way to help the child hear the messages again.

Relaxation is then induced in the child, and "conversations" are held with the bladder. Suggestions of mastery and control are included during this process:

Therapist: Before you go to sleep tonight, tell your bladder to send you a message when it feels full of pee. Tell it to say, "Wake up! I need to go to the bathroom." You will wake up dry and walk to the bathroom, where you will then pee. Your bladder can send this message as many times as it needs to during the night, and each time you will wake up dry and go to the bathroom to pee. Then think of how nice it will be to wake up in your dry bed in the morning. You will find it getting easier to hear you bladder talking to you. Pretty soon you will be able to hear it talking to you very clearly.

Before the end of the session, the child is asked to practice relaxing on his or her own.

The child is instructed to void each night before going to bed. Then the child is to spend several minutes sitting on his or her bed relaxing and talking to his or her bladder. The drawings may be used as an object upon which the child may focus attention.

A similar technique involving conversations between the child and his or her bowels may be used in the treatment of encopresis.

The length of treatment should be relatively short. Studies by Kohen et al. (1980) indicate that hypnotherapy is not likely to help such children if they have not improved within the first two or three sessions.

Speech Disorders. Stuttering (which occurs in a male-to-female sex ratio of five to one) is the speech disorder most often treated through hypnotherapy, and treatment is often effective (Less, 1990).

Crasilneck and Hall (1985) offer several useful hypnotic techniques. In order to give the child a sense of control over the condition, without placing the intimidating expectation of totally giving up the speech disorder, the suggestion may be given that the child will stutter only on the first syllable of a word and then slide through the rest of the word easily. For example, the therapist can choose a word that the child has had difficulty saying in the session:

> *Therapist*: Imagine that your speech is much more smooth than it is now. Imagine that only the first parts of words have problems coming out; the rest of the word just flows out easily. Imagine how pleased you will be to hear the last parts of the words flowing out so easily.

A second recommendation is the use of a posthypnotic cue to trigger calmness. For instance, the child is told that whenever he or she begins to speak, he or she will feel the same sense of relaxation and confidence that was felt during the hypnotic state.

> *Therapist*: Notice how nice and relaxed you feel right now. How comfortable and at ease you are. Feel your fears and worries just slip away. Imagine that whenever you feel this way your fears and worries and uneven and erratic way of talking will disappear and will be replaced by a smooth way of speaking . . . Imagine how pleased you will be to hear yourself speaking without stuttering . . . Just whisper something now and listen to how your voice sounds . . . Whenever you begin to speak, that will be a cue for you to feel relaxed and at ease like you do now, so that your voice sounds just like it did now.

Once the child (especially an older child) is hypnotized to the deepest level, suggestions may be used as possible treatment for stuttering:

> *Therapist*: Are you ready to continue? . . . (pause) When you are in a situation where there is an apprehension about speaking present, it will disappear from your mind as though it was never there . . . Any tension related to speaking will merely

signal the brain to relax . . . As sounds and words are formed, they will flow smoothly from the tongue with great ease . . . as the first word you speak rolls fluently from the mouth your confidence will increase . . . you will know that the person or people listening to you are hearing exactly what you intend them to hear . . . beautifully spoken . . . smooth . . . relaxed tones of voice . . . words pronounced perfectly . . . beautifully . . . all your fears are gone . . . swept away like writing in sand as a wave sweeps over the shore . . . it is not necessary for you to be concerned with not making a mistake . . . your subconscious mind will do that for you . . . the powerful unconscious mind will filter your words before you open your mouth . . . you will speak softly, slowly, and in a relaxed manner . . . speaking will become a source of relaxation for you . . . all emotional responses will be positive . . . speech is no longer hindered . . . it is time to speak now . . . hear how calm and relaxed your voice sounds . . .

Another technique is to record the child's improved speech while in trance. When a stutterer is asked to speak in a whisper, his or her speech usually improves. Played back to the child in the waking state, this strengthens the child's confidence in his or her abilities to accomplish the goal of improving speech.

Developmental Disorders of Adolescence

Eating Disorders. The use of hypnotic techniques in the treatment of eating disorders dates back to at least 1888 when J. Janet reportedly reinstated a normal pattern of food intake in a twenty-five-year-old woman suffering from anorexia and bulimia. A series of hypnosis sessions were conducted with suggestions of increasing the woman's attention to her tactile and visceral sensations (J. Janet, 1888; P. Janet, 1925). Since that time, many researchers have reported the successful use of hypnotic techniques in the treatment of eating disorders (Barabasz, 1990; Baker and Nash, 1987).

When discussing with the anorexic client the rationale for the use of hypnosis, hypnosis should not be presented as a means to achieve weight gain or as a way of gaining control of eating habits. These clients are often uncertain (at best) about wanting to increase their weight level and may be reluctant to undertake a treatment where this is the only goal. Instead, the explanation is offered that hypnosis is a means of weight management. Also, eating disordered persons often readily admit feelings of anxiety and feeling out of control of their lives. Framing hypnosis as a method by which the client may lessen her anxiety and increase her feelings of control is more likely to generate acceptance (Baker and Nash, 1987).

Several of the core symptoms of eating disorders appear to be responsive to hypnotic treatment and self-hypnosis. In particular, to address the anxiety and frenetic behavior that frequently accompanies eating disorders, hypnotherapy may be used to induce relaxation, slowed respiration, and appropriate heart rate. Imagery of a pleasant setting or experience may be useful to accomplish this.

In addressing distorted body image, the client may be asked to draw a picture of her body on an imaginary blackboard during trance. She can draw it as it is now, as it would be if it were ideal, as her parents see her, as men see her, and so forth. These can be discussed in therapy and manipulated via hypnotic reframing. These distortions may also be corrected by erasing and more accurately redrawing the areas, as they are presented, and again reframed in hypnosis.

Distorted interoceptive awareness may be corrected by suggesting that the communication between the mind and the body be reconnected. This communication may focus on directing attention to visceral cues such as hunger and satiety, and the association may be made between hunger and moderate amounts of food intake.

Family enmeshment issues may be addressed by giving suggestions of self-assertion and independence, helping the client to understand how she gained a sense of control in the focused area of her weight, and then helping her to transfer this control to another area. Age progression techniques may be used in which the client imagines herself as older and successfully living independently of the family. Finally, repressed traumatic events may be uncovered through age regression techniques.

Specific scripts that may be helpful for the various eating disorders follow:

For anorexia nervosa:

Therapist: From this moment on you will realize a sense of control over your life and over the wishes you have for yourself . . . you will see yourself as self-sufficient and independent . . . you and only you can control your life . . . you have been blocking the sensations from your internal organs . . . especially hunger . . . this is the source of your present difficulty regarding your body image and your health . . . I want you to visualize yourself now . . . standing fresh out of your bath . . . allow the shape of your body as you now perceive it to appear in the mirror . . . [This image should be the current negative image, so ask the adolescent to signal if this negative image is the one she sees.] Good . . . now you will see a vapor of steam clouding this image in the mirror, and as the vapor becomes thicker, the old image fades away behind the thick vapor . . . Now begin to look into the vapor . . . as you look you see a vague image beginning to appear . . . this is the body you wish to see . . . taking shape through the thick steam . . . now the vapor is beginning to fade . . . as it fades the new image begins to become clearer . . . it is very shapely . . . Think of how beautiful this new image is . . . how healthy it looks . . . strong . . . lean . . . so soft and smooth . . . it is just as you'd like it to be . . . it is the "essential you." It does not require special efforts on your part to develop . . . you will be able to keep this image in your mind . . . each time you look at yourself you will see this image and enjoy the feelings it gives you . . . Now I'm going to instruct you to forget that I have told you to replace the old image of yourself with a new one . . . you will practice this suggestion, but you will not remember getting the suggestion from me . . . the more you try to remember, the harder it will be . . . you will awaken relaxed . . . refreshed . . . and feeling great.

For bulimia:

Therapist: Would you like to continue now allowing the unconscious self to accept the importance of hunger? (pause for acknowledgment) . . . Food intake in and of itself is not very important to you any longer . . . You will avoid overeating as you have in the past . . . hurriedly and lacking in satisfaction . . . You will eat only after you have experienced the signal of hunger from your body . . . you will eat only after you have acknowledged to yourself that the experience of hunger is signaling that your body is working properly to use the stored carbohydrates and sugars that are available to it . . . that in allowing the body to use these stored nutrients you are becoming more and more healthy . . . you will feel a great overwhelming respect for your body rather than stuffing it with unhealthy foods . . . You will not be excessively hungry . . . you will be able to loose excess weight steadily . . . you will never again be fat . . . you will enjoy your food, and you will eat the least amount of food it takes to satisfy your hunger . . . eating will be a relaxing thing for you now . . . you will feel peace of mind . . . You will visualize yourself as a slender, healthy, and strong person . . . your thoughts will not be preoccupied with food any longer . . . you are free . . . calm and free from the pain food has brought you in the past.

For overeating:

> *Therapist*: In the past when you have tried to lose weight, you have denied yourself . . . you have been preoccupied with the kinds and amounts of food you desire to eat . . . Now, however, that will stop . . . you will from this day on be able to look at food in a new way . . . you will find that foods that will sustain your good health will be very appealing . . . the flavor . . . the aroma . . . the texture . . . the color . . . You will effortlessly choose those foods that are low in fat . . . savor them . . . You will eat less often and forget about eating between meals . . . eating for you will be a pleasurable time . . . the only purpose for eating being to satisfy hunger . . . You will no longer have to think about when to stop eating . . . your subconscious mind will stop you as your food intake is sufficient . . . you will allow yourself to become hungry, and the experience of hunger will not be unpleasant . . . in fact eating beyond the minimum amount necessary will become increasingly unpleasant . . . each excessive bite will decrease your enjoyment . . . You will stop eating automatically, without effort, once your body is sufficiently nourished . . . mealtime and the pleasure you will derive from your meals will be very satisfying for you . . . as you cease eating, you will notice a deep peace flooding through your being . . . calmness, tranquility, and a sense of being deeply relaxed will confirm the end of your meals . . . You will be free of anxiety . . . you will feel slim, strong, and healthy . . . you will lose all the weight you desire to lose . . . each day you will notice that the weight is leaving . . . ounce by ounce . . . pound by pound . . . letting your thin and healthy self step forward expressing itself for your pleasure.

Conduct Disorder. With delinquent and acting-out adolescents, some of the usual hypnotic techniques may need to be modified in order to alleviate the adolescents' mistrust and hostility. Benson (1984) reports the successful use of hypnotherapy with thirteen to seventeen year olds placed in a social services center for out-of-control-behavior. Following is a summary of her treatment program.

Hypnosis is introduced to the adolescent by discussing the effects of anxiety on his or her body and the usefulness of relaxation in counteracting these effects. It is presented as a method to achieve relaxation. The therapist must make it quite clear that hypnosis is a way to feel better and is not something used by the therapist to extract information. The adolescent may solve some of his or her problems in privacy, without every having to divulge private information to the therapist.

Induction techniques should not include challenges. These young people are much practiced at resisting authority and will predictably oppose the therapist's challenge. A useful induction technique, modeled on Benson (1984), is illustrated in the case of fourteen-year-old Dan:

> *Therapist*: Dan, I'd like you to close your eyes and imagine that you are watching your favorite television show. While you are doing this, I am just going to keep on talking and talking about relaxing. Pretty soon you will probably get so bored of hearing me talk that your attention may drift, and you may start to have a fantasy or daydream. You may even begin to feel like you do just before you are ready to fall asleep at night.

Treatment may address four key areas. First, treatment can focus on reducing the child's anxiety and modifying inappropriate response patterns: "While you are in this very relaxed state, you have a great deal of control over things that are usually automatic or subconscious. You may use this control to your benefit." Specific response patterns, such as getting unreasonably irritable, are addressed only if the child has agreed that he or she would like to work on that area.

A second area of treatment is to identify specific problem areas and focus on the child's own resources to resolve them. Benson suggests that the image of sorting a desk is useful for this:

> *Therapist*: Imagine a big desk in front of you. It's a big desk with plenty of places to sort and rearrange things. On that desk is everything that has ever happened to you in your life. Each thing is on a separate piece of paper. Now imagine that you are sorting through the different piles of paper. Be as thorough as you can, but only tackle the things that you feel ready to tackle right now. Take as long as you wish to sort through these things. On one side put any problems that you feel you are ready to deal with.

Finger signalling may be used for the child to indicate whether he or she wishes to discuss any of these problems with the therapist or wishes to work on these in private. The child's decision must be respected; this is an important step in building the child's trust and a sense of autonomy.

A third aim of treatment is to form realistic goals for the future. The goal is to get to the child to look ahead and make plans for the next few years:

Therapist: Although it may seem hard to look at anything except the problems and conflicts you have right now, your future is in front of you. Imagine that you have a crystal ball and that in it you can see into the future. In that crystal ball, form a picture of what you would like to be at the age of twenty-one . . . Picture that there is a path leading from where you are now to where you want to be. Picture some of the things you need to do to get down that path.

If there appears to be no way to get to that goal, the goal may need to be modified to be more realistic.

Finally, hypnotherapy may be used for ego strengthening. Benson suggests having the child imagine baking a very special batch of cookies:

Therapist: The recipe for these cookies consists of each good thing you can think of about yourself and your life. Good things like the happy relationship you have with your brother, how good you are in playing baseball, and how courageous you feel you are. You can eat these cookies whenever things aren't going so well, and you feel you need comfort or strength. And remember, you're lucky because your inner self will bake new cookies to replace any that you eat so you can eat the same ones when you need them again.

A posthypnotic suggestion should reinforce to the child that he or she will continue to have an ample supply of these cookies for use in times of stress.

Substance Abuse. Hypnotherapy appears to have limited applicability in addressing habitual drug abuse. The limited research available indicates that hypnotherapy is effective only for adolescents who are highly motivated to change and/or who fear possible harm to their physical health (Bauman, 1970). Hypnotherapy should be used only in conjunction with other, more primary interventions.

One hypnotherapeutic approach involves suggestions that the client imagine a "hypnotic high" that is even more pleasurable than the high achieved by drug use (Baumann, 1970). Another possible approach is to substitute the relaxation and well-being of the trance state for the effect of the drug. Also, hypnosis may help to increase motivation to stick with the decision to discontinue drug use.

Sexual Abuse

Hypnosis with sexually abused children may be used to help them experience a relaxed state, as an antagonist to the anxious state to which the abused child has become accustomed. This can provide the child a sense of competence and mastery over his or her environment (Friedrich, 1990, 1991). Rhue and Lynn (1991) used storytelling with sexually abused children to provide comforting hypnotic suggestions, symbolism, and metaphors that helped the children emotionally distance themselves from the trauma of the abuse. Any of the induction or therapeutic techniques outlined involving a relaxation component may be used.

Hypnosis may also be used to allow the child to build up defenses against intrusive and distracting thoughts. Suggestions are made that the child has the ability to "put the thoughts away" until an appropriate time is available to deal with them. Also, hypnosis may be used to teach the child to control the degree to which the distressing thoughts and memories occur. Suggestions may be used that give the child the control to deal with the traumatic thoughts at his or her own pace (Rhue and Lynn, 1991).

To address self-esteem issues that accompany sexual abuse, Friedrich (1990) suggests the frequent use of mastery imagery. This may involve having the child imagine participating in his or her favorite activity (such as riding a bicycle) and then having the child imagine performing great, exciting, daring (and successful) things on the bicycle. (The statement should make it clear that they will do these only in their hypnosis fantasies, and not when they actually ride their bike.) This procedure gives the child the very different feeling of having control and mastery of his or her environment.

School-related symptoms from abuse are common, in particular distractibility, poor concentration, and apathy. Self-hypnosis techniques may be taught to the child to help increase his or her ability to focus on schoolwork. Self-statements may include, "I will be able to keep my mind on my book work" or "I will not be distracted by other activities in the room."

Intrusive Medical Procedures

The apprehension that exacerbates children's pain man be related, at least in part, to the anticipatory anxiety regarding being hospitalized. Different aspects of the hospital experience are threatening to children, depending on age. Preschool children are most anxious about the medical instruments used, and school-aged children feel most threatened by the interaction with the medical staff. Adolescents are more likely to experience anxiety related to the implications of their discomfort on their future health and physical condition and on the reactions of peers.

Hypnotic techniques may focus on the features of the medical procedure that are particularly anxiety arousing for the child. An example is an eight-year-old boy who fears that his doctor is an aggressive enemy whose goal is to cause him pain. Hypnotic suggestions may involve giving the boy a sense of control of the situation and helping him to identify with the doctor in this strange experience rather than keeping the physician a mysterious and threatening stranger. An age progression technique may be used:

Therapist: Picture yourself growing up into a big, strong man. And imagine that as this big, strong man, you are a doctor who loves to help children. You are a very good doctor, and you help lots of children get better. Sometimes in order to help the children get better, you have to do things that make the children feel a little uncomfortable for a little bit. But you know that by doing this you will help the child to get all better.

The favorite-story technique has proved effective in the reduction of pain and anxiety during painful medical procedures on young children (Kuttner, 1988). The technique involves the child's telling the therapist a favorite story prior to the medical procedure. The therapist suggests to the child that when they go to the treatment room, the therapist will tell the story while the procedure is being done: "I'll bet things go a lot quicker than they usually do. And by the time we finish the story, everything will be done and the bandage will be on."

Information about the procedure and suggestions for comfort and diminished awareness of pain are incorporated into the story:

Therapist: "Winnie the Pooh tasted the honey, and it was so good. It made him feel all warm and comfortable, and now the poke is over and your leg feels all comfortable too. Winnie the Pooh kept on eating the honey and soon he felt all sleepy and comfortable.

Diverting attention from the noxious stimuli may be accomplished in other ways. Studies utilizing distraction techniques with young children have reported that the following distractors are effective:

- Relaxation and breathing exercises, such as, "Pretend you're a big round tire. Take a deep breath . . . let the air out making a hissing sound" (Jay et al., 1982, p. 9).
- Focusing on objects in the room, such as counting the number of polka dots on Dad's necktie.
- Introducing a variety of objects, such as pop-up books, puppets, and stuffed animals.
- Bubble blowing, during which the child is reinforced for counting the bubbles.

Hypnotherapy conducted separately from the invasive procedure may include the following hypnotic suggestions:

The child will experience less pain than previous times.

The child will be able to tolerate the procedure much better and with much less discomfort.

The child's "powerful, big, strong, unconscious mind" will help him or her to get better.

The child will rest well and be hungry for all meals.

The child is able to do all of the above through self-hypnosis (Crasilneck and Hall, 1985).

Pain Management

The light-switch technique is useful in the management of pediatric pain (Erickson, Hershman, and Secter, 1961). The child must be old enough to comprehend the concept of electricity traveling through wires. The technique may take the following form:

Therapist: When you flip a light switch at home, it either turns the electricity on or off. Your body is kind of like this. You have things like wires, we call them nerves, that run from your head to all the parts of your body. Some even run to [name the painful area]. When the switches in your head are turned on, you feel pain, and when they are off, you don't feel pain. In your mind right now, find the switch in your brain that is connected to [body part]. Now in your mind just reach over and turn off that switch. Notice that now that you have turned the electricity off to your [body part] you no longer feel any pain there.

Alternatively, the child can develop a "healing capsule" or "circle of light" wherein pain is diminished as the power of the capsule generator grows. Sometimes a magic wand or a "treatment laser gun" is an appealing and effective method of reducing a child's pain, especially localized pain.

Migraine Headaches. Self-hypnosis has been found to be significantly more effective than both propranolol or placebo in reducing the number of headaches in juvenile classic migraine (Olness, MacDonald, and Uden, 1987). The self-hypnosis techniques involve progressive relaxation training followed by focusing on a pleasant place or experience. Subsequent hypnotherapy sessions focus on the control of pain through the practice of isolated anesthesia. These techniques are practiced daily by the child.

Skin Problems. Hypnotic techniques have been used successfully in the alleviation of skin irritation in children with eczema (Sokel, Lansdown, and Kent, 1990). Imagery involving soothing sensations is useful. For example, a seven-year-old boy enjoys playing in the mud: "Imagine the cool rain, making wonderful puddles of water to play in. Imagine scooping up the cool mud from the puddles and spreading it gently over all parts of you that itch." Suggest that the effect will continue after the boy leaves and that he can feel this cool, comfortable relief whenever he wishes, just by imagining the rain and puddles of cool mud.

Hypnosis has been successfully used in the treatment of warts. Tasini and Hackett (1977) had children in a trance state imagine that their warts felt dry, were turning brown, and fell off. Noll (1988) suggests the following procedure. Prior to hypnotism, the child is instructed that warts are caused by viruses living inside the child's body. The child is told that he or she has "soldier and guard cells" that he or she can control by using hypnosis. During hypnosis, the child is told to set the guard and soldier cells into action and kill the viruses. The child may also imagine that a magic cream is being put on the warts by the therapist, or some device can be introduced as something like a "magic ultra-ray machine" that will cause the warts to dry up.

An Overall Mastery Procedure

With many disorders in children (and in numerous adults as well), especially in psychological as opposed to physical disorders, there is a core feeling of inadequacy. An antidote to this sense of inadequacy is a hypnotic procedure that works to develop a feeling of mastery. The following mastery procedure is adapted in part from one developed by Donna Copeland at the University of Texas M. D. Anderson Hospital and Tumor Institute (Sanders, Copeland, and Elkins, 1987). It can be adapted as an adjunct to other procedures, hypnotic or otherwise, that are focused on the specific disorder.

> *Therapist*: We've talked about how you use your imagination, sometimes to daydream and sometimes to play games. [Prepare the child by talking about activities of this sort.] So now, I want you to let your arms and legs hang loose, and let yourself take a couple of deep breaths. Maybe you can think of your arms and legs like those of a puppet and your brain is just telling them to hang loose. Or maybe you can think of yourself just lying in a warm bath or floating about in your

favorite swimming pool. Even though you are feeling looser and more relaxed, feel a sense of strength come into your muscles. Feel them becoming a little bigger, with some more power and strength

Now, your brain is continuing to control your breathing, but it's able to do it without your thinking about it, sort of like an automatic pilot or a cruise control. It's nice to know that the power to control is in there, deep inside you, and that it will take care of you and take charge of things like your breathing and heartbeat, without your having to do anything.

Now, let's move into your imagination. We're out of doors and walking along a path and we go to a place to meet Superman [or Wonder Woman or some other heroic figure the child chooses]. He's there waiting for us. He's happy to see us, and it's a good feeling to know that he'll be with us today. I believe that Superman has something to tell you about [the presenting complaint or symptom] that will help you. You may sense what that is now, or it may come to you later.

As you climb with Superman up a hill on the path, feel yourself becoming stronger, feel yourself becoming more confident in yourself and in your ability to handle your problem. Feel yourself going higher and higher up the hill, and at the same time breathing deeper, feeling stronger, and feeling safer and more confident.

Notice that you are becoming bigger, almost as big as Superman. As you do, you feel your strength growing. You are breathing deeply and confidently, and your heart is beating strongly to pump more oxygen and strength into your muscles. Notice how safe, secure, and strong you feel as this happens. [If there are any signs of anxiety now or elsewhere during the procedure, they can be reframed as signs of "readiness for action."]

Now you and Superman have reached the top of the hill. You have kept your new, growing sense of strength, and as you look off from the top of the hill, you see far in the distance. Things look so small and you begin to realize that your [presenting problem] feels less threatening than it did. You feel a much greater confidence now that you can handle things.

As you feel this, you also notice that Superman is tapping you on your shoulder. He seems to want to tell you something about [the presenting problem], and as I stay quiet for a few moments, you may want to become aware of Superman's advice, maybe by hearing your mind's voice, or having an idea, or even a short daydream. I'll now be quiet. [Stay quiet for thirty seconds to a minute.]

If your mind got the message, or even gets it later, as I talk, you may want to share it later on with me, or you may keep it a secret. It's under your control.

Now you hear or understand that Superman is offering to help you with [the presenting problem]. Using your mind, see yourself as you show him the place [where the problem most often occurs—if that is appropriate to the problem]. Now show him how well you can carry out your new skills and strengths to cope with your problems. In a few moments I'll be quiet again, and I want you to see yourself doing [the needed skill or coping strategy], see yourself doing it very well, using the power and strength you have built up. You'll see yourself doing that somehow, it doesn't have to be a clear image, but run it through your mind doing it the best way you want. And you may later want to talk about it, or wait a little longer before you share it. I'll be quiet now so let it happen. [Wait about thirty seconds to a minute.]

That was good. Maybe you had your thoughts or images way down in your unconscious where they are hard to see, or maybe they were clear images. Either way, your mind will let you do better and feel better because of them. [Consider rerunning repeats or variations of this procedure here.]

Now, before you and Superman go down the hill again, take a look out from the top of the hill, and feel how much more control you feel. Notice that Superman sort of winks or waves at you, kind of a sign that he knows you shared his strength. Now let's do down the hill, and let Superman go off on a side path where he can help others. You know you can reach him again, in your mind like we are doing now or in your dreams, if you want to make contact with him again. You know that each time you practice this mind image, you'll feel stronger and more sure of yourself. You can feel proud of yourself for your work and courage, having mastered the problem this time, just as you can in the future.

Then proceed to clear the child from the trance and obtain a report of what happened. Some children can effectively practice this on their own; sometimes (usually with older children) a tape recording will work to reinforce the effect, and occasionally parents can carry this out as a therapist surrogate (better with younger children, although the therapist always has to be careful here and closely monitor what goes on).

Conclusion

Hypnotherapy with children has received increased attention recently. This is gratifying, as children usually are good hypnotic subjects, especially if techniques are tailored to their level of functioning. As a result, numerous disorders can be helped or cured by hypnotic intervention.

16

Hypnosis and Performance Enhancement

> The cold fact is that today's players know that the fundamentals of baseball include not only hitting, fielding and running but also corking, spitting, scuffing, tarring, popping greenies, throwing shineballs, slimeballs, sleazeballs and some tricks you probably never even dreamed of.
> —Dan Gutman, *It Ain't Cheatin' If You Don't Get Caught* (1990)

The area of performance enhancement is one in which hypnosis has not been applied in any widespread and systematic fashion. For example, in their definitive textbook on exercise physiology, McArdle, Katch, and Katch (1991) do not mention hypnosis at all. This is somewhat curious, given our interest in bettering performance in such activities as sports, music, public speaking, and test taking. Indeed, many people have sought assistance for the purpose of improving their performances in such areas.

A key element in the inability of many to achieve their best performance is a high level of anxiety (Salmon and Meyer, 1992). In fact, many treatments being used to increase levels of performance have been geared to help clients relax, thus lessening anxiety levels. Biofeedback training has been used with such clients, and so has autogenic training. Hypnotherapy is a logical candidate for generating improvement in the area of performance. It is true that there may be times when the anxiety simply overwhelms preparation. For example, while filming one segment of a new show in 1991, Mike Adamle, host of the Fox Network show "The Ultimate Challenge," and a former professional football player, found himself riding a bull called Hookin' Henry at a Texas rodeo. "I went through the techniques of visualizing success you learn as an athlete," he said. "Then the paramedics dropped a rider with a compound fracture in front of me." Adamle lasted five seconds.

This chapter will deal with performance enhancement in three main areas: test performance, sports performance, and the performing arts. The suggestions about the use of hypnosis can be applied, with very minor adaptation, to diverse types of performances. For example, it has been shown that superior knowledge of the game of chess and certain personality factors, not superior memory, are what separate expert chess players from

318

novices (Trotter, 1986). Certainly hypnotic suggestions could be given to increase players' knowledge of chess and to enhance positive personality features, as well as many other types of performances.

In their study of the reading performance of fifty-two college students, Koe and Oldridge (1988) report that hypnotizable subjects scored higher than nonhypnotizable subjects on the total score and on the vocabulary score of a reading test.

Test Performance

The Problem

Inadequate test performance has prompted many people, from children through adults, to seek consultation from mental health professionals. In considering the applications of hypnosis in improving test performance, it will be assumed that a prospective client has a level of intelligence that would allow him or her to perform at a passable level on the tests concerned and adequate knowledge of the subject material covered on tests. Thus, the barrier keeping the client from performing at an adequate level is assumed to be test anxiety. That is, many people who are intelligent and have a good grasp of the subject material on a test still perform poorly because they "freeze up" in the test situation (their minds go blank, they sweat, their hearts beat rapidly), or they have so much anticipatory anxiety that they cannot prepare adequately.

Treatments in Use

Test anxiety has been treated by systematic desensitization and, to a lesser extent, relaxation training. Woods (1986) contends that the underlying rationale of these two approaches is based on three key assumptions. The first is that test anxiety differs only in degree from more specific anxieties and phobias, which are effectively treated by systematic desensitization. The second assumption is that the arousal component is the major characteristic of test anxiety. Thus, lowering arousal level should improve a student's performance. The third is that irrational cognitions or beliefs significantly contribute to the generation of anxiety.

Types of therapy that focus on replacing irrational negative cognitions with more rational thoughts may be especially applicable to the treatment of text anxiety. Boutin and Tosi (1983) point to rationale emotive therapy (RET) and cognitive behavior therapy (CBT) as two approaches that might be particularly helpful. Both view emotional and behavioral problems such as test anxiety as resulting from a person's irrational beliefs about self and the test-taking situation. Also, both give special consideration to the restructuring of a client's irrational beliefs that underlie emotional disturbance and self-defeating behavior.

Advantages of Hypnosis

Enabling clients to relax and decrease tension levels is often a focal point of hypnotherapy, so it is a logical treatment for test anxiety (Salmon and Meyer, 1992). Posthypnotic suggestions can also be used; they seem to be more effective for those who can reach a deep level of trance (Berrigan et al., 1991). Stanton (1988) has reported promising results when using hypnosis to treat test-anxious middle and high school students. Stanton's clenched fist technique has the added advantage of being easy for students to learn. An additional benefit of using hypnosis in such a population is that young people might be more eager to try out hypnosis than they would be to participate in more conventional therapies.

Hypnosis is economical in terms of time and effort, which is usually important to performance enhancement clients. Spies (1979) states that both hypnosis and biofeedback were equally effective in reducing test anxiety in his study of college students, but the time involved for hypnosis subjects was two and one-half hours per subject, while biofeedback ranged from seven and one-half hours to almost twelve hours per subject.

Finally, favorable results in terms of general classroom performance have been achieved. Galyean (1985) has reported several positive outcomes in using imagery with school children. She states that students seemed to:

- Be more attentive and less distracted.
- Be more involved in work being done in class.
- Learn more of the material being taught.
- Enjoy their learning experiences more than before imagery was introduced to them.
- Do more original and/or creative work.
- Get along better with their classmates.
- Be kinder and more helpful to one another.
- Feel more confident.
- Be more relaxed.
- Do better on tests.

Clearly, that students do better on tests is the primary goal, but these other outcomes are also desirable and may contribute to the likelihood of performing better on tests.

Suggested Hypnotic Techniques

Changing Personal History. This technique contains three steps (Stanton, 1984). First, the clinician helps the client identify a response (such as debilitating anxiety) he or she wishes to change. The patient then sits with eyes closed, recreating the unpleasant feelings associated with the unwanted behavior pattern. Usually the clinician will see visible signs (such as facial changes or altered breathing) that the client is reexperiencing the negative situation. The clinician then anchors this negative feeling, often by touch, for example, by a touch on the right shoulder.

Second, the client explores the experience to discover a resource she or he now possesses that could be "taken back" into the past to change the unpleasant feelings. Examples of such resources are increased confidence, higher self-esteem, or more maturity. The client can be encouraged to identify such resources by being instructed to think of a recent instance in which she or he acted in a calm, mature, and confident manner. A subject who cannot think of a resource that would have helped bring about a more acceptable outcome in the situation is encouraged to think of how a person she or he admires would have handled the situation. As the positive resource is brought out, it is anchored, perhaps with a touch on the left shoulder.

Third, the clinician touches the first anchor to recreate the unpleasant situation. As the client reexperiences this, the clinician touches the second anchor, brining in the positive feelings of the resource. The patient takes as long as is necessary for the negative feelings to change under the influence of the positive feelings. The patient "sees" herself or himself responding successfully, thus creating a new history.

This process can then be generalized to situations the client meets in the future. The clinician simply touches the anchor for the positive feelings and suggests that when the client undergoes anything similar to the unpleasant situation in the future, she or he is to experience the positive feelings.

The procedure is carried out during the trance state. Various methods of induction can be used to reach the trance state. (Several are described in chapters 3 and 4.) Also, Stanton (1984) describes an induction in which he has his subject close her or his eyes, relax in a chair, and concentrate on breathing rhythms, allowing each exhalation to carry away some of the tenseness.

The case of Larry concerns a common phenomenon: a hard-working intelligent student who has no problem learning course material but performs below his capabilities on tests.

> Larry, a nineteen-year-old college sophomore, went to the university counseling center to seek some relief for the anxiety he experienced during exams. He had recently received his grades for the fall semester's midterm examinations. Again, he could not believe how poorly he had done, considering that he had understood the material covered in his courses and had spent plenty of time preparing for the examinations. He had always done well on tests in high school. Larry knew that something had to be wrong. He also

322 · *Practical Clinical Hypnosis*

knew that there was no way he would get into medical school if he kept getting such grades. Dr. Z decided to use the changing personal history technique with Larry:

Dr. Z: So, what is it that you would like to change about the way you are responding in test situations?

Larry: It's just this incredible feeling of anxiety. I just can't control it.

Dr. Z: I would like you to experience right now those anxious feelings you experience when taking an exam. [touches Larry's right shoulder when it is obvious that he is feeling anxious]

Dr. Z: Larry, I would now like you to identify some resource you have, something that might help you in dealing with your anxiety during tests.

Larry: Well, I guess my confidence in myself would be considered one of my best assets.

Dr. Z: Okay, Larry, I want you to experience that feeling of confidence *right now.* [touches Larry's left shoulder, which will serve as an anchor of the feeling of confidence; touches Larry's right shoulder to bring out the anxious feelings he has while taking tests and gives Larry time to let his feeling of confidence affect his anxiety.] Now, I would like you to picture yourself taking a test. You are feeling calm and confident. [pauses to allow Larry to picture the test-taking situation; then, while touching his left shoulder] When you feel these anxious feelings in the future, you will experience a feeling of confidence and feel comfortable about and desirous of tackling the tasks you need to work on.

Clenched Fist Technique. This technique is quite similar to the changing personal history technique. Stanton (1988) suggests using a clenched fist as a trigger to bring about change of troublesome emotional states. This technique develops and uses a positive mood state within the client, which is then conditioned to the cue of a clenched fist so that it may be evoked at will. The client is shown how to release negative feelings, replacing them with this positive mood state.

The procedure begins with a hypnotic induction in which the subject is encouraged to relax and release tension and discomfort in each part of the body. Not only physical relaxation but mental calmness is encouraged. For example, clients can be told to imagine their minds as if they were ponds, the surfaces of which are very still.

As clients drift in this state, they are asked to remember a positive past situation in which they had experienced feelings of relaxation or confidence. As they mentally recreate these feelings, subjects are told to clench the fist of their dominant hand and are given the suggestion that, in the future, whenever they close this hand into a tight fist, they will reexperience the desired feelings. This operates as an anchor, a technique also central to the changing personal history approach.

Attention should then be turned toward an unpleasant emotional state, such as fear or anxiety, that a subject dislikes and wants to control. It should be suggested that the unpleasant feelings can be funneled down through the shoulder and arm into the nondominant fist, where they will be locked up tightly.

Subjects can link the two parts of this procedure together by simultaneously squeezing their dominant hands into strong, confident, happy fists and opening their nondominant hands, allowing the unpleasant feelings to flow away and evaporate into nothingness. Gradually subjects usually see that they can replace negative emotional states with positive ones. The clenching of the dominant hand operates as an anchor for the positive emotional state, while the opening of the nondominant hand is the anchor for the negative emotional state.

The procedure is most effectively carried out while subjects are in the trance state. To avoid disturbance to the state, subjects are shown how to use ideomotor finger signals, such as lifting a single finger, rather than words, to communicate with the clinician.

Susan's case demonstrates how the "clenched-fist technique can be used to enhance self-confidence and lessen performance anxiety.

Susan is a fourteen-year-old ninth grader who pays attention in classes, completes her homework, seems motivated, and tests out as quite intelligent. However, she receives mostly average to below-average grades due to her poor performance on tests. Susan, with the encouragement of her parents, is eager to try hypnosis in hopes that she can relax when preparing for tests and better recall the information she has studied. Dr. X first takes Susan through a hypnotic induction and then begins with the following dialogue:

Dr. X: Susan, I would like you to recall a past situation in which you felt confident, whether it was while you were taking a test, giving a speech, participating in sports, or anything else you might think of.

Susan: Okay, I remember when I was trying out for cheerleading last year. I felt really good about my chances of making the squad.

Dr. X: Did you make the squad?

Susan: Yes. I really like it . . . and everybody says I'm good at it too.

Dr. X: Good. Now, as you begin to experience again that feeling of confidence, I want you to clench the fist of your right hand . . .

that's right . . . feel how relaxed, calm, and confident you are right now . . . You can also experience that same feeling of confidence in the future whenever you close your right hand into a fist . . . okay, you can release it now.

Now, Susan, I want you to focus on the anxiety or the tension that you feel when you are taking a test. That feeling can be funneled down through your left arm into your left hand. Now, clench your left fist . . . that's right . . . see, you can grasp that tension tightly . . . you are in control of it . . . you are feeling relaxed, calm, and confident.

Clench your right fist again . . . notice how strong and confident you feel . . . Now, I want you to open your left hand, allowing your tension to disappear . . . you no longer have to grasp it, because it simply drains out of your hand, allowing you to feel relaxed, calm, and confident . . . You will be able to go through this procedure outside the session whenever you feel tense. You will always have a way of replacing that tension with this feeling of confidence.

Rational Stage Directed Hypnotherapy (RSDH). This approach is somewhat more specific that the two previous approaches. RSDH was designed specifically to integrate hypnotherapy, imagery training, and cognitive behavior therapy or rational emotive therapy (Boutin and Tosi, 1983). Clients are asked to visualize a test-taking situation and the emotional responses associated with it. Then they identify specific irrational thoughts and are directed to challenge and confront these thoughts and finally to replace them with more rational self-talk.

Subjects are then hypnotized and asked again to visualize the test-taking situation and to experience the resulting anxiety associated with it. They are asked to consider the same situation but to engage in and to try to experience more positive affect as they go through more rational self-talk. The clinician then guides the subjects through each developmental stage at the clients' own pace subjects seem to do better when given a posthypnotic suggestion, possibly buttressed by audiotapes, to practice the RSDH procedure outside the sessions.

John's case demonstrates how RSDH can help with performance anxiety.

John is a thirty-five-year-old university student who has gone back to school after working in his father's construction company for more than fifteen years after he graduated from high school. He has finally decided, with some obvioius enthusiasm, that he wants to teach health and physical education in high school, but he is having trouble with the exams in his anatomy course. Trying to remember a myriad of names of bones and muscles makes John break out in a sweat. He has identified not only a feeling of anxiety but specific self-defeating statements or thoughts that he finds himself repeating to himself when taking a test. Dr. F elected to use rational stage directed hypnotherapy with John:

Dr. F: John, you've told me that there are certain thoughts that consistently run through your mind when you are taking a test. Tell me what some of those thoughts are.

John: Okay . . . here's an example: If I don't know the answer to the first question on a test, I start to think that I will fail the test, and my wife will respect me less, my children will be ashamed of me, and my friends will make fun of me behind my back. Also, I sometimes think that if I don't make an A on this test, I won't be able to get a job, and I won't be able to support my family.

Dr. F: That's very good. We now have a good basis to work from. What we need to do next is work on getting you to confront those kinds of negative thoughts and to identify more rational statements that you can repeat to yourself when you are taking a test. Let me give you a couple of examples to get us started. When the negative thoughts come up, I want you to immediately tell yourself, whether you believe it or not—and we both understand that you may not believe it for awhile—that "I have studied this material thoroughly, and I know I can answer this question if I just stay calm," or, "This question is difficult, but I know that I can get at least partial credit if I write down what I know about it." [Encourages John to generate other positive statements, and then suggests that they go through a hypnotic induction.]

[After John is in the trance state] Now, John, I would like you to picture yourself taking a test . . . experience the feeling of anxiety you have when the test is handed to you and you do not know the answer to the first question . . . But now, repeat to yourself the positive statements we discussed earlier . . . focus on those thoughts, that you did study this material and you can answer these questions if you give yourself time . . . Repeat those over and over in your mind, until there is no room to think any negative thoughts . . . notice the feeling of confidence you have as you dwell on these thoughts . . . you feel calm and confident, and you can allow yourself to focus your attention on the questions on your exam . . . And now, you do not ex-

perience anxiety, but only confidence and a sense of being focused . . . look over the questions . . . Even better, John, you
can experience that feeling of confidence not only in our sessions, but anytime you need it, simply by allowing yourself to
dwell on these positive statements.

Sports Performance

The Problem

Performance anxiety, often generated by fear and/or guilt, is the enemy of
athletic success (McArdle, Katch, Katch, 1991). Fear or guilt can also interrupt muscle performance by inducing a greater secretion of adrenalin,
which accumulates throughout the body and adversely affects muscle performance. Howard and Reardon (1986) conclude that there is consistent
evidence that high levels of state anxiety have been demonstrated to have a
negative effect on athletic performance.

Aside from anxiety, self-concept (as well as related, or even generic,
self-talk) is another variable assumed to have an effect on sports performance (Masters, 1992). Of course, self-concept and anxiety are also often
related, in that our attitudes toward ourselves influence how anxious we feel
in confronting challenging situations. Similarly, our level of anxiety influences how we feel about ourselves.

Treatments in Use

Cognitive restructuring techniques have been the treatment of choice for
clients interested in improving their athletic performance. These techniques
have been used to facilitate self-concept, reduce anxiety, and increase performance in athletes. Structured relaxation techniques, such as autogenic
training, which combines relaxation with biofeedback (described in detail in
chapter 4), have also been used.

Advantages of Hypnosis

Hypnotic treatments usually try to emphasize to the client that attitude is as
important to success as skill level. Hypnotherapy teaches athletes how to use
positive motivation and clear thinking to direct their body's actions. It is
also an effective way of encouraging a person to focus all attention on only
one thought at a time (Martens, 1987).

Hypnosis can focus a person's awareness while, seemingly paradoxically, bringing a state of calmness and relaxation. This state of relaxation,
when combined with appropriate images or suggestions, can be a powerful
tool in motivating and helping an individual athlete achieve goals. Hypnosis

can help the athlete to use his or her ability more effectively. It shows how to use one's mind to help, rather than hurt, oneself.

Finally, hypnosis helps accelerate the learning process. An athlete can visualize herself or himself repeatedly performing a skill perfectly. This type of practice can reinforce proper techniques without time being spent actually performing the techniques. Although the actual physical performance of the skills is quite necessary, visualization can be an effective complement to such practice.

Relevant Research

Wojcikiewicz and Orlick (1987), in their study of forty-two fencers, found significantly less anxiety in the group who had been hypnotized, in contrast with the control group. However, the authors thought this finding may have resulted from the control condition's increasing anxiety rather than the hypnotic intervention's lowering anxiety.

In a study of beginning tennis players reported by Greer and Engs (1986), hypnosis was found to be no more effective than traditional coaching techniques. It was concluded that progressive relaxation and hypnosis, along with instructions for mentally practicing tennis strokes through visualization, was no more (or no less) effective than the traditional instruction through explanation and demonstration. However, it is not clear what instructions were given to subjects during the trance state.

More encouraging results were found in a study of weight lifters. Howard and Reardon (1986) report that their cognitive-hypnotic-imagery group showed a significant difference from a cognitive-restructuring-only group and a hypnosis-only group on measures of self-concept, anxiety, muscular growth, and neuromuscular performance. These improvements were sustained and even enhanced from one posttest measure (one week after the conclusion of treatment) to the next measure (one month after treatment).

Suggested Hypnotic Techniques

The following introduction, developed by sports psychologist Dr. Stan Frager, functions to prepare the client to understand the process and positively respond to it. It can be adapted to individual needs and to other performance enhancement situations. It can be presented in written form but should be supplemented by a complementary oral presentation.

Therapist: Remember that your first task as an athlete is to work hard at your sport. All the sports psychology in the world isn't a substitute for hard work and good coaching. As a basketball player, you have to first be able to stick the ball in the hole, play defense, and run.

Having worked in a variety of different sports, I have found that once you have developed your skills, you must learn to concentrate and relax to maximize your abilities. Remember that what the mind perceives, the body believes (and eventually achieves). If you believe something to be true (and it is a realistic goal), your body reacts as if it is true. Let me give you an example.

Suppose you get a note at school that says, "A member of your family has been seriously injured in an auto accident and you need to get to the emergency room of the hospital right away." You immediately would go to the principal's office, explain the situation, and somehow find a way to get to the hospital. Your heart would be beating fast, you'd be perspiring . . . your body is setting up for fight or flight. All kinds of physical things are happening to your body and your mind. You zoom over to the hospital as fast as you can, and as you run in the emergency room door and race up to the emergency room reception desk, the receptionist explains that there has been a terrible mistake. Because of a mix-up in names, it was not your family member that was hurt in the accident. No one in your family has been hurt, and they apologize for the error. You, of course, are now relieved—and probably a little angry about the mix-up.

What's important about that little example is that there was no accident and nobody was injured. However, you believed it to be true, and therefore your body reacted as if it were true. The fact that it really hadn't happened didn't matter at all. You believed it to be true, so your body acted as if it were true. That has a lot of importance in terms of how we handle ourselves in competition and practice.

You've probably heard the axiom, "Practice makes perfect." Unfortunately, that's wrong! Obviously, if you practiced wrong, you would perform wrong. So it isn't practice that makes perfect. The absolute truth is that persistent perfect practice makes you as perfect as you can get.

But it's very difficult to practice perfectly. Practice does make permanent, and that's important so that when you run a play, it's important that you be at the right place at the right time. We also know that if you practice hard, you will tend to play hard. Players who "dog it" in practice, thinking they will save it for the game, are most likely not going to be able to play their best when they need to. Working with champion athletes makes one thing clear: they all work very hard. So again, our mental preparation is not a substitute for hard work, good athletic ability, and a good coach.

Given that you have those three ingredients present, what do you do to prepare mentally?

A very powerful tool is a technique called visual imagery. We combine this with mental rehearsal of perfect performance of the skill that is desired. What you want to do is get yourself completely relaxed, and then we combine that with mental rehearsal of a desired performance skill.

Remember to picture yourself doing the activity perfectly, and remember to picture it as if you were actually doing it. You don't see yourself if you are shooting. For example, if you are shooting free throws, you might see the basket and the backboard and the other team, but you would not see yourself. Picture yourself shooting perfect free throws.

When you are in the actual situation, you are likely to perform in a way consistent with your mental rehearsal—perfect free throws. A great deal of research has shown that when you mentally practice a skill, you are actually doing motor control rehearsal. You are actually helping train your muscles to react to given situations in certain ways.

This type of practice is also very powerful in helping you to develop confidence. One of the things that we all search for is having more confidence. Just what is confidence? At its most basic level, it is the absence of tension and the recall of success. This is what we will work toward achieving.

So you need to approach the mental part of your game with the same intensity as the physical part of your game. A great time to do this kind of mental rehearsal is when you are going to bed at night. This kind of mental rehearsal every night as you are going to bed will result in fine-tuning your performance in practice in games. This is not to say that you are not going to occasionally have an off-day. That's the nature of the sport. What it does mean is that by practicing your concentration, you are going to maximize the gains of all the hard physical work you put it.

If you are serious and practice as hard as you can and then go into a game situation giving the same 100 percent, then no matter what the outcome of the game, you walk off the court with your head high, and you will never need to apologize to anyone for your effort.

Cognitive-Hypnotic-Imagery. This approach is somewhat different from others discussed in this chapter in that it incorporates more than strict hypnosis. Due to the favorable results Howard and Reardon (1986) found with the addition of cognitive restructuring, this method, rather than their hypnosis-only approach, is discussed here.

Subjects were introduced to concepts of cognitive control and restructuring. First, clients are instructed that they and not the environment are responsible for their thoughts and emotions. Then, a brief lecture is given to the clients, with an emphasis on the idea that self-concept is the summation of self-referring statements and is intricately related to performance. More specifically, it is emphasized that those statements on which clients focus during their daily activities will contribute to how they feel about themselves and how they perform. Third, clients identify negative self-referring statements. Negative ideation specifically associated with athletic performance is then identified. Finally, positive cognitive strategies are developed.

The first step in the hypnotic component is a preliminary discussion of hypnosis. Issues that should be addressed include beliefs and misconceptions about hypnosis, various depths that can be reached (or which are necessary) while in a trance, and that hypnosis is based on belief and confidence and not a sleep state.

The second step is the hypnotic induction. Any of various induction techniques can be used, but the one recommended by the original authors includes asking the client to get comfortable in the chair, close the eyes, and focus on deep breathing. Next, the client is directed through progressive muscle relaxation from the forehead to the toes. Counting associated with breathing is used as a deepening technique.

After the induction is conducted, the client is directed to experience the negative emotional states associated with the situations identified and to identify the negative and irrational cognitions. This sequence is negatively reinforced by the clinician (for example, by images of a noxious odor), who then directs the subject to refocus on relaxing thoughts and then visualize the negative sequence, visualizing himself or herself engaging in more rational self-talk and experiencing more positive affective responses. This self-enhancing sequence is positively reinforced by the clinician by a congratulatory patter and reintroduction of positive images.

The hypnosis state is used to enhance physiological processes. That is, subjects, are directed to visualize themselves performing the behavioral criterion measured while hypnotized. They are directed to visualize, among other things, the elimination of negative ideation, the attainment of proper levels of arousal, the successful performance of the athletic feat concerned, their feelings of pride and happiness about the increases achieved, and others' recognition of their higher level of performance. As with all imagery rehearsal, the greatest effect comes from imaging the desired response being performed in an optimal manner, with as vivid imagery as possible.

Scott's case demonstrates how an integration of techniques can help sport performance.

Scott, a seventeen-year-old junior, is a point guard on his school's boys' basketball team and is already considered a promising recruit by several major universities. He maintains above-average grades, has good leadership ability, and is very coachable. He shows a solid grasp of the fundamental skills of the sport, with one exception: his free throw shooting. Scott has been told by several college coaches that his foul shots need work, but hours of practice have not shown promising results. He is brought by his parents to Dr. B's clinic. Dr. B feels that Scott would be a good candidate for hypnosis but would also benefit from cognitive restructuring. Scott agrees to try cognitive-hypnotic-imagery, the treatment Dr. B suggests.

Dr. B first initiates a conversation with Scott regarding Scott's beliefs about hypnosis. Thus, Dr. B can allay Scott's fears and correct any misconceptions he has about hypnosis. Once the problem is identified, Dr. B wisely consults those who know about the skill components that are needed—in this case, Bill Olsen, a former basketball coach, now athletic director, and Denny Crum, head basketball coach, both at the University of Louisville. They emphasize that the best free throw shooters use an economical, comfortable motion, but most important, they use the exact same motion every time.

Next, Dr. B takes Scott through an induction. One option is to direct him to focus on his breathing. Dr. B can then slowly direct him through progressive muscle relaxation from his head to his toes. At this point, Dr. B can simply start naming the parts of the body in a rhythmic fashion— ". . . and now your forehead, and your neck, and your shoulders, and your chest . . ." As he names specific parts of the body, Dr. B instructs Scott to relax each part.

Dr. B then instructs Scott to experience the feelings of discouragement he has when he misses a free throw. He also instructs Scott to identify the negative irrational statements he makes to himself when he feels such discouragement, such as "I'm never going to make it as a college basketball player anyway; the competition is just too tough, and I don't have what it takes to make it,"or "It's no use trying to work on my free throws; I've already practiced so many hours on it, and it hasn't done any good; I might as well give up, because no coach wants a player who can't even make his free throws." After Scott generates such thoughts, Dr. B directs him to refocus on relaxing thoughts and then visualize his feelings of discouragement at not making his free throws. However, Scott is encouraged this time to engage in more rational self-talk, such as "My free throws may need work, but I must be a decent player, or coaches wouldn't be recruiting me," or "I have made shots from this distance hundreds of times in the past, and I know I can do it again if I relax and don't put so much pressure on myself."

Let us consider how Dr. B might have Scott imagine himself shooting free throws in the trance state, using images of the "shoot motion" Scott has already chosen:

Dr. B: Scott, while you stay in this relaxed state, I want you to visualize yourself making a free throw. Imagine that you have just been fouled as you attempted (and made) a last-second shot, and the score is tied . . . see yourself stepping up to the foul line . . . You glance at your teammates, and they look confident and determined as they watch you . . . the referee hands you the ball, and the shape and texture of it feel familiar and comfortable . . . You release your breath, you go into your shooter motion, doing it just right, doing it perfectly . . . you bounce the ball three times . . . you look up at the basket, bend your knees, let the ball glide out of your hand with just the right arc, you see it floating toward the basket and swishing through the net . . . feel the exhilaration of knowing that you have helped your team win the game . . . Your coach, your teammates and dozens of fans surround you, telling you they are proud of you and they knew you could do it . . . you feel only pride and happiness because of your newfound confidence . . . there is no room for the discouragement you felt before . . . I can tell by your facial expressions that you have visualized this quite well, Scott . . . It is important for you to know that you can do this visualization on your own, whenever you want to experience that feeling of confidence that you are experiencing right now.

As noted, it is critical to develop a correct technique, amplify it by vivid imagery, and use one that the client knows and accepts.

A Technique for Runners. It would appear that hypnotic work with runners has a great potential for success, considering that the mental phenomena reported by long-distance runners often bear a strong resemblance to hypnotic states (Masters, 1992). In fact, Cunningham (1981) states that the "running high" is just another variant of hypnosis. Channon (1984) describes a hypnotic technique she has used exclusively for runners. She has used this method with people who find running boring and with those who think that there is something they are missing about the running experience. First, hypnosis is induced by eye closure, and deepening is achieved by directing clients to imagine a pleasant sensory experience. For example, they are directed to imagine the movements of the body and the feeling of wet sand on the feel while walking along the edge of a lagoon, walking deeper into hypnosis.

Under hypnosis, clients are encouraged to set a target before beginning runs in the next few weeks. This target can be started in terms of time or in terms of distance. If they decided to run for a certain length of time, they are instructed to run until the hands of the watch have reached a certain position. If the target is one of distance, they can run past a certain number of streets or up to a certain landmark. Whatever the target is, it should be realistic. Clients are then encouraged to imagine running. They are directed not to think about how far or how long to run, since they have already established that. Rather, they are directed to become aware of two rhythms: the regular rhythm of their steps and breathing and then some other pattern that is rhythmic and regular—a song, a group of words, particular numbers, or something else. Whatever it is, they should repeat it mentally in time with the rhythm of their movements. Clients are first told that they will feel at one with their body but also somehow distanced from their body, where they are able to have some sort of "ideal perspective," and at the same time feel melded to or at one with the inner body. The clients are instructed that if there is any need to be alert to outside events, they will be able to do so but will be able to return easily to this pleasant state.

After letting clients experience this detached state, the clinician then instructs them to imagine reaching the target and can now begin to talk. The clients should feel peaceful, calm, and at ease, with a tired but healthy body. Finally, clients are instructed to let the scene fade gradually, calmly, and peacefully.

Although it was not a primary focus in the two techniques, we find that giving the subject a trigger, or cue word, can be important. It is an effective way for the clinician to turn over control of the trance state to the client. The clinician can condition the induction to a trigger and then hand over the trigger to the client. When this works efficiently, the client can trigger the whole induction process by just activating the signal. Stephanie's case demonstrates how some of the prior techniques can help with running performance.

> Stephanie is a forty-year-old advertising executive who is quite involved in running. She runs four to ten miles each day and runs a 10-kilometer (6.2 miles) race virtually every weekend. However, she has recently been more fatigued near the end of her daily runs and feels discouraged about this. She went to her physician, who found no physical basis for her fatigue.
>
> Although the hypnotic technique for runners is most often used

with people who find running boring, it can be equally useful with Stephanie's problem. Dr. P induces a trance in Stephanie, and then proceeds as follows:

Dr. P: I would now like you to imagine taking a slow drive in the country . . . there are no other cars around . . . you feel a soft, warm breeze . . . the wind is blowing through your hair, and you feel relaxed and carefree . . . I want you to see this drive as a journey deeper into relaxation . . . I know that you have been having trouble running as far as you would like to. What I would like you to do is to set yourself a goal each day for how far you would like to run.

Stephanie: Well, a good goal for me right now is probably eight miles a day.

Dr. P: Okay. Now I want you to think of a landmark that is about four miles away from your house, so that when you reach that landmark, you will know that you have completed one-half of your eight-mile run. If you need to pick out a specific landmark later, that's fine, but I want you to imagine one right now . . . and now, imagine that you are running, but do not think about how far you have to run, since you have already worked that out . . . Notice how relaxing it is not to have to worry about how far you will run today . . . your mind does not have to be occupied with that at all . . . instead, you can now become aware of the rhythm of your steps and of your breathing . . . You notice that both of these rhythms are showing a steady pattern, so steady that you could sing the words of a song in time with the rhythm of your steps and your breathing . . . think of your favorite song, one you like to sing along with . . . repeat the words of the song over and over in your mind, noticing how well they fit with the rhythm of your steps and breathing . . . Notice how you feel so in tune with your body . . . experience the pleasure of being in control of your body and in tune with it . . . experience a pleasant feeling of anticipation, knowing that you can easily return to such a state in your next run . . . And now, imagine that you have reached your target . . . you can now begin to slow to a relaxed jog, and finally begin walking . . . you feel so good that you were able to achieve your goal . . . you feel confident, strong, and peaceful . . . You do notice a feeling of fatigue, but it is not nearly as overwhelming as it was before . . . Now you can let the image fade from your mind gradually and peacefully, again knowing that you can easily achieve such a state of confidence in the future.

Self-Hypnosis. The popularity of this technique for performance enhancement was probably first aided by the publication of two popular books on learning to bowl better and learning to play better golf. In these books, Heise (1961a, 1961b), extensively describes induction techniques for self-hypnosis. In adapting a version of these techniques (Heise, 1961a), the clinician instructs the client to turn the lights out, lie down on a bed, and close his or her eyes. He or she then gives a script for the clients to recite, which goes through progressive muscle relaxation in a detailed manner.

After a state of relaxation has been attained, it is suggested that the athlete open his or her eyes and focus on an object above eye level. The athlete is instructed to try to get his or her eyelids to close at a specific count, such as the count of three. If the athlete has an irresistible urge to close the eyes on or before reaching the completion of the count, he or she is in a heightened state of suggestibility or self-hypnosis. Specific self-suggestions are given for this eye closure test, and when the client is in the self-hypnotic state can give himself or herself whatever posthypnotic suggestions are desired.

At this point, the client can feel free to give himself or herself specific suggestions for improving performance—shooting a perfect foul shot, for example, or kicking the perfect field goal. When the client has finished implanting suggestions for better performance in the subconscious mind, he or she should then give himself or herself a posthypnotic suggestion that the next time during self-hypnosis he or she will enter a deeper state more quickly.

We will consider two cases under the domain of self-hypnosis, since it is a technique that may be met with more enthusiasm and acceptance by athletes than is formal hypnosis with a clinician. Tennis and golf are examples of two sports in which the importance of the mental aspect of the game has been widely recognized, so we will consider cases in those sports.

> Jill is a sophomore at a private liberal arts college. She was expected to become the star of the school's women's tennis team when she arrived on campus. She had won several regional junior tournaments and had been highly recruited by Division I universities. However, her play has been inconsistent since she began her freshman year, and she has won only about 50 percent of her matches. She has practiced diligently and cannot pinpoint specific weaknesses in her game but says that she just does not feel confident in her ability anymore.
>
> At the suggestion of her coach, Jill consults with Dr. C, who is trained in hypnotic techniques. He sees that Jill is quite motivated and intelligent, and he suggests that she try self-hypnosis. He holds a preliminary session with her in order to give her specific sugges-

tions as to how to implement self-hypnosis. Let us consider what tips he might give to Jill:

Dr. C: Jill, what I would like to do is tell you some specific things you can do that will help you to become relaxed and to be able to visualize yourself playing tennis in an optimal fashion. First, you need to turn the lights out in your room, then lie on your bed, and close your eyes. You can then concentrate on your breathing, noticing how deep and cleansing each breath is. Note the effortless, soothing rhythm that your breathing has. As you find yourself in tune with that rhythm, begin to relax your muscles gradually. Just feel them going loose and comfortably slack. Start with the muscles in your face, then those in your neck, your chest, your arms, your thighs, your calves, and your feet. You can even break these areas down further, focusing on each muscle that you are aware of. When you do feel completely relaxed, open your eyes. Focus on an object above eye level. Try to get your eyelids to close at the count of three. If you have an urge to close them before you count to three, you are in a state of self-hypnosis. If not, do not become anxious. It will probably take a few times practicing this for you to reach that hypnotic state.

When you feel that you have reached a hypnotic state, you can give yourself some specific suggestions about your tennis game. For example, visualize yourself serving a perfect ace. See the motion that is effective and just feels right. You can break that skill down into parts, so that you see yourself standing at just the right distance from the endline and at just the right angle to the net, tossing the ball at just the right height and distance from your body, contacting the ball at just the right place on the head of the racket and at just the right point in your motion, and finally you can see yourself following through perfectly, watching the ball go bounce on the opponent's side of the court, out of her reach. You can even give yourself the suggestion that the next time you practice self-hypnosis you will achieve a trance state earlier and get to a deeper level of trance.

Doug is a golfer who has been on the professional tour for about three years. He enjoyed substantial success in his first year on the tour but has struggled with a "sophomore jinx" since then. Many golf analysts have touted him as having incredible natural talent but not being able to complement that with good decision making and levelheadedness. Doug admits that he does get "a little rattled" in the heat of competition and wants some help in dealing with that.

He consults a clinician, Dr. Y, who advises Doug to go through a similar hypnotic induction as that recommended to Jill. The major difference would be in the area of specific suggestions. Dr. Y recommends visualizing the perfect drive, which might go something like this:

Dr. Y: You select the perfect club for the distance you would like to hit the ball . . . you focus your eyes on the point at which you are aiming, and then you step to the ball . . . now, focus on the ball . . . your hands are in precisely the right grip, your feet are exactly the right width apart, and you are perfectly balanced in your stance . . . you swing your arms back to precisely the right height. The word *ready* will stay in your mind as the marker for this part of the swing. The word *hit* is the marker in your mind from this part of the swing on through to the finish. Now, from the top point of your swing, swing your arms through the ball at the same time as you drive with your legs, and you follow through with your swing, aiming straight toward the green . . . you hear the crowd cheer as they see the flight of the ball and realize that you have hit the green . . . you feel confident that you will do well on this hole . . . most important, you realize that you can capture that feeling of confidence anytime you need to, just by going through a visualization such as this.

The client can later be instructed to anchor this by using the markers "ready" and "hit" as self-instructions when actually playing golf. This type of procedure can be easily adapted to a wide variety of behaviors in the other sports. The client is instructed to focus on using these marker words, which acts to block distracting thoughts.

Performing Arts

The Problem

Many actors, dancers, musicians, and vocalists have sought help for a lack of creativity or originality in their performances (Salmon and Meyer, 1992). Often these performers have possessed creative skill but have lost some of that skill for some reason. Another problem is that a number of performers are highly skilled in the technical aspects of their performance but do not show a high level of creativity in artistic expression.

Advantages of Hypnosis

It has often been proposed that hypnosis and creativity involve similar phenomena (those people who are highly hypnotizable are highly creative, and vice versa). Both hypnosis and creativity may be facilitated by fantasy (Jackson and Gorassini, 1989). Therefore, a client with some creative ability may show fantasy-proneness, which is a good indicator for hypnotherapy.

Hypnosis can also enable performers to assess their own performances. There are several problems with relying solely on feedback from critics or teachers, such as obtaining conflicting information from different sources and depriving oneself of the opportunity to develop informed opinions about one's skills (Salmon and Meyer, 1992). Hypnosis can help one to tune into the quality of one's performance and evaluate it accordingly, rather than relying on potentially inaccurate feedback from others.

Relevant Research

Much of the research that has been performed concerning the relationship between hypnosis and creativity does not deal with creative performances in terms of the performing arts. Rather, studies have often used pools of students in introductory psychology courses and assessed performances on such tasks as figure drawing or verbal creativity. For example, Jackson and Gorassini (1989) found greater figural-spatial creativity in a hypnosis condition than in a waking condition. However, Ashton and McDonald (1985) found that hypnotherapy was ineffective in augmenting creativity (as measured by tests of verbal creativity) in highly hypnotizable subjects. Overall, results of using hypnotherapy with individuals who would like to increase their creativity have been mixed.

Suggested Techniques

Due to the dearth of literature concerning hypnosis and creative performance, very few hypnotic techniques have been outlined in the literature. However, with only a minimal amount of adaptation, one can use techniques mentioned earlier in this chapter.

Self-Hypnosis. The clinician can follow the lead of Heise (1961a) and teach performance enhancement clients self-hypnotic techniques. The eye closure test can be used to test for trance depth. The client can then give himself or herself specific suggestions concerning creative performance—for example, playing an overture or delivering lines with perfect expression. Although it sounds simple, such an approach can be very powerful when practiced during a trance state.

> Jack is a twenty-eight-year-old actor currently working as a waiter and attending any auditions for which he might be even remotely qualified. He is hopeful that he will get his big break one day and launch a successful acting career. However, in the past two years, his efforts have led to only a couple of parts in local commercials

and two small parts in little-known plays. Jack has no problem learning his lines. Rather, his difficultly is in expressing the desired amount of emotion in delivering his lines. Thus far, Jack has maintained a hopeful attitude that he can overcome this problem. He presents to Dr. V as someone who is eager to enhance his creativity and who feels that hypnosis might benefit him in achieving that.

Jack appears quite motivated and thus is seen by Dr. V as someone who might be a good candidate for self-hypnosis. Dr. V instructs Jack to go through progressive muscle relaxation, in which he will recite a script to himself of the body parts he intends to relax. Following this, Jack is instructed to do an eye closure test. When Jack is satisfied that he has reached a hypnotic state, he is to give himself suggestions for improving his acting. Dr. V suggests the following:

Dr. V: What you then need to do, Jack, is picture yourself delivering your lines in an optimal manner . . . you pay keen attention as the lead actress speaks to you . . . you respond almost spontaneously to her . . . the words that you have memorized so painstakingly are spoken by you as if they are coming straight from your heart. They become a part of you as you practice, and then they flow out naturally and easily. See it clearly and fully. You instinctively display the necessary amount of emotion, with seemingly no effort on your part . . . you speak your lines flawlessly . . . afterward, the audience applauds and cheers loudly when you come out for your curtain call . . . reviews in the paper the next morning laud your performance as inspiring and powerful . . . you feel very confident, and you realize that you have the range that you need to have as an actor . . . you can then suggest to yourself that the next time you do self-hypnosis that you will enter a deeper state of trance, and reach it more quickly than you did this time.

Stanton's Techniques. The changing personal history and the clenched fist technique are easily adapted to work with performance anxiety. An adaptation of Stanton's changing personal history technique (1984) includes having clients identify and experience a situation in which anxiety had caused them to perform badly or uncreatively. The clinician then anchors this experience by touching the client's right knee, for example. A positive resource that the client possesses and could be "taken back" to the negative situation is then identified by the client. For example, the client may have recently gained confidence because of feedback concerning his or her performance. This resource is then anchored, perhaps by a touch of the left knee. The first anchor point is activated, followed by activation of the second anchor point. The client can then let the positive feelings associated with a sense of confidence overcome the sense of anxiety. Finally, the suggestion should be given that the client's positive feeling will gradually emerge and then displace anxiety in future occurrences of the negative feeling.

Julia is a thirty-six-year-old cellist with a well-known metropolitan orchestra. She has gradually moved her way up in the cello section so that she recently became first chair. While she is excited about the success she has achieved, she is also quite anxious about the increased expectations of a first chair, such as frequently playing solo parts of symphonies. She has come to Dr. T seeking relief from this anxiety, as it has been a detriment to her musical expression.

In using the changing personal history technique, Julia could be instructed by Dr. T to identify a situation in which she had performed poorly. Julia might identify a particular practice in the past in which her unimaginative reading of the music was the only variable that kept her from being promoted within the cello section. Dr. T could anchor that experience by touching Julia's right knee. Julia's general feeling of confidence in her musical ability might be identified as a positive resource, which could be taken into the practice setting. This confidence would then be anchored by touching Julia's left knee.

The next step would be for Dr. T to touch the first anchor point, followed by activation of the second anchor point. He should then give Julia time for her confidence to overcome her negative feelings surrounding her bad practice session. Finally Dr. T can give the suggestion that Julia will feel confidence return in future practice and performance situations.

17
Forensic Hypnosis

> In a November 1989 interview, Jessica Hahn, the victim and/or
> participant of a sexual assault by evangelist Jim Bakker, was quoted
> as saying, "If I weren't moving into show business right now, I
> would go to college and study law and psychology."
> —*Expert Opinion* 3, no. 2 (1990)

Since forensic hypnosis combines the controversies of two disparate areas, it is replete with challenge and contention. This chapter presents accepted procedures and techniques of forensic hypnosis, as well as an overview of the psychology of hypnosis and the hypnotic phenomena as it relates to forensic applications.

Hypnosis and the Legal System

For more than half of the twentieth century, hypnosis was of little concern to judges, lawyers, and the police. In 1897, the California Supreme Court announced that "the law of the United States does not recognize hypnotism" (*People v. Ebanks*, p. 1053). There the matter remained until the late 1960s, when a few courts were willing to soften the judicial hard line against the admissibility of hypnotically refreshed testimony. Since then the renaissance of interest in hypnosis has proceeded at an astonishing pace (Levitan, 1991). Today many mental health professionals (and, unfortunately, law enforcement personnel, poorly trained therapists, and laypersons as well) utilize hypnosis and related techniques for a variety of purposes.

The fields of law and psychology have not always blended easily. Practitioners from each discipline approach problems from distinctly different orientations with different goals. The veracity of accounts is less important in clinical work than in legal work. Clinically, hypnotherapists are interested in recovering memories to aid in patients' insight, current functioning, and/or comfort, especially as it relates to trauma experienced during the commission of a crime. In the legal setting, hypnosis is used to find or help determine facts that establish guilt or innocence in accordance with accepted evidentiary rules.

Most cases involving hypnotically refreshed testimony have been criminal ones. In *Rock v. Arkansas* (1987), the U.S. Supreme Court held that a state could not enforce a blanket prohibition (a "per se" exclusionary rule) on a defendant's presenting her own testimony even though it had been refreshed through hypnosis. Nevertheless, the states continue to vary considerably on whether, and under what circumstances, other witnesses in criminal trials may present hypnotically refreshed testimony. It is important to remember that similar questions of admissibility may arise in civil cases, which *Rock v. Arkansas* did not speak to. Again, there is considerable variation by state in civil cases as well.

The legal implications of hypnotherapeutic interventions are being scrutinized more closely today by the courts than at any other time. Hypnotherapists are required to exercise extraordinary sensitivity to meet dual, and occasionally conflicting, responsibilities. Therapists who use hypnosis with clients need to be aware of the legal status of hypnosis and the legal responsibilities of those who utilize it.

A special consideration may arise when hypnosis is used on a victim of rape or another form of intrusive violence. Because of legal rulings that limit or even disqualify the testimony of previously hypnotized subjects, the use of hypnosis for therapeutic purposes may deprive the client of the legal right to testify in subsequent court actions. Despite intentions of operating in good faith, a hypnotherapist may have innocently violated the client's right to informed consent. Thus, even the therapeutic use of hypnosis may have unexpected legal consequences.

Struggle toward a Definition

Courts and hypnotherapists strive to define clearly what hypnosis is and what it is not, but the vast array of definitions—an "altered state," a "trance," "role enactment," and no "state" at all—provides more problems than solutions. To most clinicians involved in using hypnosis as a therapeutic tool, the precise definition of hypnosis is secondary to the functionality of the procedure. If a procedure works in providing relief from pain or discomfort, the process of change is generally irrelevant. In the legal setting, the court is less concerned with pragmatics than in a clear definition of what the hypnotherapist did and its implications for due process.

For therapists engaged in forensic hypnosis, Scheflin and Shapiro (1989) present an operational definition of hypnosis:

> Hypnosis is an altered state or consciousness, characterized by intensified concentration of awareness on certain suggested themes, along with diminished interest in competing perceptions. Subjects who are hypnotized experience perceptual and sensory distortions and enhanced abilities to utilize normally unconscious mental mechanisms. (p. 134)

Forensic Applications of Hypnosis

There are two main interfaces between hypnosis and law: the use of hypnosis as a tool in legal controversies and the definition of legal rights and liabilities arising from the misuse of hypnosis. The first area has received more attention. Hypnosis has been used or advocated for all of the following (Udolf, 1983):

1. As an investigative technique to obtain leads to independent evidence.
2. To enhance the memory of victims or witnesses of crime.
3. To enable a defendant to break through an amnesia.
4. To aid in the preparation of the defense.
5. As a technique by which an expert evaluates a defendant's sanity, state of mind, or criminal intent (mens rea).
6. As a defense in a criminal case.
7. To obtain confessions from defendants.

In the past few years, there has been a dramatic increase in the use of hypnosis by the criminal justice system for the purposes of investigation and memory enhancement of victims, witnesses, and defendants. Its proponents argue that hypnosis lifts amnesia and provides valuable leads or new information in cases in which it is employed (Kroger and Duce, 1979; Reiser, 1989). Others have grave concerns about the possibility of the potential misuses of hypnosis. They note that the resulting memories are actually confabulations and that hypnotized witnesses have a false sense of confidence in the veracity of memories refreshed by hypnosis (Orne et al., 1984; Diamond, 1980).

There are two quite distinct ways that hypnosis is used for memory enhancement within the criminal justice system. One use is to obtain leads to independent corroborative evidence. In a number of celebrated cases, such as the Chowchilla kidnapping case and the Boston Strangler case, hypnosis was used to elicit information that led to other physical evidence and eventually facilitated apprehension of the criminals (Orne et al., 1984). The second way is to refresh memories of potential witnesses who may have repressed or forgotten details of certain events. Problems have arisen, however, in situations in which sworn courtroom testimony is based solely on a memory that was refreshed by hypnosis. The problem becomes acute when there is no additional evidence to confirm the accuracy of such memories. Critics of this second use of hypnosis have worried that it is difficult, if not impossible, to determine whether hypnosis has produced bona-fide memories of forgotten events or whether it alters the veracity of memories and results in unreliable testimony (Spanos et al., 1989; Orne et al., 1984).

This chapter addresses the use of hypnosis as a memory enhancement technique and reviews the current state of knowledge as to the reliability and accuracy of hypnotically assisted recall.

Hypnosis as an Investigative Technique

Perhaps the least controversial use of forensic hypnosis is as a discovery procedure, that is, as a means of obtaining new, independent evidence. The rationale for the use of hypnosis as an investigative method comes from the traditional understanding that it can facilitate memory retrieval. Typically this process involves the use of hypnosis to uncover crucial facts and details that have been forgotten by the witness, victims of crime, or parties in civil action. If the subject never has to be called as a witness in subsequent court proceedings because the information is either unimportant or redundant or because the hypnosis leads to the discovery of independent evidence, then there would be few, if any, problems with preliminary hypnotic investigation.

This section will address the area of investigative hypnosis that is not likely to be used by a witness in subsequent trial. However, it is impossible to determine whether a subject hypnotized during the investigative stage of a legal proceeding will not be needed later as a subsequent witness. If it seems at all probable that the subject will be needed as a witness, decisions about which witnesses should be subjected to investigative hypnosis should be deferred until this issue has been determined or else undertaken with extreme caution.

The legal rules regarding the testimony by a witness who was previously hypnotized vary from state to state. Because a violation of the state's rules may severely limit a witnesses's later in-court testimony, consultation with legal authorities is well advised before the hypnosis is undertaken.

Investigative hypnosis, like many other applications of hypnosis, is more likely to be effective with volunteer and highly motivated subjects (Gravitz, 1985). It is a fundamental mistake to assume that investigative hypnosis ensures the truth. Even hypnotic subjects deep in trance are capable of lying if they are so motivated, as well as following calculated or inadvertent suggestions or simply making honest errors. What hypnotic investigation actually produces is a mixture of fact and fantasy in indeterminate proportions (Gravitz, 1985; Udolf, 1981). But the fact that much of it may be in error is not crucial. Such inaccuracies merely increase the cost of the investigation. Although some of the clinical material may be inaccurate in whole or in part, it may lead to the discovery of new information and evidence.

Applications of Investigative Hypnosis

Hypnosis has been used in an attempt to uncover crucial facts and details that have been forgotten by witnesses and victims of crime. In *Rock v. Arkansas*

(1987), hypnosis enabled Vickie Rock to remember she did not have her finger on the trigger when the gun went off, killing her husband. This memory led her counsel to have a gun expert examine the handgun. The inspection revealed the gun was defective and prone to fire when hit or dropped.

In *Zani v. State* (1988), a construction worker, only after a hypnosis session, was able to identify Zani thirteen years after a murder. In the infamous Ted Bundy case (*Bundy v. Dugar*, 1988) an eyewitness was hypnotized and was able to identify Bundy in a lineup.

One of the most dramatic applications of hypnosis occurs when it is used to lift retrograde amnesia. In March 1987 a twenty-five-year-old pilot flying three passengers to Miami crashed upon approach to the runway, and two passengers died. The pilot was charged with vehicular manslaughter. Following hypnosis, he relayed many details about the situation. Afterward, a reconstruction expert took these details and examined the carburetor. He found a piece of metal blocking the fuel line, and the pilot avoided a conviction for vehicular homicide.

In a case involving a woman who was too intoxicated at the time of her boyfriend's murder to remember any details of the event, Reiser and Nielsen (1980) report she was able to recover them under hypnosis. This case is particularly interesting because research in memory suggests that alcohol or physical trauma may prevent a memory from forming, and a nonexistent memory trace should be unrecoverable by any means. This type of hypnotic recall should be subject to careful scrutiny by corroborating information with other facts of evidence to ensure that it is not fantasy or confabulation. If there are inconsistencies, the data retrieved should be considered questionable, if not unreliable. In theory at least, the examiner should not be concerned with the outcome of the case, for that is a matter for the judge and jury to decide.

Hypnosis has been employed in the investigation of many well-publicized crimes. Perhaps the most celebrated case cited as evidence of the effectiveness of investigatory hypnosis is the Chowchilla kidnapping case (Reiser, 1989) in which a school bus was hijacked by masked gunmen. Twenty-six children and the bus driver were abducted at gunpoint and imprisoned in an underground tomb in a remote rock quarry. After everyone had escaped, the bus driver was questioned in his normal waking state and was unable to recall anything of significance. Under hypnosis, he was able to remember seven of eight digits of a license plate, which provided police with the necessary leads to apprehend the kidnappers.

On the surface, these anecdotal accounts are persuasive of the effectiveness of hypnosis. Indeed, any hypnotist working with a patient who recalls an event with appropriate affective abreaction, followed by symptom relief, cannot help being impressed with the vividness and apparent accuracy of the memory. However, there are numerous critics of these individual case reports.

Frequently there is no means of objectively verifying the findings. In cases like the Chowchilla kidnapping, the recall of the suspects' license number proved to be fairly accurate; in other cases, license number recall have proved completely wrong. In fact, Franklin Ray, the bus driver, recalled one incorrect license plate number as well as the correct one (Kroger and Duce, 1979). The results in this case seem to be typical of the nature of hypnotic memory recovery in that they were a mixture of correct and incorrect information.

The Effectiveness of Investigative Hypnosis

The statistics reported by law enforcement personnel are generally impressive if taken at face value. Kleinhauz, Horowitz, and Tobin (1977) note the reports of a significant increase in information in twenty-four of forty cases as a result of investigative hypnosis. In sixteen of twenty-four cases, the quality of the information was assessed as to whether it led to uncovering of the evidence or to apprehension of the criminal. They found that in fourteen of the sixteen cases, there was a "significant" increase in accurate information, and in the other two cases, the memories contradicted other available evidence.

Kroger and Duce (1979) reported that in twenty-three cases involving fifty-three witnesses and victims, new information was developed in 60 percent of the cases. Between 1976 and 1979, the Los Angeles Police Department (LAPD) conducted roughly 350 hypnotic investigations. Reiser (1980) reports that in one sample of seventy cases from the LAPD, additional information, not obtained through interrogation procedures, was obtained in fifty-four cases and that eleven cases were solved solely through the use of hypnosis. In a later report, Reiser and Nielsen (1980) noted that in a new sample of 374 cases involving hypnotic sessions conducted by the LAPD (through March 1979), 31 percent of the cases were solved and hypnosis was considered valuable in 65 percent of these. In 1989, Reiser reported a general estimate of a 77 percent increase in usable information where hypnosis was used.

Despite the compelling nature of such reports, caution is warranted in accepting the efficacy of this technique based on these findings. Most of these reports are too general to be used as a critical evaluation of hypnosis. The percentage of new information is not necessarily synonymous with the value of hypnosis in solving a case. These reports offer no operational definition for terms such as "extremely useful" and "success." Additionally, there is no way of determining if the information could have been elicited by other investigative techniques. Clinically there are many ways of resurrecting historical information from a patient, and hypnosis has not been clearly demonstrated to be superior for this purpose (Spanos et al., 1989).

In addition to these definitional problems and lack of experimental rigor, empirical data indicating the veridicality of hypnotically obtained information are meager and inadequate. For example, Reiser (1980) reported that of those hypnoinvestigative cases conducted by the LAPD in which follow-up information was available, 90.1 percent of the hypnotically elicited information was verified. The nature of this information and the methodology used for verification was not described.

For these reasons, all hypnotically generated information should be independently verified before it can be regarded as reliable. Some authors suggest that hypnotically obtained information should be corroborated by independent evidence (Kleinhauz, Horowitz, and Tobin, 1977) while others go on further and maintain that corroboration is insufficient and what is needed is independent proof of the facts so that hypnotically refreshed memories need not be offered as evidence at all (Udolf, 1987).

The only conclusion that can be validly made from the data reported by law enforcement personnel is that police officers associated with hypnotic investigations generally have positive feelings toward the usefulness of the procedure. This may be because hypnosis was actually a superior method in certain cases, but officers may also simply find it more dramatic and interesting and/or it may increase feelings of potency and control in their investigational work.

The Accuracy of Hypnotically Enhanced Memories

Memory is normally considered to be the capacity and faculty to retain information, thoughts, feelings, and other experiences in the mind and to recall what is past. Consensual definitions of memory involve three mental processes, learning, retention, and retrieval. It is clear that a stimulus must occur that forms a lasting imprint, and that imprint must be stored in order for it to be retrieved and remembered.

Loss of memory preceding and following trauma is different from amnesia due to drug or alcohol blackouts. In the trauma situation, it is assumed that the conscious memory traces are lost. However, because of the number of perceptual processes involved, some representation of events has entered long-term storage and subsequently can be retrieved. In such cases, long-term memory may have initially suffered from retrieval problems because the short-term trace has been destroyed. By contrast, during a blackout, the drugged state interferes with consolidation into long-term memory; thus, only sensory registers and short-term memory stores are involved, and no learning remains to be remembered. Retrieval strategies, such as hypnosis, can be expected to work only on trauma-induced amnesia.

Most clinicians and laypersons believe that the use of hypnosis will aid in the production of recall. But there are two crucial questions: Is it hypnosis itself that produced the enhanced recall? Are the retrieved memories accurate? Addressing the first question, Smith (1983) writes, "If an individual is suddenly able, under hypnosis, to remember important details of a crime that were not reported earlier, the assumption was that it was hypnosis that was responsible for the improved recollection" (p. 390).

For the courts, the second question of the difference between real and pseudomemories is more central. Sensational reports from nonlaboratory situations suffer from lack of control groups and fail to meet the criteria for accuracy necessary in forensic settings.

There is an extensive experimental literature dealing with the effects of hypnosis on learning and recall, and it has been reviewed critically. It is difficult to summarize this literature as a whole because the effect of hypnosis was often confounded with the effect of susceptibility, the necessary control groups were absent, or the instructions given to subjects were inadequately reported or not compatible from across studies (Watkins, 1989). Also some results that appeared impressive have proved difficult to replicate. Nevertheless, subject to the sources of error, the weight of the experimental literature appears to support the following conclusions (Spanos et al., 1989; Sheehan, 1987; Udolf, 1987):

1. The amount and quality of recalled material produced by suggestions of enhanced ability is a function of the kind of material to be recalled and the meaningfulness of the material. There is clear evidence that hypnosis does not aid in the recall of nonmeaningful or nonsense material. This is precisely what we would expect. There is no reason to anticipate that nonmeaningful stimuli would be transferred into long-term memory. Because hypnosis serves as an aid to retrieval, it would not have an impact on any memory that is not stored. With meaningful material, hypnosis can affect the quality and quantity of the remembrance.
2. The greatest production (and distortion) of material obtained under hypnosis is material that is both personally meaningful and anxiety producing.
3. Many police officer hypnotists are taught that memory is like a video recorder that provides an exact copy of every stimulus it has been exposed to. This view is highly inaccurate. Most of the stimuli entering the initial sensory register have never been noticed or perceived in the first place. Furthermore, even if every stimulus is noticed and recorded, retrieval is most appropriately conceived of as a reconstructive process that involves some type of distortion rather than a process that facilitates direct access to information as encoded originally.

Pseudomemories

Researchers and legal experts have expressed concern over the notion that deliberate and inadvertent suggestions given during the postevent hypnotic interrogations can lead to the creation of pseudomemories—false memories that subjects cannot distinguish from real memories and that are believed in and treated by subjects as real memories. Investigators (Spanos et al., 1989; Diamond, 1980) have argued that highly hypnotizable subjects are particularly attuned to cues provided by the hypnotist in the form of leading questions (for example, "Did you see the scar on the offender's face?") and other subtle suggestions. Such subjects incorporate the false memories into their memories (a scar in their image of the suspect), become unable to distinguish their false memory from what they actually witnessed, and, subsequent to the hypnotic session, report and act upon their distorted memory (pick out a suspect in a line up with a scar on his face). Thus, hypnotically refreshed memories may actually contain a mixture of confabulations, fantasy, personal abreactions, and accurate events, with no reliable means of distinguishing among these. In such circumstances, injustice may occur.

Experimental evidence concerning the effects of hypnotic procedures on pseudomemory reports is sparse. Work conducted in both hypnotic contexts and nonhypnotic contexts indicates that subjects provided with misleading information during the postevent interview frequently incorporate the misleading information into their recall (Loftus, 1989; McCann and Sheehan, 1987).

The Dilemma of Confidence and Accuracy

The question of whether doubt vanishes as an artifact of hypnotic retrieval is based on the claims that hypnosis may not affect recall as much as it does one's confidence in the accuracy of the memory. This distinction is particularly important in a courtroom, since witnesses who are more confident appear more believable to a jury (Smith and Meyer, 1987; Wells, Ferguson, and Lindsay, 1979). Moreover, the separation of confidence and accuracy, it is argued, may make a witness impervious to cross-examination. Such a witness would be unshakable, for she or he would truly believe in the accuracy of the memory, without being aware that it was merely an artifact created by hypnosis (Diamond, 1980).

The summary of the experimental evidence on the confidence of hypnotically retrieved memories has yielded mixed results. Several studies (Labelle, Lamarche, and Laurence, 1990; McCann and Sheehan, 1987) suggest that hypnotized subjects do have more confidence in their responses than do control subjects, regardless of accuracy, with the effect of confidence greatest for highly hypnotizable subjects. Other studies found no significant difference between waking and hypnotized subjects on confidence ratings. Taken together, because there have been a number of instances in which hypnotically refreshed memories did not result in an increase in confidence, it appears that the concretization of hypnotically refreshed memories is a potential, though not inherent, aspect of hypnosis. Equally clear is that enhanced confidence unrelated to accuracy can be readily demonstrated. The important question then becomes whether there is a greater threat of misplaced confidence with hypnotic methods of memory refreshment than other investigative procedures.

Waking Eyewitness Recall versus Hypnotic Recall

Eyewitness testimony is regarded by many in the judicial system as the best type of evidence, though the relevant studies suggest that it may not be (Scheflin and Shapiro, 1989; Loftus, 1979). Are hypnotically refreshed memories different from normally refreshed waking recall? Several empirical investigations (Putnam, 1979; Zelig and Beidleman, 1981) have demonstrated that waking subjects were more accurate than hypnotized subjects on leading questions and that subjects highly responsive to hypnosis have a tendency to be just as confident in their responses, even when such confidence is not warranted. Yet potential jurors indicate that they would probably place more faith in hypnotically enhanced recall (Labelle, Lamarche, and Laurence, 1990). Taken together, these studies underscore the need for caution in the use of forensic hypnosis.

Following is a summary and commentary of a case conducted by the noted forensic hypnotist Melvin Gravitz (1986) that illustrates appropriate guidelines, procedures, and precautions.

> The automobile of a married woman in her mid-thirties was found abandoned on a lonely country road at night. Several hours later, the woman was found wandering in a dazed condition along another road several miles from her vehicle. A medical examination revealed that she had been assaulted, but she was virtually amnesic for any useful details regarding the incident. After several weeks of unsuccessful police investigations, she was referred to a Ph.D.-level clinical psychologist to assist in memory retrieval, with a special request for any description of her assailant or his automobile.
>
> Prior to the hypnotic interview, the subject was contacted by telephone to verify that she was agreeable to the interview of her own volition and to discuss questions she might have about the process. Upon meeting the subject, the psychologist ascertained she was still agreeable to the hypnosis and had her sign a statement to that effect. This release indicated that she understood that a feedback report was to be provided to the police and a recorder would be used throughout the interview. Throughout the interview, which was conducted with only the subject and psychologist present, the subject reclined on a couch.
>
> The early part of the interview was spent engaging in small talk to develop rapport, after which an optical fixation procedure and

suggestions for relaxation were implemented. She was then regressed to the evening in question. In this procedure, she was asked to visualize the single pages on a day calendar being added one day at a time at her own pace until she arrived at the date of the abduction, at which point she gave a prearranged ideomotor finger signal.

She was asked to picture herself as she was driving along the country road prior to the location of where her car was found. Then, using free recall, she was asked to describe everything that was occurring, under the concept that it is best to obtain as much broad-based information as possible before getting to the specifics. Later the subjects was asked for specific details, such as, "Tell me what he looks like."

Speaking from the past tense, the subject reported that another vehicle from behind pulled up alongside her car and forced her off the road. While she was in a stunned condition, the male driver of the other car had pulled her from her car, forced her into his, and drove away. At this point the examiner stopped her stream of visualization for a moment to ask several questions designed specifically to elicit a description of the vehicle: Excerpts from the taped interview follow (Gravitz, 1986):

Examiner(E): What does the other car look like?
  Subject(S): He pulled me out of the car. I took my purse. I was begging him to let me go. Seems like I took a step or two. Then he said, "Shut up. Shut up." Then he smacked me. He smacked me two or three times. I didn't dare look at him. I'm so scared.
E: Tell me what the other car looks like. Tell me what is happening.
S: It was dark. I couldn't see. I'm frightened.
E: It's all right. Tell me what it looks like.
S: It was an awfully old car. It was dark looking. It was an old dark blue. I don't know. It was so foggy . . . The windshield was all one piece, and there were two windshield wipers. They're noisy . . . He used his hands to shift. There was a gear shift on the steering wheel. The steering wheel has a rim around it. You know, a shiny metal rim that was the horn . . . It was a noisy car . . . On the road we ran into a big curvy bank. He hit it with a jolt and sure did bang up his car. He must have damage to his car . . . on the right side . . .

On the basis of this testimony and additional information elicited by the hypnosis, the investigating authorities covered automobile service stations in the general area and discovered a mechanic who was familiar with an older-model dark blue sedan that had been brought in for repair of a fresh dent in the right front fender.

The work order listed the suspect's residence, and a subsequent search warrant of the suspect's car turned up the victim's purse on the back seat of his car. The interior of the vehicle matched in significant detail the description given by the victim under hypnosis. When confronted with the evidence, the suspect admitted his role in the crime, and he was subsequently tried and convicted.

General Procedural Recommendations

A number of guidelines have been advocated to ensure credibility of investigative procedures using hypnosis (Udolf, 1987; Scheflin and Shapiro, 1989; Orne, 1979). The following recommendations represent an integration of the relevant aspects of the major recommended guidelines.

Prehypnotic Phase

Initial Contact. When an attorney contacts an expert hypnotherapist to examine a client for the purpose of hypnotic investigation, the attorney should be cautioned to provide only the client's name, age, charges, and date of alleged offense. A written contract should be executed after the initial communication to ensure a work product and privileged communication. The attorney should be advised there is no guarantee that valid data will be retrieved, and information elicited may be detrimental to the client's case.

If the attorney is present during sessions, she or he should be seated directly behind the subject so that there is eye contact. A preferable arrangement is to place the attorney in a nearby room, where she or he can observe the session by a video monitor. She or he may then formulate questions during the inquiry and retrieval phase.

The expert should be an independent practitioner who has no vested interest in the outcome of the case. He or she should be aware of any personal dynamics and biases that could influence production of material or the opinions rendered and willing to accept the possibility that these efforts may be nonproductive.

A video recording of all interaction between the hypnotist and the subject (before, during, and after the hypnosis) should be routinely required. Without such a recording it is impossible to evaluate the relative probability that factual error has been introduced into the testimony as a result of faulty technique (Orne, 1979). Audio recordings or written transcripts of the sessions are often an inadequate basis for such a review, for they fail to disclose subtle cueing by tone of voice, facial expression, body language, and so on.

Clinical Evaluation. The clinical evaluation is a crucial part of the prehypnotic phase of interrogation. It is important to establish some rapport with the defendant. Personality structure and dynamics should be assessed through at least a brief mental status examination in order to guide subsequent interrogation. Medical and psychiatric histories and legal and family histories should also be incorporated. Misconceptions of hypnosis should be explained to the subject prior to enacting the trance. Quite often the subject becomes very relaxed, and spontaneous recall may occur, precluding the need for further investigation. If hypnotic investigation is to be pursued, written consent should be obtained from the subject.

Initial Interview. In the initial interview, the hypnotherapist determines if hypnosis has reasonable potential for use in the case. Except for intense priority concerns such as the possibility of imminent loss of life, hypnosis should be considered only after all other traditional law enforcement investigative methods have been unsuccessfully used. Hypnosis is not a short cut; it is intended to provide information obtainable by no other means.

In any memory-refreshing procedure, the first step for all clinicians is to establish a base rate for the memory via free recall report. This prehypnotic questioning informs the therapist of the current recollections and provides an opportunity to explore the incident in detail without hypnosis. The clinician should be careful not to provide information or prompting, except for indications to continue. The subject is asked what he or she is able to recall about the alleged offense. In addition, the subject should be questioned about what he or she has been told by others and has read in the newspapers or seen on television to determine if erroneous imprints have been formed.

There should be an indication that further recall may be possible. The witness must have been able to perceive details that have the potential for enhancement. One way to assess this is to note carefully what would be reasonable to expect in the field of vision while the subject is reenacting the event.

A final consideration in deciding to use hypnosis is that there must be some means of independently validating the information accessed through hypnosis, such as other witness testimony or physical evidence. Without some potential for independent corroboration, hypnosis is all too likely to be relied upon as the trier of fact.

Hypnotic Phase

Induction Procedures. The selection of induction techniques is based on the dynamics of the subject. If the subject is authoritative and hypercritical, direct and demand inductions are usually of little value, and indirect techniques should be used. If the subject appears to be highly motivated and compliant, direct techniques are most often used. The subject should be deepened as much as possible.

Regression Procedures. Any number of techniques may be used to regress the subject to a time just prior to the event in question. The subject is then gradually brought forward to the event. Age regression is usually produced by progressively suggesting disorientation as to the year, the month, and the day; then by appropriate suggestions, an earlier age level is reached. One way to obtain regression is for the operator to identify himself or herself with a surrogate figure the subject once knew. For example, if the operator plays the role of a friendly person, he or she can remark, "You are now in the fourth grade. I happened to be talking with your teacher, and she told me how well you were doing in school." Typically good subjects act in a manner indicating that, at least on some level, they are subjectively reexperiencing these early events as if they are real.

In most age regressions there is a form of role playing rather than actual revivification of the past (Orne, 1979). That is, subjects try to imagine themselves in the past and attempt to behave as they believe they did then. In contrast, a revivification means that subjects perceptually experience the past, and all memories of the event in question have been temporarily suspended. Actual revivification rarely, if ever, occurs. Most police officers mistakenly equate age regression with revivification. The problem with the age regression technique is that because memory is a selective process, even an event experienced as vivid revivification would have to include some confabulation for details.

Test for Trance. Besides observing signs for trance and depth, specific tests can be utilized to determine if the subject is actually in trance. (See chapter 2.) A suggestion for anesthesia of the subject's hand and subsequent application of a hemostat to demonstrate trance is one technique that can be performed. It is difficult for a simulator to tolerate this test because of the degree of discomfort evoked by this stimulus (Mutter, 1980).

An occasion may arise when the subject is not able to recall anything during the retrieval phase, and at this point, further deepening may be helpful, avoiding direct demands for information since this would tend to produce confabulation. Should repeated attempts at retrieval prove unsuccessful, posthypnotic dreams of the event may be suggested. The subject's attorney who is monitoring the interview may furnish written questions for the purpose of gathering information about the offense since the examiner would normally not have been privy to the details about the case.

Data Retrieval: Investigative Techniques. Whether hypnosis causes confabulation can depend on the manner in which the questions are asked. Many writers have suggested that the method of interrogation may be important in controlling the amount of suggestion given to the subject (Smith and Meyer, 1987; Loftus, 1979). There is potential danger in asking leading questions to a subject in even a moderately suggestible state. Hilgard and

Loftus (1979) and Gieselman et el. (1985) have proposed investigative methods designed to decrease the possibility of inaccuracies in all types of eyewitness procedures.

The data retrieval phase is one of the most critical in the investigative procedure. The examiner should be cautious in proceeding with the method of interrogation. The subject should be told, "Soon I am going to ask you some questions. You will say the first thought that comes into your mind. You may be surprised at your responses, but you will not be judgmental or censor those thoughts. If you do not know an answer, you will say for, for that is an acceptable response." The final statement is intended to minimize the demand characteristics of the inquiry.

The retrieval process begins by regressing the subject back to a time just prior to the incident and asking him or her to describe what he or she perceives in a narrative form. Very little should be verbalized by the examiner other than, "What is happening now?" or, "We are moving forward in time . . . you can see, hear, and feel what is happening . . . what is happening now?" After the responses are elicited, the process is repeated to gain further detail. The examiner should not lead the subject but merely parrot any responses or remain silent, allowing spontaneous verbalizations to occur.

Two variations of the interrogations technique may be used. The first is a flooding procedure in which the subject is asked, "What is happening now?" with the responses parroted without any pause, to prevent the subject from analyzing the answers. This technique may be useful for subjects who tend to give self-serving replies. In the second variation, a suggestion is given that the subject return to the event and review it from beginning to end while the examiner remains silent for a period of time such as five minutes. The subject is asked to verbalize what he or she has experienced. This method may be used when the subject claims that to remember nothing, as it facilitates memory search.

Television Technique. The most widely practiced method used in investigative hypnosis is the highly controversial television technique favored by many police hypnotists (Reiser, 1980). After inducing an apparently sufficient hypnotic trance, the hypnotist suggests to the subject that he or she will be watching a documentary on television that can be speeded up, slowed down, stopped, or reversed, with close-ups and volume control also possible. Proponents argue that this technique spares victims the trauma of re-experiencing the criminal event without sacrificing the accuracy of recall. Opponents, most notably led by Orne (1979), persuasively argue that the television technique by its very nature encourages guessing and creativity in the absence of actual memories, leading to false memories that have the potential of hardening. The television technique is likely to contaminate memories and increase the likelihood that the witness will believe in the truth of something that is actually false. For this reason, Relinger (1984) and this author strongly recommend at least initially using the free recall method, both to enhance accuracy and to reduce the extra influence of bias.

Posthypnotic Phase. Before termination of the trance, the subject should be asked for permission to have him or her remember the experiences described during the regression in order to discuss them with the attorney. If the experience has been so traumatic that the subject wishes not to remember, he or she is told, "You will remember only that which you are able to deal with emotionally." The client is then time progressed to the present and gradually brought out of trance. If suggestions for anesthesia were used to test a trance, the posthypnotic suggestion is given to extinguish the anesthesia.

Maximizing Accurate Recall

Investigative hypnosis, like most other hypnotic applications, is more likely to be effective with volunteer and highly motivated subjects (Gravitz, 1985, 1986). Accurate recall seems most probable when events to be recalled are of somewhat recent origin and as many aspects of the individual's life are included. The greater the number of visual, auditory, and kinesthetic modalities involved, the greater is the likelihood of reliable recall. The closer the reinstatement is to the original setting, the more likely successful hyperamnesia is. The major problem is standardizing an acceptable procedure that will maximize credibility. Often conditions are uncontrolled due to the variance in subject-examiner interaction, the subject's credibility, the examiner's credibility, and the lack of standard guidelines in the procedures itself (Watkins, 1989).

The law permits a wide range of devices to be used for enhancing memory, and as a general matter, as long as witnesses testify that their memory has been restored and that they are now testifying from present memory, they are permitted to do so. However, hypnosis is an exception to this general rule in many states. Because courts recognize the danger that hypnosis may produce memory distortions and may alter witnesses' ability to recognize these distortions, many courts impose significant limits on how the hypnosis of potential witnesses may be conducted, so as to minimize these risks.

Improper and Unethical Uses of Hypnosis

The cases of the improper application of forensic hypnosis include inducing confessions, bolstering testimony, and involuntary induction. These misuses are improper from a legal standpoint because they jeopardize due process and violate evidentiary standards. The alleged unethical uses of hypnosis occasionally reported generally involve (perhaps fictionally in most instances) the use of hypnosis as a means to induce a subject to commit a crime or to victimize a subject (see also chapter 18) (Scheflin and Shapiro, 1989; Udolf, 1983, 1987).

Hypnotically Induced Confessions

A confession is a statement made by a defendant in a criminal action that admits all or some of the allegations that the prosecution must prove in order to secure a conviction of a crime. For a variety of psychological reasons and legal mandates, hypnosis has no legitimate use in the interrogation of subjects for the purpose of obtaining confessions.

An unusual case in this genre originated in Indiana on September 2, 1982, when a shooting occurred at the home of Cathy Burns. Under the name Cathy Sells, she told police that an intruder had shot and wounded her two children, Eddie and Penny, while they slept and knocked her unconscious. Two police officers found no evidence of forced entry or other physical evidence and began to suspect Burns. The officers asked her to undergo hypnosis, but one officer remembered from his three-day course that hypnotizing suspects was unacceptable. They asked the deputy prosecutor for his advice, and he said, "If you've got nowhere else to go you might as well do that [hypnosis]." When under hypnosis, she first identified the assailant as her father, but then said it was "Katie," which was interpreted by a psychologist as an indication of split personality, which the police officers took as a confession. She was later cleared by psychiatrists, who concluded she did not have a split personality. A judge eventually threw the case out of court. But in the process Cathy Burns lost her job as a police dispatcher, lost custody of her children, and was ostracized socially.

The lure of hypnosis to both the uniformed and the uninformed is that it seems to be a way of selectively compelling the guilty, but not the innocent, to confess. In actuality, hypnosis cannot do that anyway. It is generally accepted that hypnosis is not able to prevent defendants from lying if they are motivated to do so (Scheflin and Shapiro, 1989; Udolf, 1983). Additionally, hypnotized subjects are hypersuggestible and more easily led, and even an honest examiner may inadvertently cue subjects in a manner that may influence their responses. For these reasons, the U.S. Supreme Court, in *Leyra v. Denno* (1954), barred the use of hypnosis to elicit confessions if it was used to coerce a confession because it violates the defendant's right of due process under the Fifth and Fourteenth amendments.

Hypnosis Used to Bolster Witness Testimony

The deliberate creation, shaping, or distortion of testimony established by the opposing party is not only unethical but also constitutes the crime of subornation or perjury, or tampering with evidence. Hypnosis calculated to give potential witnesses more confidence in the belief of their memories is unethical because it renders them less resistant to cross-examination.

Involuntary Induction

In view of the fact that hypnosis requires the cooperation of the subject, the question arises how it could be considered to be involuntary. The answer is that "involuntary" does not mean "against one's will" but "without the consent of the subject." It would appear improbable to hypnotize a subject who actively resists hypnosis. However, it is quite possible to induce hypnosis and get the subject's cooperation in a setting that he or she does not recognize as hypnosis, for example, describing the procedure as relaxation instead of hypnosis.

Claims of involuntary hypnotic induction by the police are rare but do appear from time to time. One such case involved a fifty-year-old male defendant accused of murdering his parents. The police questioned him in marathon shifts, denying him food, water, and sleep for extended periods of time. They called in a physician who specialized in psychoanalysis under the guise of examining his sinus condition. Gradually the questions turned to the criminal offense. Using a combination of relaxation, regression, and sympathy, the doctor's inquiries produced a confession, which resulted in a conviction (Levy, 1955).

Victimization during the Trance

The most commonly reported type of victimization involves seduction or sexual abuse (Hoencamp, 1990), but allegations of theft or undue financial influence are occasionally reported (Solomon, 1952). Kline (1972) cites two cases in which subjects have been sexually abused by psychopathic hypnotists. One case involves an obstetrician who used hypnosis to take sexual advantage of his patients, and the other case was of a graduate psychology student who used hypnosis to molest young boys sexually while babysitting for them.

In the civil realm, it is speculated that a unscrupulous hypnotist could influence a person to make a will listing the hypnotist as a beneficiary or sign a contract, deed, or other legal documents against the subject's best interest. Few actual cases have been reported (Antich, 1967; Udolf; 1987).

Modern authorities do not dispute the fact of victimization; they dispute its explanation. Some plausible hypotheses have been offered (Watkins, 1989; Venn, 1988; Orne, 1972):

> That the idea of hypnotic coercion is used by some subjects as justification for actions that they would have committed anyway.

That a coerced person's behavior may be attributable to nonhypnotic coercive factors such as alcohol intoxication, an authority relationship, or a close interpersonal relationship with the hypnotist.

That hypnotic coercion is possible only if the subject believe that it is, in which case the subject is responding not to hypnosis but to self-fulfilling prophecy.

That hypnotic coercion is possible but through such methods as creating delusions, activating latent motivations, or giving suggestions that are followed compulsively.

There is likely some truth in each position.

Practitioners who engage in this victimization are subject to civil liability and, in many states, may be guilty of a form of criminal sexual assault. Taking advantage of a client who is hypnotized is at a minimum negligence in that the professional breached a duty to the client to act as a reasonably prudent practitioner to avoid injury to the patient. Furthermore, such conduct would violate the ethical standards of the profession, which prohibits sexual contact with patients. Therefore, the practitioner would be liable for any damages (including pain and suffering) caused to be client. Contact with a patient who is hypnotized is almost surely to be viewed by courts as physical contact without consent, which is civil battery. In addition to actual damages, such conduct could well lead to awarding punitive damages.

A number of states have recognized by statue that sexual conduct with a client who has not voluntarily and knowingly consented is a form of sexual assault. Contact with a patient who is hypnotized would almost surely fall in that category.

Hypnotically Induced Crime

The potential for whether hypnosis can be used to make a subject commit a crime has been debated by psychologists and legal writers from the time of Mesmer. Those who believe that a hypnotized subject can be induced to commit a crime through coercion or deception generally cite that the hypersuggestibility of the subject and compliance or the desire to please the hypnotist make it easy to instill false beliefs. The suggestion of posthypnotic amnesia would make the subject unaware of the real motivation for the criminal acts and hence protect the hypnotist from detection.

Experimental evidence of the ability of hypnosis to cause criminal behavior has generally taken the form of demonstrations of a subject's willingness to commit antisocial, immoral, or self-injurious behaviors while under hypnosis. Orne (1972) reports a demonstration in which a young woman readily accepted a suggestion to stab people with a pseudodagger and to poison them with sugar, but she refused a suggestion to undress.

Experts generally agree that subjects will not violate their ethical codes or do something that they would not normally do in a waking state (Orne, 1972). But it is clear that hypnotic subjects can be induced to perform dangerous and antisocial behaviors. Nevertheless, there is considerable doubt whether hypnosis is doing this. Subjects who know that they are in experimental situations presume that the hypnotist will assume responsibility for their actions. Indeed, when told that they are in an experiment, it is possible to get subjects to engage in almost any type of dangerous or antisocial behavior.

The use of hypnosis to induce antisocial behavior has received scant attention because the vast majority of courts have given little credence to the defense that the defendant acted under hypnotic influence. The American Law Institute's Model Penal Code provides that a defendant whose acts result from hypnosis or posthypnotic suggestion is not guilty of a "voluntary act" that would support a criminal conviction. Such research is seldom easily approved or funded. Any such claim appears to be more of a theoretical than a practical matter; no American case has been found in which a defendant successfully raised such a defense. Two cases in which the defendant tried to raise this are *People v. Marsh* (1959) and *People v. Worthington* (1894). In those rare cases in which actual crimes have been committed under hypnotic influence, the relationship between the hypnotist and subject, rather than the hypnosis, has been found to account for the subject's compliance.

Ethical Considerations

Today, therapeutic or forensic work with hypnosis is judged not only by the ethical standards of one's own profession but also by the local legal requirements of one's practice.

Informed Consent or Duty to Warn

In cases where there is some reason to believe the contents of a hypnotherapy session may later be brought into the legal arena, the therapist has a duty to inform clients that hypnosis might place their legal rights in jeopardy. Although undoubtedly rare, such a situation would pose an ironic dilemma. On one hand, the practicing hypnotherapist can forgo the use of hypnosis to protect the legal interests of the client, at the expense of not being able to provide therapeutic relief. On the other hand, the therapist may have to determine, prior to using hypnosis, whether the therapeutic gain from the use of hypnosis will outweigh the potential loss of legal redress. If hypnosis is to be used, the client should give written informed consent certifying that she or he has been informed about the potential legal consequences of hypnosis and still desires that it be undertaken.

Legal Regulation of Hypnosis

Because the induction and suggestions procedures common to hypnosis are easy to learn and implement, these techniques are often portrayed as deceptively simple and unrealistically powerful. This deception, along with the public's increasing interest in miracle cures, has led to the proliferation of the popularity of hypnosis.

To date, the practice of hypnosis has not been effectively restricted by legislatures of the courts. While the use of hypnotism is not in and of itself the illegal practice of medicine or psychology without a license, when a practitioner claims to use it for the treatment of physical or mental disorders, then this should constitute the illegal practice of medicine or psychology without a license (or, depending on the state, another licensed full-spectrum treatment discipline). Therapists should also be able to support their use of hypnosis by a training background that includes formal coursework (not just a weekend workshop or two), a period of intensive supervision, and a subsequent period of monitoring-supervision. Unfortunately, states have seldom dealt effectively with this, and related criminal prosecutions are few and far between. Two such cases are *People v. Cantor* (1961) and *Masters v. State* (1960).

The professional psychotherapist who utilizes hypnosis is faced with debunking the myths of the magical cure quality of hypnosis and simultaneously employing the powerful placebo and treatment effects that are possible. Effective hypnotherapy in the legal system involves a comprehensive understanding of human functioning and pathological states, cognizance of the current literature on hypnotically refreshed memory, sufficient training in hypnosis and therapy, and an understanding of the current status of the local laws regarding hypnosis. It is a job that requires a great deal of skill and training, although proficiency in hypnosis alone is not sufficient.

18

The Hypnotherapist in Court

Reply to a plaintiff who claims his cabbages were eaten by your goat: You had no cabbages. If you did they were not eaten. If they were eaten, it was not by a goat. If they were eaten by a goat, it was not my goat. And, if it was my goat, he was insane.
—Quoted by J. W. McElhaney, *Trial Notebook*

Hypnosis may enter the legal arena in several ways: as a defense for criminal acts supposedly committed by a hypnotized individual (more as a matter of fiction within their reality), as an alleged cause or factor in malpractice, as an investigatory device, or as an aid to the examiner in determining the subject's state of mind (either at the time of examination or at a previous time). Hypnosis may also be important in considering the admissibility of confessions induced by hypnosis or of evidence from a witness whose memory has been refreshed under hypnosis.

Cases involving defendants allegedly hypnotized at the time they committed a crime are rare (Scheflin and Shapiro, 1989). Although some debate continues as to the coercive power of hypnosis, both mental health professionals and courts have considered the likelihood of crimes being committed under hypnotic suggestion to be small and have not been persuaded by such a defense.

Perhaps most surprising about hypnosis in court is the absence of many officially reported cases. In only one area has there been much legal activity regarding hypnosis: the effect of hypnosis on the admissibility of the testimony of a witness. In other areas, among them malpractice, defense to criminal charges, and coerced confessions, the cases are few and far between. Overall, courts have been avoidant of issues related to hypnosis.

Historically courts have seldom permitted the use of hypnosis in the open courtroom, and it is virtually unheard of in modern times. Such use appears unnecessary and may influence a jury unduly. Confessions induced by hypnosis are highly suspect because they are not highly reliable, and yet they are powerful evidence. Whether hypnotic coercion of confession can indeed occur is related to the question of whether any forms of coercion may be induced by hypnosis. The evidence is unclear, though there appears to be more support for the position that they can be induced, faked, or influenced. The conclusion that confessions resulting from the use of hypnosis should be inadmissible seems reasonable (Scheflin and Shapiro, 1989).

Certainly clinicians using any theory or technique can end up in court,

362

either as an expert witness or, much less desirably, as a party to a malpractice action. The clinical use of hypnosis is an additional factor that can spur such participation in either role. By following these guidelines, the hypnotherapist will not only function more efficiently but will significantly lessen the probability of being accused of malpractice. After discussing malpractice and hypnosis, and malpractice and professional liability suits in general, and how to deal with media inquiries, the first set of guidelines is concerned with case preparation in general, followed by guidelines for entering into a case as an expert witness, preparing for a deposition, and preparing for the actual courtroom appearance, if that is actually required.

Malpractice and Hypnosis

There are few reported malpractice cases directly involving hypnosis. One recent case (*Plunto v. Wallenstein*, 1989) involved performance hypnosis in which the subject fell to the stage and was injured. Other claims have been made. For example, in *Lebbos v. Heinrichs* (1988), this civil case claimed a failure to use hypnosis as a form of therapy; the physician committed malpractice, it was claimed, by failing to treat the patient's psychogenic amnesia with hypnosis. The case was dismissed for failure to pursue the claim vigorously. In *Dockweiler v. Wentzell* (1988) it was claimed that a psychologist used "methods of hypnosis and transference" to obtain sexual contact with a client. In *Johnson v. Gerrish* (1986) it was alleged that hypnosis used in a stop-smoking program facilitated an acute psychotic break, and that a registered nurse had allowed a licensed practical nurse to administer such treatment, even knowing that the latter was not authorized to give such treatments, but the jury found the plaintiffs had more of the fault than the defendants. These are among the very few cases making claims of civil liability that directly involve hypnosis. For a variety of reasons, few subjects (plaintiffs) recovered in these cases.

The absence of officially reported cases, however, does not mean that there are not malpractice claims related to hypnosis. Many cases, even those that go to trial, are not officially reported. Generally only appellate cases are reported (although some trial court decisions in the federal system are reported). In addition, claims may be made and settled without the filing of formal court cases. Despite the fact that it is nearly impossible to know how many civil liability claims are made in which hypnosis played a role, it is reasonable to guess that such cases are relatively rare.

The reasons for so few reported malpractice cases bearing on the use of hypnosis are several. First, the level of claims against mental health professionals is small generally (Smith, 1991). Furthermore, malpractice that might be committed as a part of psychotherapy is likely to be related to some other form of liability associated with the treatment, such as negligent diagnosis or the failure to refer to a specialist. Finally, the use of hypnosis is relatively low risk, and therefore even its misuse is often not associated with catastrophic injuries.

In the absence of a large body of reported cases, it is possible to apply general legal principles that would govern such malpractice cases. Most malpractice cases are based on claims of negligence. The plaintiff must demonstrate that a client was injured because a practitioner failed to exercise reasonable care in providing professional services. That means that the practitioner did not act as a reasonably prudent practitioner would have acted under the circumstances; the practitioner was careless in a professional sense, and as a result a client was injured. Except in unusual cases, whether a practitioner acted reasonably depends on whether he or she followed the custom of the profession in providing services.

Defining the standard of care for a hypnotist is difficult because of the absence of generally accepted national standards for hypnosis and because of the enormous diversity in the people who perform hypnosis. The qualifications of those doing hypnosis range from the rank amateur, to the barely trained police officer, to the extremely well-trained professional with doctoral-level education. It is not at all clear whether they all should be held legally to the same level of competence and care. Certainly each practitioner at a minimum should be held to that level of care he or she claims to have. Someone who claims to be doing therapy with hypnosis, for example, at least implicitly claims a level of expertise that the public should be able to rely on.

Problems that may lead to malpractice claims from hypnosis include the following:

1. Inadequate training to do hypnosis or the form of therapy that is undertaken.
2. Failure to do a proper history or background information gathering if this leads to injury.
3. Failure to refer a patient to another practitioner when formal consultation is necessary.
4. Failure to obtain informed consent.
5. The release of confidential information without patient consent.
6. Taking unfair advantage of a client.

Any activity that is considered unethical by the profession to which the specific hypnotist belongs also has a significant potential for liability.

Taking advantage, particularly sexual advantage, of clients, is among the most troublesome and fastest growing areas of malpractice liability in the mental health professions. Whether based in negligence or an intentional tort such as battery, any sexual contact between a hypnotherapist and a client represents the legal basis for a successful malpractice claim. Certainly such contact originating while the client is under hypnosis or a posthypnotic suggestion would be a matter of clear civil liability and probable criminal action.

Malpractice considerations have been increasing for all health professionals. Although some malpractice claims have been based on intentional torts (such as battery, false imprisonment, or intentional infliction of mental distress), most are based on the torts of negligence and/or contract liability. Overall, claims commonly arise from concepts such as unfair advantage (such as sexual improprieties), incorrect or inadequate treatment or diagnosis, failure to obtain informed consent, breach of confidentiality, wrongful involuntary commitment, failure to prevent suicide, nonfulfillment of contract (implicit or explicit), defamation, or failure to refer and/or to avoid practicing in a specific area where competence is lacking. Sexual impropriety claims and payouts and those for incorrect treatment are the most common.

The guidelines discussed throughout this chapter will help avoid the specter of malpractice, as well as promote effective and efficient clinical functioning. In addition, several specific steps may be taken to lessen malpractice probabilities:

1. Think of records as eventual legal documents.
2. Unless necessary, avoid touching clients, especially of the opposite sex.
3. Avoid dual relationships to the degree possible, especially business relationships that involve clients, which easily lead to later lawsuits.
4. Get written releases.
5. Do not collect overdue bills from clients whom you could reasonably expect to be litigious and/or who expressed disappointment with their treatment.
6. Avoid, to the degree feasible, high-risk clients (paranoid, borderline, or narcissistic clients, chronic legal offenders, sexual problems in a fragmenting marriage, the seriously depressed, and/or suicidals).
7. If you are supervising students or other clinicians, make sure communication and insurance liability issues are covered and clear.
8. Maintain and document colleague counsel and supervision where necessary (for example, if you feel a client is attracted to you and/or vice versa).

If a malpractice, ethics, or licensing complaint has become active, the following actions are suggested by professional activity groups in the various mental health professional organizations:

1. Consider seeking legal assistance except for the most trivial issues. If any formal action is taken (any lawsuit is filed or a formal complaint

lodged with a licensing authority), contact an attorney for advice and, probably, to handle the case.

2. Inform your malpractice insurance. If you do not have malpractice insurance or you cannot get such insurance, you should not be using hypnosis in any fashion—or any other therapeutic technique, for that matter. Your malpractice insurance policy probably requires that you make this disclosure fairly quickly in the event of any form of liability claim. An attorney will be able to interpret your malpractice policy to determine just when and how you must provide information to the insurance company.

3. Consider the merits of the complaint. If the complaint is well founded, it may make sense to settle the matter early. Your attorney and insurance company are critical here, and you should discuss the matter openly with them.

4. Cooperate with the ethics committee or licensing board in their investigation of the complaint. Become familiar with their rules and procedures. Provide the documentation they request. Contact the chair of the ethics committee or licensing board if you have any questions regarding their investigation. Seek legal advice before releasing information to anyone.

5. Gather all relevant documents and records but do not show them to anyone except your attorney and, with his or her advice, the ethics committee or licensing board.

6. Do not destroy or alter any documents.

7. Prepare additional documents, such as chronicles of events to refresh your memory.

8. Remember that professional case consultation with colleagues is not generally considered privileged information.

9. Be familiar with all the issues in your case.

10. Do not attempt to resolve or settle the case yourself.

11. Provide copies of your files, calendars, notes, and other materials as advised by your attorney. Keep the originals.

12. Avoid any public comments, and do not make self-incriminating statements. Generally do not talk to anyone about this matter. Most professional liability policies do not cover ethics committee or licensing board complaints, since malpractice coverage is usually restricted to lawsuits. But consider consulting with an attorney before responding to an ethics committee or licensing board complaint.

Professional Liability Suits

If you become aware of the possibility that a suit may be filed against you, gather all available information on the matter, meticulously follow all of the relevant steps noted above, and take the following additional steps:

1. Keep in contact with your attorney.
2. Contact the attorney assigned to handle your case by the insurance company. Follow his or her advice.
3. Do not attempt to resolve or settle the case yourself or with the plaintiff's attorney while not working with your own attorney.
4. Provide the insurance carrier with all the written information you have regarding the allegations.
5. Do not panic or discuss the situation with anyone not directly representing your interests except for privileged conversations with your attorney.
6. Prepare any additional documents needed to refresh your memory.
7. Do not distribute any documents without your attorney's approval, and refer all communications from the plaintiff or plaintiff's attorney to your attorney.

Response to Public or Media Inquiries

These kinds of issues, especially when they involve hypnosis, often bring inquiries from the public and/or media. A good rule of thumb is to say "no comment." If you fear that one or two of your comments will be taken out of context and at the same time do not want to be portrayed as avoiding making a comment, state that you would be willing to comment as long as it is stipulated that the interview as a whole will be broadcast or published. You could then challenge, in whatever fashion seems appropriate, a later published statement suggesting or stating that you were unwilling to make any comment. But if you do speak out (on this, or just in response to inquiries in general from the media), observe the following guidelines to minimize complications:

1. Try to make sure the reporter is reputable.
2. Ask that quotations be read back to you as a condition of talking, if possible.
3. When reporters call, tell them you want to think over their questions and will call them back.
4. Think about the context of your comments within the article and how controversial the topic is. Will your comments hurt anyone?
5. Ask the reporter what assurances can be given that he or she will not draw conclusions you are not making.
6. Ask yourself if you are violating anyone's confidentiality in speaking to the media and if you need a signed waiver. Often the client must consent to the public release of any information. In other instances, there are court limits on the release of information.

7. Consider making an audiotape of any interview, and inform the reporter that you are taping it.

General Principles for Case Preparation

Hypnotherapists can take a number of measures to insure that their procedures are ethical, appropriate, and expert. This first set of suggestions concerns general issues with which most clinicians would concern themselves; later, we discuss the preparations for depositions and the courtroom appearance. The general suggestions for case preparation are as follows:

1. Do not take on a case in which you do not have a reasonable degree of expertise. There are numerous examples of health professionals taking on cases in which they have only a passing awareness of the issues or the requirements of practice. If your are trying to branch into a new area, make sure that you receive appropriate background education and supervision. Even the best and most experienced clinicians continue to use colleague consultation throughout their careers. It is also appropriate to inform the client, in a nonthreatening fashion, that this is a new area for you and to tell the client what the limits are that can be expected from your participation.

2. Establish a clear contract with your client. At the very least, make a thorough oral presentation in a contractual manner of what the client can expect from you and also of what you will expect from the client. It is advisable to put this in writing. The contract should clearly cover the issues of confidentiality (especially when seeing a child or adolescent) and compensation.

3. Keep meticulous notes on your encounter with the client and on related events. Make sure that when you return to the case after a lengthy period of absence from it, you will be able to reconstruct what occurred between you and the client and can report clearly what the client told you.

4. Observe relevant guidelines in keeping records. A record should contain, at a minimum, identifying data, dates of services, types of services, and, where appropriate, a record of significant actions taken. Providers should make all reasonable efforts to record essential information within a reasonable time of their completion. If treatment is involved, a treatment plan should be included. The guidelines for retention of records are governed by state, federal, and professional regulations. From a conservative perspective, the full record should be maintained intact for three years after the completion of planned services or after the date of last contact with the user, whichever is later; a full record or a summary of the record should be maintained for an additional twelve years; the record should be disposed of no sooner than fifteen years after the completion of planned services or after the date of last contact, whichever is later. If those records are subsequently

submitted to another professional or an agency, the records should be accompanied by an indication of whether the clinician considers the information (especially any assessment data) to be obsolete.

5. Make sure your relevant history is a thorough one. Many cases have related issues that occur in the history of the client. The relevance of these issues may not be apparent at the time. Make sure that you have looked at all of the potential issues that are possibly relevant.

Expert Witness Case Preparation

While these suggestions and principles are important for virtually any professional in the health professions, there are several other suggestions that become important if you eventually become directly involved in the judicial process in a client's case:

1. Take some time to observe courtroom procedures in general, and try to observe various professionals in the role of an expert witness to help you become familiar and comfortable with courtroom process.
2. Although experts who are called by one party should be an advocate for their opinions and not for the party, they still must operate within the adversary legal system. Therefore, you should not discuss the case with anyone other than the court or the party for whom you have conducted an evaluation without the knowledge or permission of the court or that party.
3. Once the opinion has been formed, insist that the attorney who employs you provide the basic facts of the case and the relevant statutory and case law and that he or she explains the theory under which the case is to be pursued. Understanding of these issues is crucial to your preparation for the case, and reports and testimony should specifically address these legal issues.
4. Prepare your case in language that will be meaningful to the court. Remember that jurors are going to be put off by jargon, or they may misunderstand it and not give proper weight to your testimony.
5. Prepare yourself to give a thorough overview of all the examination devices that you will be referring to. In the courtroom, you may be asked about the reliability and validity of these devices, about how they were derived, or about what they are purported to measure or treat. You should be ready to answer in a crisp, efficient fashion, easily understandable manner.
6. Make sure ahead of time of the role and position you will take in the courtroom situation, and communicate this to the attorney who has brought you into the case.
7. When you are close to presenting the case in deposition or in court,

make sure you can be comfortable with your knowledge of the client. This may entail bringing the client in for visits shortly before the court testimony. In many court cases, the professional's last contact may have been many years before actually going into court. In such a case, it is helpful to see the client again, if at all possible, to check on prior data that were collected and to update impressions and inferences.

Deposition Preparation and Presentation

In virtually every case that takes on a legal dimension, there is a strong likelihood that the hypnotherapist will be deposed (usually civil cases; depositions are used less often in criminal cases). Indeed, in many cases there may be no courtroom appearance after a deposition, either because the case is settled out of court or the material that came to the light in the deposition eliminated the need or desire to have the hypnotherapist testify in person.

Many of the suggestions already mentioned as critical in general and in expert witness case presentation are relevant to the deposition as well. However, the following are more specific to preparation for a deposition:

1. Organize and review all materials pertinent to the case, and request a predeposition conference with the attorney.
2. Bring to the deposition only those records, notes, and other materials that you are willing for all involved parties to be aware of or, in many cases, to gain access to.
3. Be aware that there are two types of subpoenas. The first, the *subpoena ad testicandum*, is what most people assume—a summons to appear at court at a specified date and time. The second, the *subpoena duces tecum*, requires the clinician to bring specific materials to the court.
4. Just because a particular set of records has been requested or even subpoenaed does not mean they must be released. If in doubt, insist that the attorney requesting the information provide a valid authorization from the affected person, request a court order before releasing the information (in some jurisdictions, even a court order is not sufficient), and seek independent legal counsel before acting. The attorney representing the client should be informed so that she or he may challenge the request.
5. Bring an extra copy of your curriculum vitae; it is likely that it will be incorporated into the record at this time.
6. Be courteous, and speak in a voice that is audible to everyone, especially the stenographic reporter.
7. Be honest in all responses, but do not provide information that is not requested. Avoid elaboration.
8. Think before you respond. You can take as much time as you wish to

think out your response, since there is no issue of conveying a confused or tentative image to the jury, as there may be in the courtroom.

9. If an attorney objects, stop talking. It is best to let the attorneys deal with the point in question.

10. Remember that the opposing attorney will be evaluating you as a witness and may try many things in deposition that will not be used in trial, e.g., possibly letting you sit for a long time as a ploy to make you nervous, or appearing to get extremely angry or disdainful, to elicit a desired response.

11. Thoroughly read and check the deposition when a copy is sent to you for your signature; do not waive your right to sign it. Correct any errors in it as your attorney instructs. Keep a copy of the deposition with your other records pertaining to that case.

12. Prior to going to court, review your copy of the deposition, and take it with you to the witness stand.

Courtroom Presentation

While all cases in which the clinician is deposed do not result in a court appearance, many do. The following suggestions are useful when presenting testimony in the courtroom:

1. Be honest in all of your testimony. If you do not know the answer, say so, and offer to give related information that may clarify the question. Do not try to answer questions when you do not know the answer. Aside from the ethical issues, it is likely that you will be tripped up later in the cross-examination.

2. Do not be overly reluctant to admit limitations in your expertise or in the data available. If the cross-examining counsel presents a relevant and accurate piece of datum, acknowledge this in a firm and clear fashion, and do not put yourself into a defensive position.

3. Acknowledge, by eye contact, the person who has requested your statement, be it the judge or one of the attorneys. At the same time, maintain eye contact with the jury as much as possible.

4. Be aware of the three classic errors of the expert witness: becoming too technical, too complex in discussion, or condescending and/or too simplistic. Any of these approaches is likely to lose the attention of the jurors and may also turn them against you and the content of your testimony.

5. Avoid long, repetitive explanations of your points. If at all possible, keep your responses to two or three statements. If you feel more is needed, try to point our that you cannot fully answer the question without elaborating.

6. Never answer questions that you do not understand. If you are uncomfortable with the wording of the question, ask to have it restated and, if need be, describe your problems with the question as originally posed.

7. Listen carefully to what is asked in each question before answering. If there is a tricky component to the question, acknowledge that, and then try to deal with it in a concise fashion. If the attorney has made an innuendo that is negative to the case or to you, respond, if you feel it is appropriate, without becoming adversarial. Keep your response unemotional. This may be a good time to bring in a bit of humor; however, the use of humor requires great caution.

8. If you feel the attorney has misstated what you have just said, when he or she asks a follow-up question, take the time to clarify unemotionally what you actually did say and then answer the next question.

9. Speak clearly, fluently, and somewhat louder than you would normally speak. Make sure the jury hears you. Speak when spoken to, and avoid smoking or chewing. Avoid weak or insipid speech patterns, commonly marked by formal grammar; hesitation forms, such as "Uh," "You know," "Well"; hedges, such as "sort of," "I guess," "I think"; overly polite speech; and the use of a questioning form of sentence structure rather than straightforward sentences. Communicate a confident, straightforward attitude.

10. Avoid using graphs, tables, or exhibits that are not easily visible, readable, and comprehensible by the average juror.

11. Be prepared for questions about journal articles, books, and other materials relevant to issues in this particular case. This is more important now than it was at the deposition stage. You cannot check up on all of the relevant literature, but by familiarizing yourself with some key recent articles, you can more easily blunt an attack.

12. Be prepared to be questioned about the issue of fees. Attorneys may ask questions like, "How much are you being paid to testify for this client?" You need to correct that and state what you were asked to do, then give your full and honest opinion to the best of your knowledge, and that it was then up to the attorney to decide whether to use you in the courtroom. Also, make sure that you state that you are not being paid for your testimony but that you are being paid for the time that you put into this trial, no matter what testimony would emerge from that time spent. For that reason, you probably will look better to the jury if you charge by the hour rather than a flat fee for a case.

13. Be professional in dress and demeanor. Informal dress is seldom appropriate in a courtroom. Reasonably conservative attire makes a more positive impression on the jury. Similarly, your demeanor should be professional, and you should avoid becoming involved in any kind of tirade or acrimony.

14. Never personalize your interactions with an attorney who is attempting to disrupt you. If you become emotional and make any kind of personal attack, you will likely taint the value of your testimony. There may be times when you do need to express some emotion in giving an opinion in order to emphasize that opinion, but make sure the emotion is properly placed on the opinion and not as a defensive or attacking response toward the court, jury, or a cross-examining attorney.

Just as the clinician is organizing to make an effective presentation to the court, at least one attorney is usually preparing to devalue any or all parts of the clinician's testimony. The well-prepared clinician reminds himself or herself of the strategies that he or she is likely to encounter.

Anticipating the Cross-Examination

Cross-examination is designed to challenge or discredit those data and opinions that have been presented by the hypnotherapist that are inconsistent with that attorney's case. There are a variety of ways in which the cross-examining attorney will attempt to challenge this testimony:

1. One primary target for examination is often the expert's qualifications. Two kinds of questions concerning qualifications are whether a witness is sufficiently qualified to be permitted (by the judge) to testify as an expert and the weight that should be given (by the judge or jury) to the expert's opinion. Presumably, the more highly qualified the expert is, the greater is the weight that should be given that professional's opinion. The expert's experience in the area and the credentials and level of relevant education are common targets.

2. Another common way to challenge the expert witness is through contradictory testimony from other experts in the field. These experts may testify in the trial, or the challenge may be in the form of a book or article submitted as written authority. A favorite approach is to attempt to lead the witness by asking if such-and-such a source is authoritative and then presenting the contradictory testimony from that source. When an expert is asked if this book or person is authoritative, it may be wise to make a disclaimer that, "Dr._____ does write in this field. Other experts might agree with some of the things he says, but he's not my authority [or the only authority]."

3. A third technique is to attack the procedures used by the expert witness. A classic instance is the discovery that the expert spent a very short period of time with the client.

4. Another area in which the hypnotherapist can be impeached is through bias, for example, by attacking the expert witness as a hired gun and asking a variety of questions about how the individual has been paid.

It is probably wise for the expert to bill on an hourly basis rather than through a flat fee because this seems to communicate to jurors a more professional approach. Also, the expert should be prepared to note that it was his or her work that was paid for, not any outcome or particular slant to the testimony.

5. Another potential point of attack is any special relationship to the client. If there is any sense in which the expert is a friend of the client, is doing the client a favor, or in turn is receiving favors for the testimony, the expert's testimony is likely to have a less positive impact on the jury.

6. Expert witnesses are occasionally cross-examined on their personal vulnerabilities or deficiencies. Any general indications of instability or deviation in the history of the expert witness may be brought out if they can be discovered. Persons who have obvious vulnerabilities—possibly a history of alcoholism or hearing or vision problems (which may in some instances be relevant)—should consider a means of handling such an attack.

7. Just as attorneys will try to challenge the sources of an inference, they will also try to discredit the process of deriving the inference or opinion. They may try to introduce at least apparently contradictory data or may simply ask, "Isn't this alternate idea possible?" It is important for the expert witness not to become too defensive. There may be a reasonable admission that other interpretations are possible. The expert witness needs to define that we are in a world of probabilities, possibly stating something to the effect, "Yes, almost anything is possible, but I feel that the bulk of evidence supports the opinion I have rendered."

8. An excellent way to discredit an expert witness is to disclose prior reports or transcripts of court testimony given by the same expert that are at least apparently contradictory to the present testimony. The expert should be aware of this possibility, and experts who publish are even more vulnerable. They need to be able to explain this situation reasonably—that opinions do change over time and that they may have made a statement some time before with which they do not wholly agree now, or they need to point out why the earlier comments do not exactly apply here. Defensiveness is a bad strategy. Openness can be the best method of handling this type of attack.

At its root, cross-examination is a process of searching for the truth by challenging the ideas and conclusions of the expert. In this sense, it compresses into a short time the long process of challenge to publication and research. Cross-examination is not a perfect process of truth finding. The presentation of information to a lay jury may cause obfuscation through cross-examination. Some attorneys unfairly attack or even badger witnesses. The fact that some attorneys try these tactics, however, does not mean that they have succeeded; such tactics often backfire. If an expert has drawn reasonable conclusions based on thorough procedures and has avoided exaggerated statements and emotional responses to cross-examination, the expert will have succeeded in making his or her point to the jury. A dry run with a practice cross-examination can be especially helpful, particularly for the expert who has not testified before.

Hypnosis in an Investigation

Persons who work with hypnosis may enter the legal arena in an investigative or testamentary capacity, for example, by helping a witness to enhance the memory of a relevant incident. It is in this area that most legal activity has occurred.

Simply aiding in an investigation usually brings up less complex legal ramifications. For example, I was asked to help a young woman who had been raped to recall the license plate of her attacker's car. After raping her, he had thrown her from the car. As she rolled over, she had a glimpse of the licence plate. When she stood up, she happened to see a police car and finally got the attention of the police. But in this period of stress and frenzy, she had forgotten the license plate. The rapist had made one big mistake: she was the niece of a police detective. He was willing to try anything, even hypnosis, to nail this fellow. Her uncle brought her to me, and she proved to be a good subject. In the second session she was able to recall five of the six digits. By a process of elimination and stakeouts, the perpetrator was caught and convicted, but without any necessity for me to make a court appearance in this case.

Hypnosis and Witnesses

When hypnosis is used to enhance the memory of a witness, a court appearance is almost a certainty if the case goes to trial. The hypnotist is then virtually assured of a legal battle over the admissibility of hypnotically enhanced evidence in general and such evidence in this specific case. There has been a plethora of legal cases challenging the admissibility of such testimony. The legal highlights of this controversy are as follows:

> 1897, *People v. Ebanks*: This is the first clearly documented specific forensic application of hypnosis in the United States. Ebanks, while intoxicated, allegedly murdered two elderly citizens. His attempted defense was based on testimony obtained under hypnosis suggesting that Ebanks's alleged amnesia regarding the events of the murder was due to the fact that he did not commit these crimes. The court denied the

admissibility of such evidence, and Ebanks was convicted and eventually executed.

1923, *Frye v. United States*: Referring to the use of the polygraph, the Frye rule sets the standard, subsequently applied to many other procedures, including hypnosis, that in order to admit the results of a scientific or mechanical method or technique, "the thing from which the deduction is made must be sufficiently established to have gained general acceptance in the field in which it belongs" (Frye, 58 at 523).

1969, *Harding v. State*: This Maryland case established the modern precedent for the concept that the trier of fact should decide the weight to be given to hypnotically influenced testimony: thus, it may be admitted.

1981, *State v. Hurd*: The New Jersey Supreme Court, recognizing the hazards of hypnotically influenced testimony and influenced by noted hypnosis researcher and therapist Martin Orne, adopted a set of six procedural safeguards, which are still highly influential: (1) the session should be conducted by a licensed psychologist or psychiatrist, (2) the hypnotist should be independent of and not responsible to the prosecutor, investigator, or defense, (3) prior information provided to the hypnotist should be in writing, (4) before inducing hypnosis, the facts the subject has should be obtained and recorded, (5) the sessions should be recorded, (videotaping is desirable but not mandatory), and (6) only the hypnotist and subject should be present during prehypnotic testing, the session itself, and the posthypnotic interview.

1980, *State v. Mack*: The Minnesota Supreme Court, applying the 1923 Frye rule, held hypnotically refreshed testimony to be inadmissible.

1982, *People v. Shirley*: The California Supreme Court, without reference to *Frye*, at least until appeal, rejected the Hurd rules as "pretense" and applied a sweeping rule of inadmissibility to hypnotically influenced testimony.

1987, *Rock v. Arkansas*: the U.S. Supreme Court held that it is a violation of constitutional rights to prevent arbitrarily *in a criminal action* the defendants from presenting hypnotically refreshed testimony. They held that the difficulties stemming from this kind of testimony from the defense can be handled by the process of cross-examination or by rules of evidence.

In *Rock v. Arkansas*, the Supreme Court considered a narrow but important issue regarding the presentation of testimony "refreshed" by hypnosis. In that case, Vickie Rock could only partly remember the acts that gave rise to her being charged with shooting her husband. She was hypnotized to enhance her memory and under hypnosis remembered that the gun had misfired because it was defective. The trial court applied the Arkansas rule prohibiting testimony that resulted from matters recalled under hypnosis. The U.S. Supreme Court overturned her conviction, however, holding that an absolute ban on such testimony from the defendant violated the constitutional right to testify in her own defense. It was the absolute rule preventing the defendant from presenting hypnotically enhanced testimony that the Court struck down.

The Supreme Court noted that many states had limited the use of hypnotically enhanced testimony and that the effect of hypnosis probably increases both the correct and incorrect memories. The Court felt, however, that this difficulty could be cured with good cross-examination or rules regulating hypnotically enhanced testimony. It was unnecessary to have an absolute rule that prohibited it altogether. In all likelihood, a state could generally enforce the procedural safeguards proposed by Orne and discussed elsewhere in this book without violating the constitutional right of the defendant.

Several of the limits of this case should be noted. First, it applied only to testimony from the defendant: it did not automatically give the prosecution the same right to present hypnotically refreshed testimony. (A state would be free to permit the prosecution to present such testimony, but it is not required to do so.) Second, it was the defendant herself who was going to testify, and it is not clear that a state would always be constitutionally required to permit the defense to present hypnotically refreshed testimony by someone else on behalf of the defense. Third, this was a criminal case: it would not apply to civil cases. The trend in civil cases is toward a "safeguard rules" approach, similar to the Hurd rules, following a leading precedent case (*Lemieux v. Superior Court*, 1982), which states, "Few dangers so great as in the search for truth as man's propensity to tamper with the memory of others." Finally, this case was a five-to-four decision in 1987, with the "liberal" justices of the time making up the majority. Between 1987 and 1992, most of the justices who made up that majority left the Court, so its continued vitality must be questioned.

There are substantial experimental data to suggest that memories can be influenced by suggestion. A landmark study by Loftus and Palmer (1974) that received much attention points to how easily memory can be influenced even without hypnosis. These researchers found that subjects remembered broken glass more than twice as often in films of an auto accident they had viewed. In this film, no broken glass was ever present. They were apparently cued only by the experimenter's differential use of descriptors (for example,) "smashed into" versus "hit" in referring to the accident to be recalled.

Subsequent research (Laurence and Perry, 1988; Scheflin and Shapiro,

Figure 18–1.
Consent Form for Hypnosis Investigation*

I,_____ , hereby agree voluntarily and freely, to undergo hypnosis and be interviewed under hypnosis in order to assist with an investigation. I understand that either an audio or video tape recording will be made of the entire interview and that this method of preservation of the interview may be used, as to be determined by my attorneys, for any lawful purpose connected with this investigation.

_____ , a mental health professional, with experience and training in hypnosis, has explained the procedures to be used during the course of this hypnosis session and any questions I had concerning this procedure have been answered to my satisfaction. The purpose of this interview under hypnosis is to assist my memory in recalling_____

_____

_____

Possible Additions:
[For potential defendant or other parties]
  I have specifically consulted with my attorney regarding the legal consequences of undergoing hypnosis. I understand that (mental health professional's name) is not an attorney and cannot be responsible for the legal consequences of undergoing hypnosis.
[For possible prosecuting witnesses]
  I have consulted with the prosecutor's office regarding the possible legal consequences of undergoing this hypnosis, and those consequences have been explained to me by the prosecutor or my own attorney to my satisfaction. I understand that (mental health professional's name) is not an attorney and cannot be responsible for the legal consequences of undergoing hypnosis.

_____
Interviewee   Date
Witnesses:

_____
Hypnotist-Interviewer   Date

_____
Witness   Date

* Adapted in part from Wester (1987)

1989) has consistently found that both perceptions and memories can be changed by suggestions made during hypnosis. Just as imagined events can mimic the authenticity of true events in people's recall, hypnotized persons can report fantasized occurrences as compellingly as if they were real. The Labelle et al. (1990) study is one of the more recent demonstrations of the ability to create pseudomemories through hypnosis.

If a hypnotist chooses to help enhance the memory of a witness, it is advisable to follow a set of procedures, like the Hurd rules, as well as using a consent form. The form in figure 18–1 is adapted in part from Garner (1987) and should be adapted by users to fit the specific credentials, criteria, and case information.

References

Chapter 1: Introduction

Levitan, A. (1991). Hypnosis in the 1990s—and beyond. *American Journal of Clinical Hypnosis, 33,* 141–149.

Morgan, J., Darby, B. and Heath, A. (1992). The future of hypnosis through the remainder of the decade: A Delphi poll. *American Journal of Clinical Hypnosis, 34,* 149–157.

People v. Ebanks. 117 Cal. 652, 49P. 1049 (1897).

Rock v. Arkansas. 107 S. Ct. 2704 (1987).

Sarbin, T. (1991). Hypnosis: A fifty year perspective. *Contemporary Hypnosis 8,* 1–15.

State v. Hurd. 86 N.J. 525, 432 A.2d 86 (1981).

Wester, W. (Ed.) (1987). *Clinical hypnosis.* Cincinnati: Behavioral Science Centers.

Wolberg, L. (1972). *Hypnosis: Is it for you?* New York: Harcourt Brace Jovanovich.

Yapko, M. (1990). *Trancework: An introduction to the practice of clinical hypnosis* (2d ed.). New York: Brunner/Mazel.

Chapter 2: Hypnotic Sensibility and Preliminary Considerations in Hypnosis Cases

Baker, E. (1987). The state of the art of clinical hypnosis. *International Journal of Clinical and Experimental Hypnosis 35,* 203–214.

Balthazard, C. & Woody, E. (1992). The spectral analysis of hypnotic performance with respect to absorption. *International Journal of Clinical and Experimental Hypnosis 40* (1), 21–43.

Barber, T. (1964). Hypnotizability, suggestibility, and personality: V. A critical review of research findings. *Psychological Reports 14,* 299–320.

Bates, B. L., and Brigham, T. A. (1990). Modifying hypnotizability with the Carleton Skills Training Program: A partial replication and analysis of components. *International Journal of Clinical and Experimental Hypnosis 38,* 183–195.

Bergerone, C., Cei, A., and Ruggieri, V. (1981). Suggestibility and cognitive style. *International Journal of Clinical and Experimental Hypnosis 29,* 355–357.

Bramwell, J. M. (1903/1956). *Hypnotism: Its history, practice and theory.* New York: Julian Press.

Crasilneck, H. B., and Hall, J. A. (1985). *Clinical hypnosis: Principles and applications* (2d ed.). Orlando, Fla.: Grune & Stratton.

Crawford, H. J. (1982). Hypnotizability, daydreaming styles, imagery vividness, and absorption: A multidimensional study. *Journal of Personality and Social Psychology 42,* 915–926.

Edmonston, W. (1986). *The induction of hypnosis.* New York: Wiley. Gfeller, J. D., Lynn, S. J., and Pribble, W. E. (1987). Enhancing hypnotic susceptibility: Interpersonal and rapport factors. *Journal of Personality and Social Psychology 52,* 586–595.

Gorassini, D. R., and Spanos, N. P. (1986). A social-cognitive skills approach to the successful modification of hypnotic susceptibility. *Journal of Personality and Social Psychology 50,* 1004–1012.

London, P. (1962). *Children's Hypnotic Susceptibility Scale.* Palo Alto: Consulting Psychologists Press.

Lubar, J., Gordon, D., Harrist, R., Nash, M. et al. (1991). EEG correlates of hypnotic susceptibility based upon Fast Fourier Power Spectral Analysis. *Biofeedback and Self-Regulation* 16(1), 75–85.

MacHovec, F. (1988). Hypnosis complications, risk factors, and prevention. *American Journal of Clinical Hypnosis 31,* 40–49.

Malott, J. M., Bourg, A. L., and Crawford, H. J. (1989). The effects of hypnosis upon cognitive responses to persuasive communication. *International Journal of Clinical and Experimental Hypnosis 37,* 31–40.

Morgan, A. H., and Hilgard, J. R. (1978/1979). The Stanford Hypnotic Clinical Scale for adults. *American Journal of Clinical Hypnosis* 21(2,3), 134–147.

Nadon, R., Laurence, J., and Perry, C. (1987). Multiple predictors of hypnotic susceptibility. *Journal of Personality and Social Psychology 53,* 948–960.

Nadon, R., Hoyt, I., Register, P., and Kihlstrom, J. (1991). Absorption and hypnotizability. *Journal of Personality and Social Psychology 60,* 144–153.

Pereira, M., and Austrin, H. R. (1980). Locus of control and status of the experimenter as predictors of suggestibility. *International Journal of Clinical and Experimental Hypnosis 28,* 367–374.

Plotnick, A., Payne, P., and O'Grady, D. (1991). The Stanford Hypnotic Clinical Scale for Children—Revised: An evaluation. *Contemporary Hypnosis* 8(1), 33–40.

Radtke, H., and Stam, H. (1991). The relation between absorption, openness to experience, anhedonia, and hypnotic susceptibility. *International Journal of Clinical and Experimental Hypnosis* 39(1), 39–56.

Saavedra, R. L., and Miller, R. J. (1983). The influence of experimentally induced expectations on responses to the Harvard Group Scale of Hypnotica Susceptibility, Form A. *International Journal of Clinical and Experimental Hypnosis 31,* 37–46.

Shor, R. E., and Orne, E. C. (1962). *Harvard Group Scale of hypnotic susceptibility.* Palo Alto: Consulting Psychologists Press.

Spiegel, H. (1974). *Manual for the Hypnotic Induction Profile.* New York: Soni Medica.

Tellegen, A., and Atkinson, G. (1974). Openness to absorbing and self-altering experiences ("absorption"), a trait related to hypnotic susceptibility. *Journal of Abnormal Psychology 83,* 268–277.

Weitzenhoffer, A. M. (1980). Hypnotic susceptibility revisited. *American Journal of Clinical Hypnosis 22,* 130–146.

Weitzenhoffer, A. M., and Hilgard, E. R. (1959). *Stanford Hypnotic Susceptibility Scale, Forms A and B.* Palo Alto: Consulting Psychologists Press.

Weitzenhoffer, A. M., and Hilgard, E. R. (1962). *Stanford Hypnotic Susceptibility Scale, Forms C.* Palo Alto: Consulting Psychologists Press.

Weitzenhoffer, A. M., and Hilgard, E. R. (1963). *Stanford Profile Scales of Hypnotic Susceptibility.* Palo Alto: Consulting Psychologists Press.

Wickless, C., and Kirsch, I. (1989). Effects of verbal and experiential expectancy manipulations on hypnotic susceptibility. *Journal of Personality and Social Psychology 57,* 762–768.

Wilson, S. C., and Barber, T. X. (1978). The Creative Imagination Scale as a measure of hypnotic responsiveness: Applications to experimental and clinical hypnosis. *American Journal of Clinical Hypnosis 20,* 235–249.

Wright, M., and Wright, B. (1987). *Clinical practice of hypnotherapy* New York: Guilford.

Chapter 3: Induction Techniques

Bramwell, J. (1903/1956). *Hypnotism: Its history, practice and theory.* New York: Julian Press.

Chiasson, S. (1973). *A syllabus on hypnosis.* Des Plaines, Ill. American Society of Clinical Hypnosis, Foundation of Education and Research.

Edmonston, W. (1986). *The induction of hypnosis.* New York: Wiley.

Erickson, M. (1964). The confusion technique in hypnosis. *American Journal of Clinical Hypnosis 4,* 183–210.

Gravitz, M. (1991). Adverse behavior associated with the eye-roll of hypnotizability. *Psychotherapy 27* 267–270.

Jencks, B. (1984). Using the patient's breathing rhythm. In W. Wester and A. Smith (Eds.), *Clinical hypnosis: A multidisciplinary approach.* Philadelphia: J. B. Lippincott.

Kroger, W. (1977). *Clinical and experimental hypnosis* (2d ed.). Philadelphia: J. B. Lippincott.

London, P. (1963). *Children's Hypnotic Susceptibility Scale.* Palo Alto: Consulting Psychologists Press.

Page, R., and Handley, G. (1991). A comparison of the effects of standardized Chiasson and eye-closure inductions on susceptibility scores. *American Journal of Clinical Hypnosis 34*(1), 46–50.

Perry, C. (1979). Hypnotic coercion and compliance to it: A review of evidence presented in a legal case. *International Journal of Clinical and Experimental Hypnosis 27,* 187–218.

Saavedra, R., and Miller, R. (1983). The influence of experimentally induced expectations on responses to the Harvard Group Scale of Hypnotica Susceptibility, Form A. *International Journal of Clinical and Experimental Hypnosis 31,* 37–46.

Schumaker, J. (1991). The adaptive value of suggestibility and dissociation. In J. Schumaker (Ed.), *Human suggestibility.* New York: Routledge.

Strauss, B. (1991). The use of a multimodal image, the Apple Technique, to facilitate clinical hypnosis. *International Journal of Clinical and Experimental Hypnosis 39*(1), 1–5.

Venn, J. (1984). The spiral technique of hypnotic induction. *International Journal of Clinical and Experimental Hypnosis 32,* 287–289.

von Kirchenbaum, C., and Persinger, M. (1991). Time distortion—a comparison of hypnotic induction and progressive relaxation procedures. *International Journal of Clinical and Experimental Hypnosis 39*(2), 63–66.

Weitzenhoffer, A. (1980). Hypnotic susceptibility revisited. *American Journal of Clinical Hypnosis 22,* 130–146.

Wright, M., and Wright, B. (1987). *Clinical practice of hypnotherapy.* New York: Guilford.

Chapter 4: Deepening Techniques.

Bates, B. (1990). Compliance with the Carleton skill training program. *British Journal of Experimental and Clinical Hypnosis 7*(3), 159–164.

Bates, B., and Brigham, T. (1990). Modifying hypnotizability with the Carleton Skills Training Program. *International Journal of Clinical and Experimental Hypnosis 38*(3), 183–195.

Berrigan, L., Kurtz, R., Stabile, J., and Strube, M. (1991). Durability of "posthypnotic suggestions" as a function of type of suggestion and trance depth. *International Journal of Clinical and Experimental Hypnosis 39*(1), 24–38.

Dember, W. (1991). Personal communication.

Edmonston, W. (1986). *The induction of hypnosis.* New York: John Wiley.

Hammond, D., Haskins-Bartsch, C., McGhee, M., and Grant, C. (1987). The use of fractionation in self-hypnosis. *American Journal of Clinical Hypnosis 30,* 119–124.

Kleinhauz, M. (1991). Prolonged hypnosis with individualized therapy. *International Journal of Clinical and Experimental Hypnosis 39*(2), 82–92.

Korn, E. (1984). Altered states of consciousness. In G. Pratt, D. Wood, and B. Alman, *A clinical hypnosis primer.* LaJolla, Calif.: PCA Press.

Kuriyama, K. (1968). Clinical applications of prolonged hypnosis in psychosomatic medicine. *American Journal of Clinical Hypnosis 11,* 101–111.

Luthe, W. (1969) (Ed.). *Autogenic therapy.* Vols. 1–6 New York: Grune & Stratton.

Schultz, J., and Luthe, W. (1959). *Autogenic training: A psychophysiological approach to psychotherapy.* New York: Grune and Stratton.

Silva, C., and Kirsch, I. (1987). Breaching hypnotic amnesia by manipulating expectancy. *Journal of Abnormal Psychology 96,* 325–329.

Spanos, N., DeBrevil, S., and Gabora, N. (1991). Four-month follow-up of skill-training-induced enhancements in hypnotizability. *Contemporary Hypnosis 8,* 25–32.

Van Dyck, R., Zitman, F., Linssen, C., and Spinhoven, P. (1991). Autogenic training and future-oriented hypnotic imagery in the treatment of tension headache. *International Journal of Clinical and Experimental Hypnosis 39,* 6–23.

Walker, W. (1991). Music as a pathway for self-hypnosis. *Australian Journal of Clinical and Experimental Hypnosis 18*(1), 57–59.

Chapter 5: Indirect and Ericksonian Techniques

Brown, D. and Fromm, E. (1987). Hypnodiagnosis. In J. Gordon (Ed.), *Handbook of Clinical and Experimental Hypnosis* Hillsdale, N.J.: Lawrence Erlbaum Associates.

Erickson, M. (1967). "An introduction to the study and application of hypnosis for pain control." In J. Lassner (Ed.), *Proceedings of the International Congress on Hypnosis and Psychosomatic Medicine.* Berlin: Springer-Verlag.

Erickson, M., Hershman, S., and Sector, I. (1961). *Practical application of medical and dental hypnosis.* Brunner/Mazel: New York.

Erickson, M., and Rossi, E. (1976). Two level communication and the microdynamics of trance and suggestion: In E. Rossi (Ed.), *The nature of hypnosis and suggestion.* New York: Irvington.

Erickson M., and Rossi, E. (1979). *Hypnotherapy: An exploratory casebook.* New York: Irvington.

Erickson, M., and Rossi, E. (1980). *The collected papers of Milton Erickson on hypnosis I. The nature of hypnosis and suggestion.* New York: Irvington.

Erickson, M., and Rossi, E. (1981). *Experiencing hypnosis: Therapeutic approaches to altered states.* New York: Irvington.

Erickson, M., Rossi, E., and Rossi, S. (1976). *Hypnotic realities: The induction of clinical hypnosis and forms of indirect suggestion.* New York: Irvington Publishers.

Erickson, M., and Zeig, J. (1948/1980). *The Collected Papers of Milton Erickson on Hypnosis IV.* New York: Irvington.

Freud, S. (1938). "The interpretation of dreams." In A. Brill (Ed.), *The Basic Writings of Sigmund Freud.* New York: Modern Library.

Gilligan, S. (1988). Symptom Phenomena as Trance Phenomena. In J. Zeig and S. Lankton (Eds.), *Developing Ericksonian therapy.* New York: Brunner/Mazel.

Haley, J. (1973). *Uncommon therapy: The Psychiatric techniques of Milton H. Erickson, M.D.* New York: Norton.

Klein, R. (1990). "Pain control interventions of Milton H. Erickson." In J. Zeig and S. Gilligan (Eds.), *Brief therapy: Myths, methods, and metaphors.* New York: Brunner/Mazel.

Lankton, S., and Lankton, C. (1983). *The answer within: A clinical framework of Ericksonian hypnotherapy.* New York: Brunner/Mazel.

Lankton, S., and Zeig, J. (Eds.) (1988). *Research, comparisons and medical applications of Ericksonian techniques.* Ericksonian Monographs No. 4. New York: Brunner/Mazel.

Masters, K. (1992). Hypnotic susceptibility, cognitive dissociation, and runner's high in a sample of marathon runners. *American Journal of Clinical Hypnosis, 34,* 193–201.

Otani, A. (1990). Characteristics of change in Ericksonian hypnotherapy. *American Journal of Clinical Hypnosis 33*(1), 29–39.

Rosen, S. (1982). *My voice will go with you: The teaching tales of Milton Erickson, M.D.* New York: Norton.

Rossi, E. (1986). *The psychobiology of mind-body healing.* New York: Norton.

Zeig, J., and Lankton, S. (1988). *Developing Ericksonian therapy: State of the art.* New York: Brunner/Mazel.

Zeig, J. (1982). *Ericksonian approaches to hypnosis and psychotherapy.* New York: Brunner/Mazel.

Chapter 6: Direct Suggestion and Posthypnotic Techniques

Berrigan, L., Kurtz, R., Stabile, J., and Strube, M. (1991). Durability of "posthypnotic suggestions" as a function of type of suggestion and trance depth. *International Journal of Clinical and Experimental Hypnosis 39,* 24–38.

Brown, D., and Fromm, E. (1987). *Hypnosis and behavioral medicine*. Hillsdale, N.J.: Lawrence Erlbaum Associates.

Cheek, D., and LeCron, L. (1968). *Clinical hypnotherapy*. New York: Grune and Stratton.

Critenbaum, C., King, M., and Cohen, W. (1985). *Modern clinical hypnosis for habit control*. New York: W. W. Norton & Co.

Dorcus, R. (1956). *Hypnosis and its therapeutic applications*. New York: McGraw-Hill.

Edmonston, W. (1986). *The induction of hypnosis*. New York: Wiley.

Erickson, M., Hershman, S., and Sector, I. (1961). *Practical application of medical and dental hypnosis*. New York: Brunner/Mazel.

Erickson, M., Rossi, E., and Rossi, S. (1976). *Hypnotic realities: The induction of clinical hypnosis and forms of indirect suggestion*. New York: Irvington Publishers.

Goodwin, J., Hill, S., and Attias, R. (1990). Historical and folk techniques of exorcism. *Dissociation* 3(2), 94–101.

Hilgard, E. and Hilgard, J. (1975). *Hypnosis in the relief of pain*. Los Altos, Calif.: William Kaufmann.

Koe, G. (1989). Hypnotic treatment of sleep terror disorder: A case report. *American Journal of Clinical Hypnosis* 32(1), 36–39.

MacHovec, F. (1985). Treatment variables and the use of hypnosis in the brief therapy of post-traumatic stress disorders. *International Journal of Clinical and Experimental Hypnosis* 33(1), 6–14.

Meyer, R. and Tilker, H. (1976). The clinical use of direct hypnotic suggestion: A traditional technique in the light of current approaches. In *Hypnosis and behavior therapy*. Edited by Edward Dengrove. Springfield, Ill.: Charles C. Thomas.

Patterson, D., Questad, K., and de Lateur, B. (1989). Hypnotherapy as an adjunct to narcotic analgesia for the treatment of pain for burn debridement. *American Journal of Clinical Hypnosis* 31, 156–163.

Prior, A., Colgan, S., and Wherwell, P. (1990). Changes in rectal sensitivity after hypnotherapy in patients with irritable bowel syndrome. *Gut* 31(8), 896–898.

Trenerry, M., and Jackson, T. (1983). Hysterical dystonia successfully treated with post-hypnotic suggestion. *American Journal of Clinical Hypnosis* 26(1), 42–44.

Weitzenhoffer, A. (1953). *Hypnotism: An objective study in suggestibility*. New York: Wiley.

Yapko, M. (1983). A comparative analysis of direct and indirect hypnotic communication styles. *American Journal of Clinical Hypnosis* 25(4), 270–275.

Chapter 7: Hypnotic Age Regression

Anderson-Evangelista, A. (1980). *Hypnosis: A journey into the mind*. New York: Arco Publishing.

Bodden, J. (1991). Accessing state-bound memories in the treatment of phobias. *American Journal of Clinical Hypnosis* 34(1), 24–28.

Coons, P. (1988). Misuse of forensic hypnosis: A hypnotically elicited false confession with the apparent creation of a multiple personality. *International Journal of Experimental and Clinical Hypnosis 36*, 1–11.

Denburg, E. (1990). Hypnotic age regression and the autokinetic effect. *American Journal of Clinical Hypnosis 33*, 50–55.

Eisel, H. (1988). Age regression in the treatment of anger in a prison setting. *Journal of Offender Counseling, Services and Rehabilitation 13*(1), 175–181.

Fuhriman, N., Zingaro, J., and Kokenes, B. (1990). A preliminary comparative study of drawings produced under hypnosis and in a simulated state by both MPD and non-MPD adults. *Dissociation 3*(2), 107–112.

Gibson, H., and Heap, M. (1991). *Hypnosis in therapy*. Hillsdale, N.J.: Laurence Erlbaum.

Gross, M. (1983). Hypnoanalysis and the treatment of bulimia. *Medical Hypnoanalysis 4*(2), 77–82.

Goldberg, B. (1990). The clinical use of regression and progression in psychotherapy. *Psychology: A Journal of Human Behavior 27*(1), 43–48.

Hadley, J., and Staudacher, C. (1985). *Hypnosis for change*. New York: Ballantine.

Horton, A. (1991). *Neuropsychology across the life-span*. New York: Springer.

Hynes, J. (1982). Hypnotic treatment of five adult cases of trichotillomania. *Australian Journal of Clinical and Experimental Hypnosis 10*(2), 109–116.

Jue, R. (1988). Regression therapy as a transpersonal modality. *Journal of Transpersonal Psychology 20*(1), 4–9.

Kohut, H. (1971). *The analysis of the self: A systematic approach to the psychoanalytic treatment of narcissistic personality disorders*. New York: International Universities Press.

Lawrence, J. (1986). Duality, dissociation and memory; creation in highly hypnotizable subjects. *International Journal of Clinical and Experimental Hypnosis 32*(4), 295–310

Nash, M. (1987). What, if anything, is regressed about hypnotic age regression? A review of the empirical literature. *Psychological Bulletin 102*(1), 42–57.

Nash, M. (1988). Hypnosis as a window on aggression. *Bulletin of the Menninger Clinic 52*(5), 383–403.

Oystragh, P. (1988). Vaginismus: A case study. *Australian Journal of Clinical and Experimental Hypnosis 16*(2), 147–152.

Piaget, J., and Inhelder, B. (1969). *The psychology of the child*. New York: Basic Books.

Price, R. (1986). Hypnotic age regression and self-reparenting technique, 22 and 25 and 29 year old females with depression and anxiety vs. substance abuse and sexual inhibition vs. depression. *Transactional Analysis Journal 16*(2), 120–127.

Scott, J. (1984). Hypnosis and regression, patients with emotional disorder. *Medical Hypnoanalysis 5*(1), 17–33.

Spiegel, D., and Rosenfeld, A. (1984). Spontaneous hypnotic age regression: Case report. *Journal of Clinical Psychiatry 45*(12), 522–524.

Stolorow, D., and Lachmann, F. (1980). *Psychoanalysis of developmental arrests: Theory and treatment*. New York: International Universities Press.

Vanderlinden, J., and Vandereycken, W. (1988). The use of hypnotherapy in the treatment of eating disorders. *International Journal of Eating Disorders* 7(5), 673–679.

Chapter 8: Self-Hypnosis

Braun, B. G. (1984). Uses of hypnosis with multiple personality. *Psychiatric Annuals* 14, 34–40.

Cheek, D., and LeCron, L. (1968). *Clinical hypnotherapy.* Orlando: Grune & Stratton.

Fromm, E., and Kahn, S. (1990). *Self-hypnosis: The Chicago paradigm.* New York: Guilford Press.

Hammond, D. C., Haskins-Bartsch, C., Grant, C. W., and McGhee M. (1988). Comparison of self-directed and tape assisted self-hypnosis. *American Journal of Clinical Hypnosis 31,* 120–135.

Hammond, D. C., Haskins-Bartsch, C., McGhee M., and Grant, C. W. (1987). The use of fractionation in self-hypnosis. *American Journal of Clinical Hypnosis 30,* 119–124.

Hilgard, E. R. (1979). Divided consciousness in hypnosis: The implications of the hidden observer. In *Hypnosis: Developments in research and new perspectives.* Edited by Erika Fromm and Ronald E. Shor. New York: Aldine.

Kline, M. V. (1976). The effect of hypnosis on conditionability. In *Hypnosis and behavior therapy.* (Edited by Edward Dengrove.). Springfield, Ill.: Charles C. Thomas, Publisher.

Kluft, R. P. (1988). Autohypnotic resolution of an incipient relapse in an integrated multiple personality disorder patient: A clinical note. *American Journal of Clinical Hypnosis 31*(2), 91–96.

Kohen, D. P. (1986). Applications of relaxation/mental imagery (self-hypnosis) in pediatric emergencies. *International Journal of Clinical and Experimental Hypnosis 34*(4), 283–293.

Kohen, D. P., and Botts, P. (1987). Relaxation-imagery (self-hypnosis) in Tourette syndrome: Experience with four children. *American Journal of Clinical Hypnosis 29*(4), 227–237.

Kroger, W. S., and Fezler, W. D. (1976). Hypnotic techniques. In *Hypnosis and behavior modification: Imagery conditioning.* Philadelphia: J. B. Lippincott Company.

Large, R. G., and James, F. R. (1988). Personalized evaluation of self-hypnosis as a treatment of chronic pain: A repertory grid analysis. *Pain 35,* 155–164.

Levitan, A. (1991). Hypnosis in the 1990s—and beyond. *American Journal of Clinical Hypnosis 33*(3), 141–149.

Lombard, L. S., Kahn, S. P., and Fromm, E. (1990). The role of imagery in self-hypnosis: Its relationship to personality characteristics and gender. *International Journal of Clinical and Experimental Hypnosis, 38*(1), 25–37.

London, P. (1967). The induction of hypnosis. In *Handbook of clinical and experimental hypnosis.* (Edited by Jesse E. Gordon.) New York: Macmillan.

McConkey, K. M. (1986). Opinions about hypnosis and self-hypnosis before and after hypnotic testing. *International Journal of Clinical and Experimental Hypnosis 34*(4), 311–319.

Neufield, V., and Lynn, S. J. (1988). A single-session group self-hypnosis smoking cessation treatment: A brief communication. *International Journal of Clinical and Experimental Hypnosis 36*(2), 75–79.

Orian, C. (1989). Self-injurious behavior as a habit and its treatment. *American Journal of Clinical Hypnosis* 32(2), 84–89.

Raskin, M., Bali, L. R., and Peeke, H. V. (1980). Muscle biofeedback and transcendental meditation. *Archives of General Psychiatry 37*, 93–97.

Rothman, I., Carroll, M. L., and Rothman, F. D. (1976). Homework and self-hypnosis: The conditioning therapies in clinical practice. In *Hypnosis and behavior therapy.* (Edited by Edward Dengrove.) Springfield, Ill.: Charles C. Thomas, Publisher.

Sanders, S. (1987). Styles of clinical self-hypnosis. In *Clinical hypnosis: A case management approach.* (Edited by William C. Webster II.). Cincinnati: Behavioral Science Center, Publications.

Sanders, S. (1991). *Clinical self-hypnosis.* New York: Guilford.

Shapiro, M. (1991). Bandaging a "broken heart": Hypnoplay therapy in the treatment of a multiple personality disorder. *American Journal of Clinical Hypnosis* 34(1), 1–10.

Soskis, D. A., Orne, E. C., Orne, M. T., and Dinges, D. F. (1989). Self-hypnosis and meditation for stress management: A brief communication. *International Journal of Clinical and Experimental Hypnosis* 37(4), 285–289.

Walker, W. (1991). Music as a pathway for self-hypnosis. *Australian Journal of Clinical and Experimental Hypnosis* 18(1), 57–59.

Chapter 9: Hypnosis and the Habit Disorders

Agee, L. (1983). Treatment procedures using hypnosis in smoking cessation programs: A review of the literature. *Journal of the American Society of Psychosomatic Dentistry and Medicine 30,* 111–126.

Anderson, M. (1985). Hypnotizability as a factor in the hypnotic treatment of obesity. *International Journal of Clinical and Experimental Hypnosis 33,* 150–159.

Baer, L., Carey, R., and Meminger, S. (1986). Hypnosis for smoking control cessation: A clinical follow-up. *International Journal of Psychosomatics 33,* 13–16.

Barabasz, A., Baer, L., Sheehan, D., and Barabasz, M. (1986). A three-year follow-up of hypnosis and restricted environmental stimulation therapy for smoking. *International Journal of Clinical and Experimental Hypnosis 34,* 169–181.

Barabasz, M., and Spiegel, D. (1989). Hypnotizability and weight loss in obese subjects. *International Journal of Eating Disorders 8,* 335–341.

Carlson, J. (1989). Brief therapy for health promotion. *Individual Psychology Journal of Adlerian Theory, Research and Practice 45,* 220–229.

Carnes, P. (1989). *Contrary to love: Helping the sexual addict.* Minneapolis: Comp-Care Publishers.

Citrenbaum, C., King, M., and Cohen, W. (1985). *Modern clinical hypnosis for habit control.* New York: W. W. Norton.

Cochrane, G. (1987). Hypnotherapy in weight-loss treatment: Case illustrations. *American Journal of Clinical Hypnosis 30,* 20–27.

Crasilneck, H. (1990). Hypnotic techniques for smoking control and psychogenic impotence. *American Journal of Clinical Hypnosis 32,* 147–153.

Davidson, G. (1985). Smoking control: Audiotaped self-hypnosis as adjuvant treatment in a clinical series. *Australian Journal of Clinical and Experimental Hypnosis 13,* 107–112.

Edmonston, W. (1981). *Hypnosis and relaxation: Modern verification of an old equation.* New York: Wiley.

Frischholz, E., and Spiegel, D. (1986). Adjunctive use of hypnosis in the treatment of smoking. *Psychiatric Annals 16,* 87–90.

Golan, H. (1991). Treatment of tongue thrust with hypnosis: Two case histories. *American Journal of Clinical Hypnosis 33*(4), 235–240.

Holroyd, J. (1990). How hypnosis may potentiate psychotherapy. In M. Fass and D. Brown (Eds.), *Creative mastery in hypnosis and hypnoanalysis: A festschrift for Erika Fromm.* Hillsdale, N.J.: Laurence Erlbaum.

Horowitz, M., Hini-Alexander, M., and Wagner, T. (1985). Psychosocial mediators of abstinence, relapse, and continued smoking: A one-year follow-up of a minimal intervention. *Addictive Behaviors 10,* 29–39.

Hull, W. (1986). Psychological treatment of birth trauma with age regression and its relationship to chemical dependency. *Pre- and Peri-Natal Psychology Journal 1,* 111–134.

Hyman, G., Stanley, R., Burrows, G., and Horne, D. (1986). Treatment effectiveness of hypnosis and behavior therapy in smoking cessation: A methodological refinement. *Addictive Behaviors 11,* 355–365.

Jordan, T. (1989). Did he fall or was he pushed? Thoughts on habits and hypnosis. *British Journal of Experimental and Clinical Hypnosis 6,* 122–125.

Lambe, R., Osier, C., and Franks, P. (1986). A randomized controlled trial of hypnotherapy for smoking cessation. *Journal of Family Practice 22,* 61–65.

Maxmen, J. (1986). *Essential psychopathology.* New York: W. W. Norton.

Mott, Jr., T., and Roberts, J. (1979). Obesity and hypnosis: A review of the literature. *American Journal of Clinical Hypnosis 22,* 3–7.

Orman, D. (1991). Reframing of an addiction via hypnotherapy. *American Journal of Clinical Hypnosis 33*(4), 263–271.

Resnick, R., and Resnick, E. (1986). Psychological issues in the treatment of cocaine abuse. *National Institute on Drug Abuse Research Monograph Series 67,* 290–294.

Ronan, W. (1988). Hypnoanalysis and eating awareness training (H.E.A.T.). *Medical Hypnoanalysis Journal 3,* 137–149.

Spiegel, H., and Spiegel, D. (1978). *Trance and treatment: Clinical uses of hypnosis.* New York: Basic Books.

Vandamme, T. (1986). Hypnosis as an adjunct to the treatment of a drug addict. *Australian Journal of Clinical and Experimental Hypnosis 14,* 41–48.

Walker, W., Collins, J., and Krass, J. (1982). Four hypnosis scripts from the Macquarie Weight Control Programme. *Australian Journal of Clinical and Experimental Hypnosis 10,* 125–133.

Chapter 10: Hypnotherapy and Psychological Disorders, I

Araoz, D. (1983). Hypnosex therapy. *American Journal of Clinical Hypnosis 26,* 37–41.

Bodden, J. (1991). Assessing state-bound memories in the treatment of phobias: Two case studies. *American Journal of Clinical Hypnosis 34*(1), 24–28.

Crasilneck, H. (1982). A follow-up study in the use of hypnotherapy in the treatment of psychogenic impotency. *American Journal of Clinical Hypnosis 25,* 52–61.

Der, D., and Lewington, P. (1990). Rational self-directed hypnotherapy: A treatment for panic attacks. *American Journal of Clinical Hypnosis 32,* 160–167.

DeRoos, Y., and Johnson, D. (1983). Hypnosis and rational-emotive therapy as used in teaching improved auto suggestion. *College Student Journal 17,* 68–75.

Domangue, B. (1985). Hypnotic regression and reframing in the treatment of insect phobias. *American Journal of Psychotherapy 39,* 206–214.

Eichelman, B. (1985). Hypnotic change in combat dreams of two veterans with post-traumatic stress disorder. *American Journal of Psychiatry 142,* 112–114.

Ellis, A. (1962). *Reason and emotion in psychotherapy.* New York: Lyle Stuart.

Gilmore, L. (1987). Hypnotic metaphor and sexual dysfunction. *Journal of Sex and Marital Therapy 13,* 45–57.

Golden, W., Dowd, E., and Friedberg, F. (1987). *Hypnotherapy: A modern approach.* New York: Pergamon Press.

Gould, R., and Krynicki, V. (1989). Comparative effectiveness of hypnotherapy on different psychological symptoms. *American Journal of Clinical Hypnosis 32,* 110–117.

Haberman, M. (1987). Complications following hypnosis in a psychotic patient with sexual dysfunction treated by a lay hypnotist. *American Journal of Clinical Hypnosis 29,* 166–170.

Holroyd, J. (1987). How hypnosis may potentiate psychotherapy. *American Journal of Clinical Hypnosis 29,* 194–200.

Johnson, G., and Hallenbeck, C. (1985). A case of obsessional fears treated by brief hypno-imagery intervention. *American Journal of Clinical Hypnosis 27,* 232–236.

Kelly, S. (1984). Measured hypnotic response and phobic behavior. *International Journal of Clinical and Experimental Hypnosis 32,* 1–5.

Kingsbury, S. (1988). Hypnosis in the treatment of post-traumatic stress disorder: An isomorphic intervention. *American Journal of Clinical Hypnosis 31,* 81–90.

Lamb, C. (1985). Hypnotically-induced deconditioning: Reconstruction of memories in the treatment of phobias. *American Journal of Clinical Hypnosis 28,* 56–62.

McCue, E., and McCue, P. (1988). Hypnosis in the elucidation of hysterical aphonia: A case report. *American Journal of Clinical Hypnosis 30,* 178–182.

McGuinness, T. (1984). Hypnosis in the treatment of phobias: A review of the literature. *American Journal of Clinical Hypnosis 26,* 261–272.

MacHovec, F. (1985). Treatment variables and the use of hypnosis in the brief therapy of post-traumatic stress disorder. *International Journal of Clinical and Experimental Hypnosis 33,* 6–14.

Masters, W., and Johnson, V. (1970). *Human sexual inadequacy.* Boston: Little, Brown.

Meyer, R. (1992). *The clinician's handbook* (3d ed.). Boston: Allyn & Bacon.

Monaghan, F. (1985). The delayed stress syndrome. *International Journal of Psychosomatics 32,* 20–23.

Morgan, V., Darby, B. and Heath, A. (1992). The future of hypnosis through the remainder of the decade: A Delphi poll. *American Journal of Clinical Hypnosis 34,* 149–157.

Mutter, C. (1987). Post-traumatic stress disorder: Hypnotherapeutic approach in a most unusual case. *American Journal of Clinical Hypnosis 30*, 81–86.

Nugent, W., Carden, N., and Montgomery, D. (1984). Utilizing the creative unconscious in the treatment of hypodermic phobias and sleep disturbance. *American Journal of Clinical Hypnosis 26*, 201–205.

Obler, M. (1982). A comparison of a hypnoanalytic/behavior modification technique and a cotherapist-type treatment with primary orgasmic dysfunctional females: Some preliminary results. *Journal of Sex Research 18*, 331–345.

Palan, B., and Chandwani, S. (1989). Coping with examination stress through hypnosis: An experimental study. *American Journal of Clinical Hypnosis 31*, 173–180.

Sarbin, T. (1991). Hypnosis: A fifty year perspective. *Contemporary Hypnosis 8*, 1–15.

Seif, B. (1982). Hypnosis in a man with fear of voiding in public facilities. *American Journal of Clinical Hypnosis 24*, 288–289.

Stanton, H. (1986). The removal of phobias through ego-state reframing. *International Journal of Psychosomatics 33*, 15–18.

Stanton, H. (1989). Hypnosis and rational-emotive therapy—a de-stressing combination. *International Journal of Clinical and Experimental Hypnosis 37*, 95–99.

Stewart, D. (1986). Hypnoanalysis and orgasmic dysfunction. *International Journal of Psychosomatics 33*, 21–22.

Taylor, R. (1985). Imagery for the treatment of obsessional behavior: A case study. *American Journal of Clinical Hypnosis 27*, 175–179.

van der Hart, O., and van der Velden, K. (1987). The hypnotherapy of Dr. Andries Hoek: Uncovering hypnotherapy before Janet, Breuer, and Freud. *American Journal of Clinical Hypnotherapy 29*, 264–271.

Van Dyke, P., and Harris, R. (1982). Phobia: A case report. *American Journal of Clinical Hypnosis 24*, 284–287.

Van Dyck, R., and Hoogduin, K. (1989). Hypnosis and conversion disorders. *American Journal of Psychotherapy 43*, 480–493.

Wolpe, J. (1958). *Psychotherapy by reciprocal inhibition.* Stanford, Calif.: Stanford University Press.

Chapter 11: Hypnotherapy and Psychological Disorders, II

Brink, N. (1987). Three stages of hypno-family therapy for psychosomatic problems. *Imagination, Cognition, and Personality 6*, 263–270.

Brown, D. and Fromm, E. (1987). *Hypnosis and behavioral medicine.* Hillsdale, N.J.: Lawrence Erlbaum Associates.

Brownfain, J. (1967). Hypnodiagnosis. In J. Gordon (Ed.), *Handbook of Clinical and Experimental Hypnosis.* New York: Macmillan.

Confer, W. (1984). Hypnotic treatment of multiple personality: A case study. *Psychotherapy 21*, 408–413.

Coons, P. (1986). Treatment progress in 20 patients with multiple personality disorder. *Journal of Nervous and Mental Disease 174*, 715–721.

Culbertson, F. (1989). A four step hypnotherapy model for Gill de la Tourette's Syndrome. *American Journal of Clinical Hypnosis 31*, 252–256.

De Angelis, T. (1991). When going gets tough, the hopeful get going. *APA Monitor,* July, p. 18.

Ebert, B. (1988). Hypnosis and rape victims. *American Journal of Clinical Hypnosis* *31*, 50–56.

Eisen, M. (1989). Return of the repressed: Hypnoanalysis of a case of total amnesia. *International Journal of Clinical and Experimental Hypnosis 37*, 107–119.

Friedrich, W. (Ed.) (1991). *Casebook of sexual abuse treatment.* New York: W. W. Norton.

Frischolz, E., Braun, B., Sachs, R., Hopkines, L. et al. (1990). The dissociative experience scale: Further replication and validation. *Dissociation 3*, 151–153.

Gorton, G. (1988). Life-long nightmares: An eclectic treatment approach. *American Journal of Psychotherapy 42*, 610–618.

Heatherton, T., and Baumeister, R. (1991) Binge eating as escape from self-awareness. *Psychological Bulletin 110*(1), 86–108.

Jensen, P. (1984). Case report of conversion catatonia: Indication for hypnosis. *American Journal of Psychotherapy 38*, 566–570.

Kaszniak, A., Nussbaum, P., Berren, M., and Santiago, J. (1988). Amnesia as a consequence of male rape: A case report. *Journal of Abnormal Psychology 97*, 100–104.

Kluft, R. (1983). Hypnotherapeutic crisis intervention in multiple personality. *American Journal of Clinical Hypnosis 26*, 73–83.

Kluft, R. (1986). Preliminary observations on age regression in multiple personality disorder patients before and after integration. *American Journal of Clinical Hypnosis 28*, 147–156.

Kluft, R. (1988). On treating the older patient with multiple personality disorder: "Race against time" or "make haste slowly"? *American Journal of Clinical Hypnosis 30*, 257–266.

Kluft, R. (1992). Enhancing the hospital treatment of dissociative disorder patients by developing nursing expertise in the application of hypnotic techniques without formal trance induction. *American Journal of Clinical Hypnosis 34*, 158–174.

Kovatsch, C. (1987). Hypnosis in assertiveness and social skills training. In W. Wester II (Ed.), *Clinical hypnosis: A case management approach.* Cincinnati, Ohio: Behavioral Science Center.

Malarewicz, J. (1988). Ericksonian techniques in family therapy. In J. Zeig and S. Lankton (Eds.), *Developing Ericksonian Therapy.* New York: Brunner/Mazel.

Malon, D., and Berardi, D. (1987). Hypnosis with self cutters. *American Journal of Psychotherapy 41*, 531–541.

Murray-Jobsis, J. (1985). Exploring the schizophrenic experience with the use of hypnosis. *American Journal of Clinical Hypnosis 28*, 34–42.

Murray-Jobsis, J. (1991). An exploratory study of hypnotic capacity of schizophrenic and borderline patients in a clinical setting. *American Journal of Clinical Hypnosis 33*(3), 150–160.

Nugent, W., Carden, N., and Montgomery, D. (1984). Utilizing the creative unconscious in the treatment of hypodermic needles and sleep disturbance. *American Journal of Clinical Hypnosis 26*, 201–205.

Price, R. (1987). Dissociative disorders of the self: A continuum extending into multiple personality. *Psychotherapy 24*, 387–391.

Ross, C. (1984). Diagnosis of multiple personality during hypnosis: A case report. *International Journal of Clinical and Experimental Hypnosis 32*, 222–235.

Seif, B. (1985). Clinical hypnosis and recurring nightmares: A case report. *American Journal of Clinical Hypnosis 27*, 166–168.

Shapiro, M. (1991). Bandaging a "broken heart": Hypnotherapy in the treatment of multiple personality disorder. *American Journal of Clinical Hypnosis 34*(1), 1–10.

Somer, E. (1990). Brief simultaneous couple hypnotherapy with a rape victim and her spouse: A brief communication.) *International Journal of Clinical and Experimental Hypnosis 38*, 1–5.

van der Hart, O. (1988. An imaginary leave-taking ritual in mourning: A brief communication. *International Journal of Clinical and Experimental Hypnosis 36*, 1–5.

van der Hart, O., Brown, P., and Turco, R. (1990). Hypnotherapy for traumatic grief: Janetian and modern approaches integrated. *American Journal of Clinical Hypnosis 32*, 263–271.

Werbel, C., Mulhern, T., and Dubi, M. (1983). The use of hypnosis as therapy for the mentally retarded. *Education and Training of the Mentally Retarded 18*, 321–323.

Wilson, T., Momb, D., Hunt, R., and Heiber, R. (1989). Reparenting young schizophrenic people. *International Child Welfare Review*, 31–38.

Chapter 12: Applications in Pain Management and in Dentistry

Anderson, J., Basker, M., and Dalton, R. (1990). Suggestions with migraine. In D. Hammond (Ed.), *Handbook of hypnotic suggestions and metaphors*. New York: W. W. Norton.

Auerbach, J. (1990). Hypnotic suggestions with cancer. In D. Hammond (Ed.), *Handbook of hypnotic suggestions and metaphors*. New York: W. W. Norton.

Barber, J. (1986). Hypnotic analgesia. In A. Holzman and D. Turk (Eds.), *Pain Management*. New York: Pergamon Press.

Bishay, E., and Lee, C. (1984). Studies of the effects of hypnoanesthesia on regional blood flow by transcutaneous oxygen monitoring. *American Journal of Clinical Hypnosis 27*, 64–69.

Clarke, J., and Persichetti, S. (1990). Imagery with hypersensitive gag reflex. In D. Hammond (Ed.), *Handbook of Hypnotic Suggestions and Metaphors*. New York: W. W. Norton.

Clarke, J., and Reynolds, P. (1991). Suggestive hypnotherapy for nocturnal bruxism: A pilot study. *American Journal of Clinical Hypnosis 33*(4), 248–253.

Crasilneck, H., and Hall, J. (1985). *Clinical hypnosis: Principles and applications* (2d ed.). New York: Grune & Stratton.

DeBenedittis, G., and Panerai, A. (1989). Effects of hypnotic analgesia and hypnotizability on experimental ischemic pain. *International Journal of Clinical and Experimental Hypnosis 37*, 55–69.

Erickson, M., Hershman, S., and Secter, I. I. (1990). *The practical application of medical and dental hypnosis*. New York: Brunner/Mazel.

Ewin, D. (1990). Emergency hypnosis for the burned patient. In D. Hammond (Ed.), *Handbook of hypnotic suggestions and metaphors*. New York: W. W. Norton.

Hammond, D. (1990). Dental hypnosis. In D. Hammond (Ed.), *Handbook of hypnotic suggestions and metaphors.* New York: W. W. Norton.

Heron, W. (1990). Gagging suggestion. In D. Hammond (Ed.), *Handbook of hypnotic suggestions and metaphors.* New York: W. W. Norton.

Hilgard, E., and Hilgard, J. (1975). *Hypnosis in the relief of pain.* Los Altos, Calif.: William Kaufmann.

Kroger, W. (1990). Suggestions for operative hypnodontics. In D. Hammond (Ed.), *Handbook of hypnotic suggestions and metaphors.* New York: W. W. Norton.

Malone, M., Kurtz, R., and Strube, M. (1989). The effects of hypnotic suggestion on pain report. *American Journal of Clinical Hypnosis 31,* 221–230.

Melzack, R. (1975). The McGill Pain Questionnaire. In R. Melzack (Ed.), *Pain measurement and assessment.* New York: Raven.

Melzack, R., and Wall, P. (1965). Pain mechanisms: A new theory. *Science 150,* 971–979.

Miller, M., Barabasz, A., and Barabasz, M. (1991). Effects of active alert and relaxation hypnotic inductions on cold pressor pain. *Journal of Abnormal Psychology 100,* 223–226.

Murray-Jobsis, J. (1990). Ego building. In D. Hammond (Ed.), *Handbook of hypnotic suggestions and metaphors.* New York: W. W. Norton.

Neiburger, E. (1990). Suggestions with TMJ. In D. Hammond (Ed.), *Handbook of hypnotic suggestions and metaphors.* New York: W. W. Norton.

New Lexicon Webster's dictionary of the English language (1988). New York: Lexicon Publications.

Patterson, D., Questad, K., and de Lateur, B. (1989). Hypnotherapy as an adjunct to narcotic analgesia for the treatment of pain for burn debridement. *American Journal of Clinical Hypnosis 31,* 156–163.

Pattie, F. (1967). A brief history of hypnotism. In J. Gordon (Ed.), *Handbook of clinical and experimental hypnosis.* New York: Macmillan.

Rodolfa, E., Kraft, W., and Reilley, R. (1990). Etiology and treatment of dental anxiety and phobia. *American Journal of Clinical Hypnosis 33*(1), 22–28.

Shor, R. (1967). Physiological effects of painful stimulation during hypnotica analgesia. In J. Gordon (Ed.), *Handbook of clinical and experimental hypnosis.* New York: Macmillan.

Watkins, J., and Watkins, H. (1990). Dissociation and displacement: Where goes the "ouch?" *American Journal of Clinical Hypnosis 33,* 1–10.

Weinstein, E., and Au, P. (1991). Use of hypnosis before and during angioplasty. *American Journal of Clinical Hypnosis 34*(1), 29–37.

Chapter 13: Hypnotherapy and Medical Disorders, I

Acousta-Austan, F. (1991). Tolerance of chronic dyspnea using a hypnoeducational approach. *American Journal of Clinical Hypnosis 33*(4), 272–277.

Anderson, K., and Masur, F. (1983). Psychological preparation for invasive medical and dental procedures. *Journal of Behavioral Medicine 6*(1), 1–40.

Blankfield, R. (1991). Suggestion, relaxation, and hypnosis as adjuncts in the care of surgery patients: A review of the literature. *American Journal of Clinical Hypnosis 33*(3), 172–186.

Brady, J., Luborsky, L., and Kron, R. (1974). Blood pressure reduction in patients with essential hypertension. *Behavior Therapy 5*, 203–205.

Case, D., Fogel, D., and Pollack, A. (1980). Intrahypnotic and long-term effects of self-hypnosis on blood pressure in mild hypertension. *International Journal of Clinical and Experimental Hypnosis 28*(1), 27–38.

Collison, D. (1975). Which asthmatics should be treated by hypnotherapy? *Medical Journal of Australia 1*, 776–781.

Deabler, H., Fidel, E., Dillenkoffer, R., and Elder, S. (1973). The use of relaxation and hypnosis in lowering high blood pressure. *American Journal of Clinical Hypnosis 16*, 75–83.

Diamond, H. (1959). Hypnosis in children: The complete cure of 40 cases of asthma. *American Journal of Clinical Hypnosis 1*, 124–129.

Dunbar, H. (1938). *Emotions and bodily changes.* New York: Columbia University Press.

Finer, B. (1980). Hypnosis and anesthesia. In G. Burrows and L. Dennerstein (Eds.), *Handbook of hypnosis and psychosomatic medicine.* Amsterdam: Elsevier.

Frankel, F. (1987). Significant developments in medical hypnosis over the last 25 years. *International Journal of Clinical and Experimental Hypnosis 35*(4), 231–247.

Freeman, E., Feingold, B., Schlesinger, K., and Gorman, E. (1964). Psychological variables in allergic disorders: A review. *Psychosomatic Medicine 26*, 534.

Friedman, H., and Taub, H. (1984). Brief psychological training procedures in migraine treatment. *American Journal of Clinical Hypnosis 26*(3), 187–200.

Friedman, H., and Taub, H. (1985). Extended follow-up study of the effects of brief psychological procedures in migraine therapy. *American Journal of Clinical Hypnosis 28*(1), 27–33.

Fung, E., and Lazar, B. (1983). Hypnosis as an adjucnt in the treatment of von Willebrand's disease. *International Journal of Clinical and Experimental Hypnosis 31*(4), 256–265.

Gardner, G., and Olness, K. (1981). *Hypnosis and hypnotherapy with children.* New York: Grune and Stratton.

Gibson, H., and Heap, M. (1991). *Hypnosis in therapy.* Hillsdale, N.J.: Lawrence Erlbaum.

Gravitz, M. (1988). Early uses of hypnosis as surgical anesthesia. *American Journal of Clinical Hypnosis 10*(3), 201–208.

Jana, H. (1967). Effect of hypnosis on circulation and respiration. *Indian Journal of Medical Research 55*, 591–598.

Jencks, B. (1978). Utilizing the phases of breathing rhythm in hypnosis. In F. Frankel and H. Zamansky (Eds.), *Hypnosis at its bicentennial.* New York: Plenum.

Kagan, J., Snidman, N., Julia-Sellers, M., and Johnson, M. (1991). Temperament and allergy symptoms. *Psychosomatic Medicine 53*, 332–340.

Kroger, W., and Fezler, W. (1976). *Hypnosis and behavior modification: Imagery Conditioning.* Philadelphia: Lippincott.

LaBaw, W. (1975). Autohypnosis in hemophilia. *Hematologia 9*, 103–110.

McIntosh, I., and Hawney, M. (1983). Patient attitudes to hypnotherapy in a general medical practice. *International Journal of Clinical and Experimental Hypnosis 36*(4), 219–223.

Schultz, J. (1954). Some remarks about the techniques of hypnosis as an anesthetic. *British Journal of Medical Hypnotism 5*, 23–25.

Singh, R. (1989). Single session treatment of refractory headache: Evaluation with three patients. *Australian Journal of Clinical and Experimental Hypnosis 17*(1), 99–105.

Swirsky-Sacchetti, T., and Margolis, C. (1986). The effects of a comprehensive self-hypnosis training program on the use of factor VIII in severe hemophilia. *International Journal of Clinical and Experimental Hypnosis 34*(2), 71–83.

Turnbull, J. (1962). Asthma as a learned response. *Journal of Psychosomatic Research 6*, 59.

Wain, H., Ahmen, D., and Oetgen, W. (1983). Hypnotic intervention in cardiac arrhythmias: Advantages, disadvantages, precautions and theoretical considerations. *American Journal of Clinical Hypnosis 27*(1), 70–75.

Watkins, J. (1986). *Hypnotherapeutic Techniques.* New York: Irvington.

Chapter 14: Hypnotherapy and Medical Disorders, II

Acosta-Austan, F. (1991). Tolerance of chronic dyspnea using a hypnoeducational approach: A case report. *American Journal of Clinical Hypnosis 33*(4), 272–277.

Blankfield, R. (1991). Suggestion, relaxation, and hypnosis as adjuncts in the care of surgery patients: A review of the literature. *American Journal of Clinical Hypnosis 33* (3), 172–186.

Bowen, D. (1989). Ventilator weaning through hypnosis. *Psychosomatics 30*(4), 449–450.

Chiasson, S. (1984). Hypnosis in other related medical conditions. In W. Wester and A Smith, Jr. (Eds.), *Clinical hypnosis: A multidisciplinary approach.* Philadelphia: J. B. Lippincott.

Crasilneck, H., and Hall, J. (1985). *Clinical hypnosis: Principles and applications* (2d ed.). Orlando, Fla.: Harcourt Brace Jovanovich.

Delee, S. (1955). Hypnotism in pregnancy and labor. *Journal of the American Medical Association 159*, 750–754.

Frankl, F. (1987). Significant developments in medical hypnosis during the past 25 years. *International Journal of Clinical and Experimental Hypnosis 35*(4), 231–247.

Hadley, C. (1988). Complementary medicine and the general practitioner: A survey of general practitioners in the Wellington area. *New Zealand Medical Journal 9*, 766–768.

Hall, H. (1984). Imagery and cancer. In A. Shiekh (ed.), *Imagination and healing.* Farmington, N.Y.: Baywood.

Halley, F. (1991). Self-regulation of the immune system through biobehavioral strategies. *Biofeedback and self-regulation 16*(1), 55–74.

Harmon, T., Hynan, M., and Tyre, T. (1990). Improved obstetric outcomes using hypnotic analgesia and skill mastery combined with childbirth education. *Journal of Consulting and Clinical Psychology 58*, 525–530.

Holroyd, J., and Hill, A. (1989). Pushing the limits of recovery: Hypnotherapy with a stroke patient. *International Journal of Clinical and Experimental Hypnosis 37*(2), 120–128.

Hunter, M. (1987). Hypnosis in medical practice. In W. Wester (Ed.), *Clinical hypnosis: A case management approach.* Cincinnati: Behavioral Science Center.

Kaufman, K., Tarnowski, K., and Olsen, R. (1989). Self-regulation treatment to reduce the aversiveness of cancer chemotherapy. *Journal of Adolescent Health Care 10*, 323–327.

Kroger, W. (1977). *Clinical and experimental hypnosis in medicine, dentistry, and psychology* (2d ed.). Philadelphia: J. B. Lippincott.

McIntosh, I., and Hawney, M. (1983). Patient attitudes to hypnotherapy in a general medical practice: A brief communication. *International Journal of Clinical and Experimental Hypnosis 36*(4), 219–223.

Manganiello, A. (1986). Hypnotherapy in the rehabilitation of a stroke victim: A case study. *American Journal of Clinical Hypnosis 29*(1), 64–68.

Mehl and Lewis, E. (1988). Psychobiosocial intervention in threatened premature labor. *Pre- and Peri-Natal Psychology Journal 3*(1), 41–52.

Minichiello, W. (1987). Treatment of hyperhidrosis of amputation site with hypnosis and suggestion involving classical conditioning. *International Journal of Psychosomatics 34*(4), 7–8.

Nash, M., Minton, A., and Baldridge, J. (1988). Twenty years of scientific hypnosis in dentistry, medicine, and psychology: A brief communication. *International Journal of Clinical and Experimental Hypnosis 36*(3), 198–205.

Newton, B. (1982–1983). The use of hypnosis in the treatment of cancer patients. *American Journal of Clinical Hypnosis 25*(2–3), 104–113.

Radil, T., Snydrova, I., Hacik, L., Pfeiffer, J., and Votava, J. (1988). Attempts to influence movement disorder in hemiparetics. *Scandinavian Journal of Rehabilitation Medicine, Supplement 17*, 157–161.

Redd, W., Rosenberger, P., and Hendler, C. (1982–1983). Controlling chemotherapy side affects. *American Journal of Clinical Hypnosis 25*(2–3), 161–172.

Riley, V. (1981). Psychoneuroendocrine influences on immuno-competence and neoplasia. *Science 212*, 1100–1109.

Spanos, N., Williams, V., and Gwynn, M. (1990). Effects of hypnotic, placebo, and salicylic acid treatments on wart regression. *Psychosomatic Medicine 52*, 109–114.

Spiegel, D., and Bloom, J. (1983). Group therapy and hypnosis reduce metastatic breast carcinoma pain. *Psychosomatic Medicine 45*(4), 333–339.

Spiegel, D., Bloom, J., Kraemer, H., and Gottheil, D. (1989). Effect of psychosocial treatment on survival of patients with metastatic breast cancer. *Lancet 2*(8668), 888–891.

Stampone, D. (1990). The history of obstetric anesthesia. *Journal of Perinatal Neonatal Nursing 4*(1), 1–13.

Vollhardt, L. (1991). Psychoneuroimmunology: A literature review. *American Journal of Orthopsychiatry 61*, 35–47.

Weinstein, E., and Au, P. (1991). Use of hypnosis before and during angioplasty. *American Journal of Clinical Hypnosis 34*(1), 29–37.

Chapter 15: Hypnosis with Children

Ambrose, G. (1956). *Hypnotherapy with children: An introduction to child guidance and treatment by hypnosis for practitioners and students.* London: Staples Press Limited.

Baker, E., and Nash, M. (1987). Applications of hypnosis in the treatment of anorexia nervosa. *American Journal of Clinical Hypnosis 29*, 185–193.

Barabasz, M. (1990). Treatment of bulimia with hypnosis involving awareness and control in clients with high dissociative capacity. *International Journal of Psychosomatics 37*, 53–56.

Baumann, F. (1970). Hypnosis and the adolescent drug abuser. *American Journal of Clinical Hypnosis 13*, 17–21.

Benson, G. (1984). Short-term hypnotherapy with delinquent and acting-out adolescents. *British Journal of Experimental and Clinical Hypnosis 1*, 19–27.

Crasilneck, H., and Hall, J. (1985). *Clinical hypnosis: Principles and applications* (2d ed.). Orlando, Fla.: Grune & Stratton.

Culbertson, F. (1989). A four-step hypnotherapy model for Gilles de la Tourette's Syndrome. *American Journal of Clinical Hypnosis 31*, 252–256.

Erickson, M., Hershman, S., and Secter, I. (1961). *The practical application of medical and dental hypnosis.* New York: Brunner/Mazel Publishers.

Friedrich, W. (1990). *Psychotherapy of sexually abused children and their families.* New York: W. W. Norton & Co.

Friedrich, W. (1991). Hypnotherapy with traumatized children. *International Journal of Clinical and Experimental Hypnosis 39*(2), 67–81.

Gardner, G. (1974). Hypnosis with children. *International Journal of Clinical and Experimental Hypnosis 22*, 20–38.

Gardner, G. (1977). Hypnosis with infants and preschool children. *American Journal of Clinical Hypnosis 19*, 158–162.

Gardner, G., and Olness, K. (1988). *Hypnosis and hypnotherapy with children* (2d ed.). Philadelphia: Grune & Stratton.

Hilgard, J., and Morgan, A. (1978). Treatment of anxiety and pain in childhood cancer through hypnosis. In F. Frankel and H. Zamansky (Eds.), *Hypnosis at its bicentennial: Selected papers.* New York: Plenum Press.

Hulse-Trotter, K., and Tubbs, E. (1991). Inducing resistance to children. *Law and Human Behavior 15*(3), 273–286.

Jampolsky, G. (1975, October). Hypnosis in the treatment of learning problems. Paper presented at the meeting of the Society for Clinical and Experimental Hypnosis, Chicago.

Janet, J. (1888). Un Cas d'hysterie grave. *Revue scientifique 1*, 616.

Janet, P. (1925). *Psychological healing* (vol. 2). New York: Macmillan.

Jay, S., Elliott, C., Ozolins, M. et al. (1982). Behavioral management of children's distress during painful medical procedures. Paper presented at the meeting of the American Psychological Association Convention, Washington, D.C.

Kohen, D., Olness, K., Colwell, S., and Heimel, A. (1980, November). 500 pediatric behavioral problems treated with hypnotherapy. Paper presented at the annual meeting of the American Society of Clinical Hypnosis, Minneapolis.

Kuttner, L. (1988). Favorite stories: A hypnotic pain-reduction technique for children in acute pain. *American Journal of Clinical Hypnosis 30*, 289–295.

Lees, R. (1990). Some thoughts on the use of hypnosis in the treatment of stuttering. *British Journal of Clinical and Experimental Hypnosis 7*(2), 109–114.

London, P. (1963). *Children's Hypnotic Susceptibility Scale.* Palo Alto: Consulting Psychologists Press.

London, P. (1965). Developmental experiments in hypnosis. *Journal of Projective Techniques and Personality Assessment 29*, 189–199.

London, P., and Cooper, L. (1969). Norms of hypnotic susceptibility in children. *Developmental Psychology 1*, 113–124.

Morgan, A., and Hilgard, J. (1973). Age differences in susceptibility to hypnosis. *International Journal of Clinical and Experimental Hypnosis 21*, 78–85.

Morgan, A., and Hilgard, J. (1979). The Stanford Hypnotic Clinical Scale for children. *American Journal of Clinical Hypnosis 21*, 148–155.

Noll, R. (1988). Hypnotherapy of a child with warts. *Developmental and Behavioral Pediatrics 9*, 89–91.

Olness, K., MacDonald, J., and Uden, D. (1987). Comparison of self-hypnosis and propranolol in the treatment of juvenile classic migraine. *Pediatrics 79*, 593–597.

Plotnick, A., Payne P., and O'Grady, D. (1991). Correlates of hypnotizability in children: Absorption, vividness of imagery, and social desirability. *American Journal of Clinical Hypnosis 34*(1), 51–58.

Rhue, J., and Lynn, S. (1991). Storytelling, hypnosis and the treatment of sexually abused children. *International Journal of Clinical and Experimental Hypnosis 39*, 198–214.

Sanders, S., Copeland, D., and Elkins, G. (1987). Advanced workshop on hypnosis with children. American Psychological Association. New York.

Sokel, B., Lansdown, R., and Kent, A. (1990). The development of a hypnotherapy service for children. *Child: Care, Health and Development 16*, 227–233.

Stanton, H. (1988). Improving examination performance through the clenched fist technique. *Contemporary Educational Psychology 13*, 309–315.

Tasini, M., and Hackett, T. (1977). Hypnosis in the treatment of warts in immunodeficient children. *American Journal of Clinical Hypnosis 19*, 152–154.

Valente, S. (1990). Clinical hypnosis with school age children. *Archives of Psychiatric Nursing 4*, 131–136.

Young, M., and Montano, R. (1988). A new hypnobehavioral method for the treatment of children with Tourette's disorder. *American Journal of Clinical Hypnosis 31*, 97–106.

Chapter 16: Hypnosis and Performance Enhancement

Ashton, M., and McDonald, R. (1985). Effects of hypnosis on verbal and non-verbal creativity. *International Journal of Clinical and Experimental Hypnosis 33*, 15–26.

Berrigan, L., Kurtz, R., Stabile, J., and Strube, M. (1991). Durability of "posthypnotic suggestions" as a function of type of suggestion and trance depth. *International Journal of Clinical and Experimental Hypnosis 39*(1), 24–38.

Boutin, G., and Tosi, D. (1983). Modification of irrational ideas and test anxiety through rational stage directed hypnotherapy (RSDH). *Journal of Clinical Psychology 39*, 382–391.

Channon, L. (1984). A script for reluctant runners. *Australian Journal of Clinical and Experimental Hypnosis 12*, 139–141.

Cunningham, L. (1981). *Hypnosport*. Glendale, Calif.: Westwood Publishing.

Galyean, B. (1985). Guided imagery in education. In A. Sheikh and K. Sheikh, (Eds.), *Imagery in education* (pp. 161–177). Farmingdale, N.Y.: Baywood Publishing.

Greer, H., and Engs, R. (1986). Use of progressive relaxation and hypnosis to increase tennis skill learning. *Perceptual and Motor Skills 63*, 161–162.

Heise, J. (1961a) *How you can bowl better using self-hypnosis*. North Hollywood: Wilshire Book.

Heise, J. (1961b). *How you can play better golf using self-hypnosis*. North Hollywood: Wilshire Book.

Howard, W., and Reardon, J. (1986). Changes in the self concept and athletic performance of weight lifters through a cognitive-hypnotic approach: An empirical study. *American Journal of Clinical Hypnosis 28*, 248–257.

Jackson, L., and Gorassini, D. (1989). Artifact in the hypnosis-creativity relationship. *Journal of General Psychology 116*, 333–334.

Koe, G., and Oldridge, O. (1988). The effect of hypnotically induced suggestions on reading performance. *International Journal of Clinical and Experimental Hypnosis 36*, 275–283.

McArdle, W., Katch, F., and Katch, V. (1991). *Exercise physiology* (3d ed.). Philadelphia: Lea & Febiger.

Martens, R. (1987). *Coaches' guide to sport psychology*. Champaign, Ill.: Human Kinetics Publishers.

Masters, K. (1992) Hypnotic susceptibility, cognitive dissociation, and runner's high in a sample of marathon runners. *American Journal of Clinical Hypnosis 34*, 193–201.

Salmon, P., and Meyer, R. (1992). *Notes for the green room: Enhancing musical performance*. New York: Lexington Books.

Spies, G. (1979). Desensitization of test anxiety: Hypnosis compared with biofeedback. *American Journal of Hypnosis 22*, 108–111.

Stanton, H. (1984). Changing the experience of test anxiety. *International Journal of Eclectic Psychotherapy 3*(2), 23–28.

Stanton, H. (1988). Improving examination performance through the clenched fist technique. *Contemporary Educational Psychology 13*, 309–315.

Trotter, R. (1986, July). The mystery of mastery. *Psychology Today*, pp. 32–38.

Wojcikiewicz, A., and Orlick, T. (1987). The effects of post-hypnotic suggestion and relaxation with suggestion on competitive fencing anxiety and performance. *International Journal of Sport Psychology 18*, 303–313.

Woods, S. (1986). Hypnosis as a means of achieving modification in the treatment of academic anxiety: III. *Australian Journal of Clinical Hypnotherapy and Hypnosis 7*, 106–121.

Chapter 17: Forensic Hypnosis

Antich, J. (1967). Legal regulations concerning the practice of hypnosis. *Journal of the American Society of Psychosomatic Dentistry and Medicine 14*, 3–12.

Bundy v. Duggar, 850 F.2d 1402 (1988).

Cooper, L., and London, P. (1973). Reactivation of memory by hypnosis and suggestion. *International Journal of Clinical and Experimental Hypnosis 21*, 312–323.

Diamond, M. (1980). Inherent problems in the use of pretrial hypnosis on a prospective witness. *California Law Review 68*, 313–349.

Garver, R. (1987) Investigative hypnosis. In W. Wester (Ed.) *Clinical hypnosis*. Cincinnati, OH: Behavioral Science Center.

Gieselman, R., Fisher, R., Mackinnon, D., and Holland, H. (1985). Eyewitness memory enhancement in the police interview. *Journal of Applied Psychology 27*, 358–418.

Gravitz, M. (1985). Resistance in investigative hypnosis: Determinants and management. *American Journal of Clinical Hypnosis 28*, 76–83.

Gravitz, M. (1986). A case of forensic hypnosis: Implications for investigation. In E. Dowd and J. Healy (Eds.), *Case studies in hypnotherapy*, New York: Guilford Press.

Hilgard, E., and Loftus, E. (1979). Effective interrogation of the eye-witness. *International Journal of Clinical and Experimental Hypnosis 27*, 342–357.

Hoencamp, E. (1990). Sexual abuse and the abuse of hypnosis in the therapeutic relationship. *International Journal of Clinical and Experimental Hypnosis 4*, 283–297.

Kleinhauz, M., Horowitz, I., and Tobin, Y. (1977). The use of hypnosis in police investigation: A preliminary communication. *Journal of the Forensic Science Society 17*, 375–401.

Kline, M. (1972). The production of antisocial behavior through hypnosis: New York clinical data. *International Journal of Clinical and Experimental Hypnosis 20*, 80–94.

Kroger, W., and Duce, R. (1979). Hypnosis in criminal investigation. *International Journal of Clinical Hypnosis 27*, 358–374.

Labelle, L., Lamarche, and Laurence, J. (1990). Potential jurors' opinions on the effects of hypnosis on eyewitness identification. *International Journal of Clinical and Experimental Hypnosis 38*(4), 315–319.

Levitan, A. (1991). Hypnosis in the 1990s—and beyond. *American Journal of Clinical Hypnosis 33*, 141–149.

Levy, S. (1955). Hypnosis and legal immutability. *Journal of Criminal Law and Police Science 46*, 333–346.

Leyra v. Denno. 347 U.S. 556 (1954).

Loftus, E. (1979). *Eyewitness testimony*. Cambridge, Mass.: Harvard University Press.

McCann, T., and Sheehan, P. (1987). Confidence effects in experimental pseudomemory. In K. Bowers (Chair), Hypnosis and memory: Recent findings. Symposium conducted at the 38th Annual Meeting of the Society for Clinical and Experimental Hypnosis, Los Angeles.

Masters v. State. 341 S.W.2d 938 (Texas Crim., 1960).

Mutter, C. (1980). Critique of videotape presentation on forensic hypnotic regression: The case of Dora. *American Journal of Clinical Hypnosis 27*, 42–51.

Mutter, C. (1984). The use of hypnosis with defendants. *American Journal of Clinical Hypnosis 27*, 42–51.

Orne, M. (1972). Can a hypnotized subject be compelled to carry out otherwise unacceptable behavior? *International Journal of Clinical and Experimental Hypnosis 20*, 101–117.

Orne, M. (1979). The use and misuse of hypnosis in court. *International Journal of Clinical Hypnosis 27*, 311–341.

Orne, M., Soskis, D., Dinges, D., and Orne, E. (1984). Hypnotically induced testimony. In G. Wells and E. Loftus (Eds.), *Eyewitness testimony: Psychological perspectives*. Cambridge, England: Cambridge University Press.

People v. Cantor. 118 Cal. App. 2d Supp. 843, 18 Cal. Rptr. 363 (1961).

People v. Ebanks. 117 Cal. 652 LRA 269, 49 P. 1049 (1897).

People v. Marsh. 170 Cal. App. 2d 284, 338 P.2d 495 (4th Dist. 1959).

People v. Worthington. 105 Cal. 166, 38 P.689 (1894).

Putnam, W. (1979). Hypnosis and distortions in eyewitness memory. *International Journal of Clinical and Experimental Hypnosis 27*, 437–448.

Reiser, M. (1980). *Handbook of investigative hypnosis.* Los Angeles: Law Enforcement Hypnosis Institute.

Reiser, M. (1989). Investigative hypnosis. In D. Raskin (Ed.), *Psychological methods in criminal investigation and evidence.* New York: Springer.

Reiser, M., and Nielsen, M. (1980). Investigative hypnosis. *American Journal of Clinical Hypnosis 23*, 75–84.

Relinger, H. (1984). Hypnotic hyperamnesia: A critical review. *American Journal of Clinical Hypnosis 26*, 212–225.

Rock v. Arkansas. 107 S. Ct. 2704. (1987).

Scheflin, A., and Shapiro, J. (1989). *Trance on trial.* New York: Guilford.

Smith, M. (1983). Hypnotic memory enhancement of witnesses: Does it work? *Psychological Bulletin 94*, 387–407.

Smith, S., and Meyer, R. (1987). *Law, behavior and mental health.* New York: New York University Press.

Solomon, J. (1952). Hypnotism, suggestibility and the law. *Nebraska Law Review,* 575–596.

Spanos, N., Gwynn, M., Comer, S., Baltruweit, W., and de Groh, M. (1989). Are hypnotically induced pseudomemories resistant to cross-examination. *Law and Human Behavior 13*(3), 271–289.

Watkins, J. (1989). Hypnotic hyperamnesia and forensic hypnosis: A cross-examination. *American Journal of Clinical Hypnosis 32*, 71–83.

Wells, G., Ferguson, T., and Lindsay, R. (1979). Accuracy, confidence and juror perceptions in eyewitness identification. *Journal of Applied Psychology 64*, 440–448.

Udolf, R. (1983). *Forensic hypnosis.* Lexington, Mass.: Lexington Books.

Udolf, R. (1987). *Handbook of hypnosis for professionals* (2d ed.). New York: Van Nostrand Reinhold.

Venn, J. (1988). Misuse of hypnosis in sexual contexts: Two case reports. *International Journal of Clinical and Experimental Hypnosis 36*, 12–18.

Zani v. State. 758 S.W.2d 233 (Tex. Cr. App., 1988).

Zelig, M., and Beidleman, W. (1981). The investigative use of hypnosis: A word of caution. *International Journal of Clinical and Experimental Hypnosis 29*, 401–412.

Chapter 18: The Hypnotist in Court

Dockweiler v. Wentzell. 169 Mich. App. 368, 425 N.W.2d 468 (1988).

Frye v. United States. 293 F.1013 (D.C. Cir. 1923).

Garver, R. (1987). Investigative hypnosis. In W. Wester (Ed.), *Clinical hypnosis.* Cincinnati: Behavioral Sciences Center.

Harding v. State. 5 Md. App. 230, 246 A.2d 302 (1968), cert. denied, 395 U.S. 949 (1969).

Johnson v. Gerrish. 518 A.2d 721 (Maine 1986).

Laurence, J., and Perry, C. (1988). *Hypnosis, will, and memory.* New York: Guilford.

Lebbos v. Heinrichs. 6969 F. Supp. 1279 (N.D. Cal. 1988).

Lemieux v. Superior Court. 644 P.2d 1300, 1304 (Ariz. 1982).

Loftus, E., and Palmer, J. (1974). Reconstruction of automobile destruction: An example of interaction between language and memory. *Journal of Verbal Learning and Verbal Behavior 13*, 585–589.

People v. Ebanks. 117 Cal. 652, LRA 269 49 P.1049 (1987).

People v. Shirley. 31 Cal. 3d 18, 181 Cal. Rptr. 243, 641 P.2d 775 (1982).

Plunto v. Wallenstein. 1989 U.S. Dist. Lexis 9579 (E. Dist. Pa. 1989).

Rock v. Arkansas. 107 S. Ct. 2704 (1987).

Sheflin, A., and Shapiro, J. (1989) *Trance on trial.* New York: Guilford.

Smith, S. (1991). Mental health malpractice in the 1990s. *Houston Law Review 28*, 209–283.

State v. Hurd. 86 N.J. 525, 432 A.2d 86 (1981).

State v. Mack. 292 N.W.2d 764 (Minn. 1980).

Index

About the Author

ROBERT G. MEYER, Ph.D., is a professor in the psychology department at the University of Louisville, specializing in clinical and forensic psychology and hypnosis. He has practiced in clinical hypnosis for over twenty-five years, and is a member of The American Society of Clinical Hypnosis, The Society for Clinical and Experimental Hypnosis, and Division 30 (Psychological Hypnosis) of the American Psychological Association. In addition to *Notes for the Green Room: Enhancing Musical Performance,* he has published over fifty journal articles, is the coauthor of *Law, Behavior and Mental Health* and *Law for the Psychotherapist,* and is the author of *Abnormal Psychology* and *The Clinician's Handbook* (now in its third edition). He is also past-president of the Kentucky Psychological Association and the editor of the *Bulletin of the American Academy of Forensic Psychology.*